# Advanced Professional Skin Care
Peter T. Pugliese, M.D.

Cover design and illustration: Philip L. Huber

Editorial staff: Susan Pugliese, Gene Berube, and Susan Walmer
Art director: Maria Hollenbach
Illustrator: Philip L. Huber
Topical Agent and chapter opening cartoonist: Angelo Cupani
Photographer: Gerald Vlasak
Chemistry structures and tables: Emelie Swackhammer
Designers: Maria Hollenbach and Philip L. Huber
Topical agent narrative: Patt Pugliese

ISBN 0-9630211-0-9

Published by APSC Publishing,
Box 250, Bernville, PA 19506

This book is dedicated to Joanne, my wife, companion, and friend; to my teachers and colleagues, and to all the estheticians who have encouraged the birth of this book.

## ACKNOWLEDGEMENTS

No one brings a book into creation alone. Without the help of many talented individuals most books would remain only good intentions. My heartfelt thanks to Maria Hollenbach, Art Director, for her long hours of labor and artistic talent, and for the concept of the Topical Agent; to Philip Huber whose suggestions and deadlines helped carry the book to completion; to my daughter, Susan, who labored far into the night to edit and retype; to my daughter, Patt, for her inspired Topical Agent captions; to Gene Berube and Sue Walmer, associate editors whose eagle eyes and keen minds corrected many errors and added valuable criticism; to Diane Fenstermacher who posed as a live model for many of the drawings. To Jerry Vlasak for his photographic skills. To Emilie Swackhammer for her scientific structures and tables, and to Angelo Cupani for his clever and whimsical cartoons. Finally, to my wife, Joanne, who put up with my 5:00 AM writing sessions, proofing the first typing and offering suggestions. I must also note that without the inspiration and encouragement of many estheticians this book would never have been written.

# FOREWORD

This is a startling and, indeed, a stunning book. It is unique in many ways and cannot be compared to any previous text.

It has specifically been designed for the edification of the skin care specialist, a relatively new breed of professionals who provide a wide range of services to keep skin healthy, attractive and pleasing.

This is not a how-to-do-it handbook; rather, it teaches the scientific foundations of skin care, comprehensively covering the fundamentals of anatomy and physiology. This is done in surprising depth and detail, often exceeding what can be learned about the structure and function of skin in classic textbooks of dermatology.

Leafing through the book, one is first struck by the clever graphics which are artistic and creative cartoons that convey concise and potent messages. These are fun and light-hearted, but very instructive. These fascinating conceptions should not lead one to conclude that this is an easy book to read and understand. Indeed, this work is not for browsing or bed-time reading. It is dead serious and demanding. It contains a good deal more knowledge than anyone should store in his or her cerebral cortex, being in this respect a valuable reference source for basic knowledge of "everything you ever wanted to know about skin." Without reading the title, physicians could easily place this volume as a companion piece on the shelf alongside traditional dermatologic texts.

The writing style lightens the burden of the intellectual digging necessary to appreciate the many hard facts compressed into every page. It is breezy and snappy, using familiar, non-pedantic language, that is to say, it is reader-friendly.

The author stresses repeatedly that aestheticians provide services which beautifully complement the activities of plastic surgeons and dermatologists, making it crystal clear where the boundaries are drawn. This approach emphasizes that their specialty of skin care is part of the medical enterprise and is not simply a cosmetic gimmick pandering to the vanities of the privileged.

This handsome text should be on display in the salon setting for handy consultation. If nothing else, it will convey to the patient-client that the professional is serious and knowledgeable.

Albert M. Kligman, M.D., Ph.D.
Emeritus Professor of Dermatology
University of Pennsylvania
Philadelphia, Pennsylvania
1991

# INTRODUCTION

This book was written to fill a perceived need for a new textbook in the field of advanced nonmedical skin care. Skin care to a large measure in the United States is delivered by cosmetologists and a subdivision of cosmetologists known as **estheticians.** These estheticians are skin care specialists in their own right, however, as most are not trained as hairdressers, which make up the major number of cosmetologists. As a percentage of gross sales skin care accounts for only 3.3 % of the 41 billion dollar professional beauty care industry. Most experts in this field attribute this low level of interest to a lack of well trained skin care specialists. Indeed, there are no real skin care schools in the United States that provide the level of training that is currently available in Europe.

This then is a "bridge book". It attempts to bridge the gap between the level of training in Europe and the current level in the US. At the same time, it will help to bridge the gap between professional skin care and medicine. As a note to my medical colleagues, this book does not proport to make physicians out of estheticians, or to replace the role of the physician, rather its purpose is to help both groups serve their common client/patient better. There is little question that medicine and professional skin care are moving closer. Just as the skills of the paramedicals are accepted in medicine today, they were not so recognized 20 years ago.

No apology is given for some of the more difficult material in this text, nor is there an apology needed for some of the simplifications and omissions, as both were necessary if the book was ever to be written. As with any textbook, the views and prejudices of the author are reflected and for these I ask the reader for indulgence. I have attempted to introduce a bit of humor here and there to ease the strain of serious concentration. This is not a workbook, but rather a reference textbook; there are no lesson plans or questions at the end of the chapters. In the near future a companion book designed as a working manual will be written to outline in detail the various procedures involved in advanced skin care.

Finally, this book was written in response to requests by estheticians who have asked for more information on skin care. I have been privileged to lecture to many thousands of these skin care specialists and I am much impressed with their sincerity and zeal for learning. I hope that in some measure this book will help in their quest for that knowledge.

Our mission involves the preservation of the most complex, efficiently designed Community on the planet. Surrounding this community is a wall of protection. It keeps the inside in, the outside out, controls the climate, and receives communications. The wall protects the Community. WE protect the Wall.

It's not like the old days anymore. When Gramps was on The Force, the job was mainly just smoothing over the cracks. When Dad started, the responsibility included more activity, and some defense.

But secretly (back when Dad and Gramps were still calling me Squirt) The Force was training a future breed of reinforcement Intelligence. To make the grade required skills of performance, stability, compatibility, communication, and the scrutiny of some pretty high-ups. And I don't mind telling you, being smooth and good lookin' got you in the system quicker. I made the grade. Now they call me a Topical Agent.

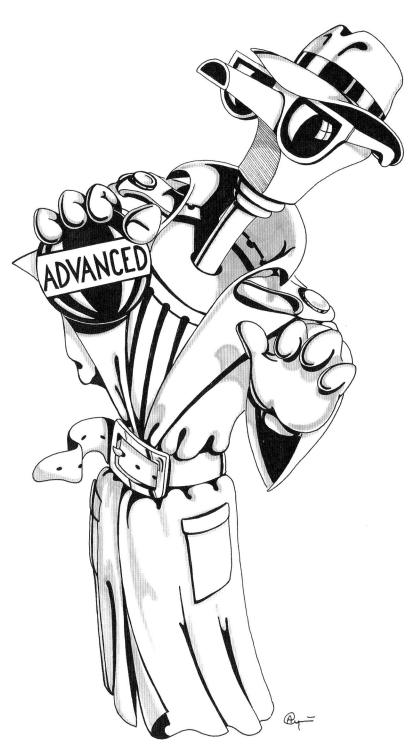

# Contents

We're going into this armed with more intelligence and skill than any team ever had. Along the way, we'll help you choose your weapons and chart your strategy. You'll have the run of the place--learn the mean streets, where the enemies hide, and who your allies are.

But, more than anything else, ya gotta know who YOU are, WHERE you are, and what your GOAL is.

Because, kid, the final report on this mission doesn't end up on somebody's desk--it becomes the blueprint for a mission you call your own.

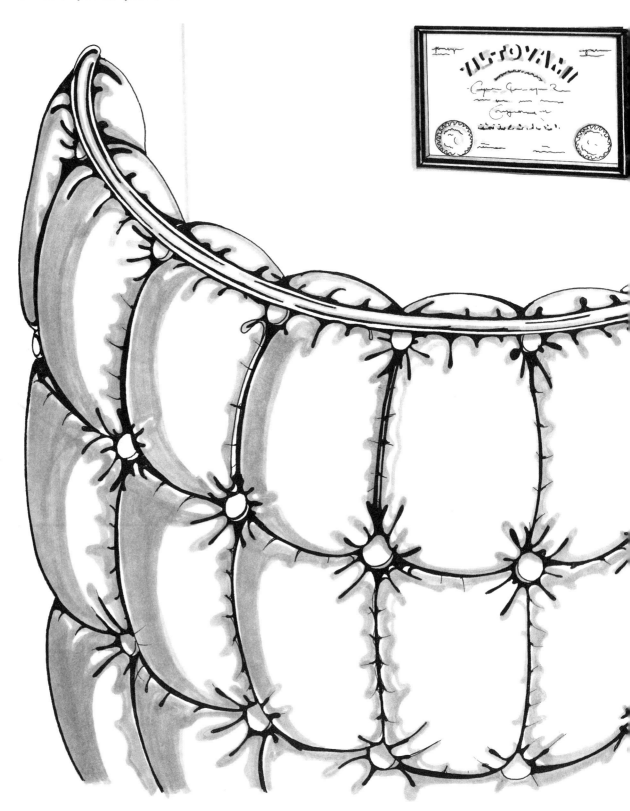

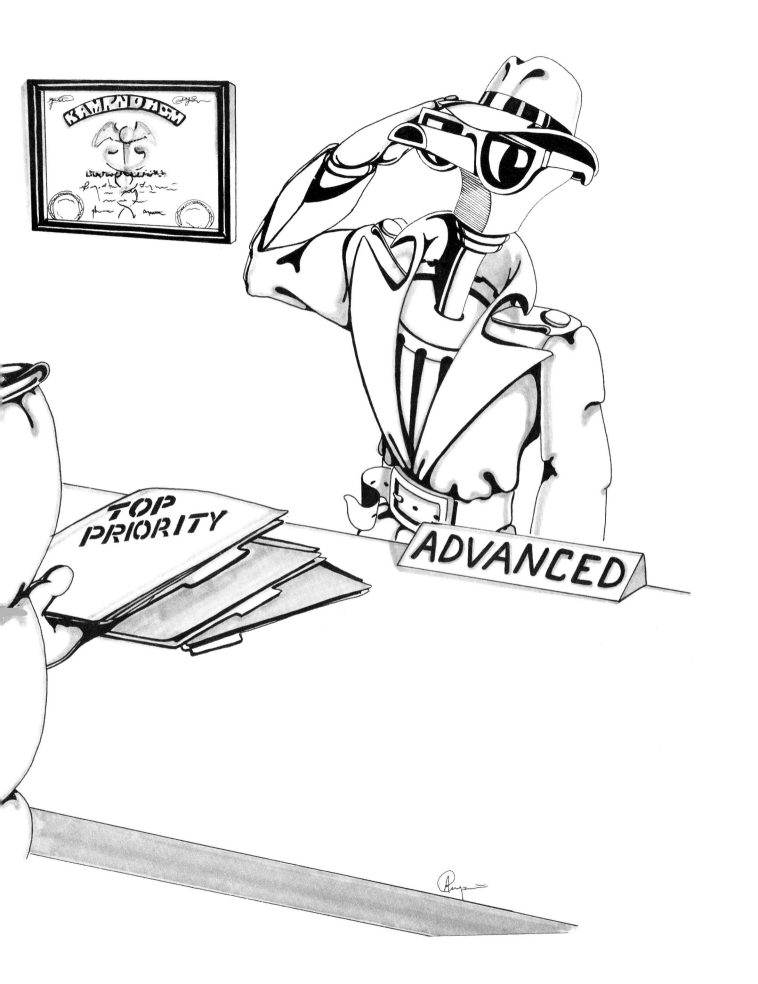

# The Skin Care Specialist

There are few joys in life greater than those derived from helping a fellow human to achieve happiness. Whether you are a parent granting the wish of a child, a physician relieving pain or attempting to save a life, or a beautician creating a new hair style, you are providing a service that is happiness-oriented. The skin care specialist has long been in a unique position to help others achieve a more attractive appearance. Today this field is expanding to encompass a wider range of services and skills.

The skin care specialist is an emerging new professsional. It was recognized in Europe that skin care and general cosmetology were difficult to master as disciplines. The rise of esthiology over the last twenty years as a separate specialty within cosmetology is evidence of the need and interest. As the esthiologist advanced in skills, there was a move toward providing assistance to physicians in the pre- and post-operative care of surgical patients. Initially this was only with patients undergoing cosmetic surgery, but now the service has increased to include general surgical patients and those patients undergoing reconstructive surgery.

The trend for the skin care specialist is to-ward a closer working relationship with the medical profession. Plastic surgeons have started to work with skin care specialists, both as a referral source and as actual office staff within the surgeon's office. Clearly, this trend can only continue to grow. The lack of trained make-up artists who are also skilled in skin care has been a stumbling block to moving this trend forward. This need is addressed in this book.

## WHAT IS A SKIN CARE SPECIALIST

I have used the term skin care specialist and esthetician almost as synonymous terms when in reality they are somewhat different. Esthetics deals mainly with beauty and relates, to a large extent, to beautiful facial skin. The skillful use of make-up is implied in this definition. When the esthetician deals with medically related problems such as acne and pigment disorders, the current level of expertise requires them to stop at this line. The skin care specialist crosses this line with a bold step. The need for the skills of a person trained in both management of skin problems and the ability to instantly change the appearance of a client's face is now evident to many medical specialists. Being aware that more and more plastic surgeons would be searching for trained skin specialists was what prompted me to write this book.

When I examine the training of most estheticians in the United States I find two main groups of estheticians, the well trained and the inadequately trained. Throughout the USA so much variation exists in the training requirements that it is quite difficult to move from state to state without a new requirement having to be met. What can we do about this? Well, first we need to look around us and see that the European estheticians are better trained, some having at least two years of training compared to a few months in the USA. Next, we need to see where we are going and what we need to do to reach that goal.

**The Definition of a Skin Care Specialist. What Are You?**

A skin care specialist is a trained professional who is well grounded in the anatomy, physiology, and pathology of the skin and in the art and science of clinical skin care. This means that the skin care specialist should be capable of working with any level of medical professional. It means that the training and background will provide sufficient knowledge to evaluate new treatments, new products, and new concepts. It means a life long dedication to continuing education and a commitment to the professional skin care society. It means you are a professional in the true meaning of the word, capable of receiving a client in a professional manner, in a professional office, and rendering professional care. This carries the obligation to observe all the professional requirements that will be discussed later.

The skin care specialist is not just a "facialist", if there is such a word. Since the skin covers the entire body, this is the area of expertise of the skin care specialist. There is a need to know how the skin on the foot is different from skin on the buttocks and on the face. What are the metabolic needs of the skin in these areas and what special attention do these areas require? A well trained skin care specialist should be able to work in the most upscale salon or the most advanced skin care clinic and feel comfortably competent. To reach this goal requires training and more training.

## THE CURRENT STATUS OF SKIN CARE IN THE USA

The estimated gross sales for the salon business in the United States for the year 1990 was 36 billion dollars. Of this, skin care represents only 0.5 billion, less than 1.5%! Nail care represents five billion or about 14% of the market. It seems incredible that hair care, which represents about 4% of the body surface, and nails, which are less than 1% of the body surface should command 98.5% of the salon business. Something is wrong, but what? Let's take a look at the present situation. Several companies in hair care have done this and have become quite successful. They have identified two problems: lack of professionalism (which means poor training) and poor management.

There were no skills in greeting and preparing clients, no uniformity in the operators' treatment skills, no selling skills, no training in how to build and maintain business or how to grow in hard times. The average hairdresser is less educated and less skilled than the average skin care specialist, yet they too have caught the spark of the new wave of salon management.

Is it possible to do in skin care what is happening in hair care? The answer is an emphatic YES. We must first realize that skin care is much more complex than hair care which is essentially cleansing, styling, perming, and coloring. We must recognize that we are in a different type of market but the same principles apply. Professional and management skills are needed for success.

Now let's look at professional skin care today. There are 50 states with licenses, with training requirements from 0 to 1 year. The requirements for teachers are quite limited. There are numerous skin care schools in the United States but not one has a curriculum that will meet the needs of the skin care specialist of the future. The lack of basic sciences, laboratory facilities, and adequate clinical material is very evident.

There appears to be little incentive for degree level teachers to enter into this field. Since most students with academic goals in teaching and research see no future in skin care, we lose this type of individual. How can we change all this?

The first place to start is with the training of estheticians. We need better schools and more of them. These schools must be designed to train future teachers in skin care as well as to train students. We need to organize the course into basic sciences with laboratory training and then add the clinical training. As the student gains skills and know-how, additional clinical skills are added, including advanced special skills such as post-surgical care, camouflage make-up, electrolysis, therapeutic massage, lymphatic drainage, hydro-therapy, and other special techniques. Pressure point therapy and modified acupuncture could also be explored. The curriculum should be standardized on a national basis as to minimal requirements. The National Cosmetology Association should be the front runner in this effort and indeed a beginning has been made. It will not be easy for many obstacles must be overcome. The course should supply the basic information needed to allow the student to go on for bachelor's and master's degrees. There must be an association with universities that will provide this type of training and which will provide credit for the basic courses already taken. I strongly believe all this will come to pass with a cooperative effort of skin care specialists.

## WHY THIS BOOK WAS WRITTEN

Over the last 10 years I have had the privilege to help in the education of many skin care specialists. The enthusiasm and eagerness of these students for new knowledge is impressive. Many times I have been asked by students for sources of reference materials to pursue specific topics in skin care and I was unable to suggest sources other than medical text books. It has taken me over four years to put together this text book. In the beginning stages I found the most difficult task was to select the material to include in the book that would be of the greatest benefit to both present and future skin care specialists. Since the trend clearly points to a closer working relationship with the medical profession I have developed this book with that in mind. At the same time I saw the need to provide a good background in science, allowing the student to keep abreast of new develop-

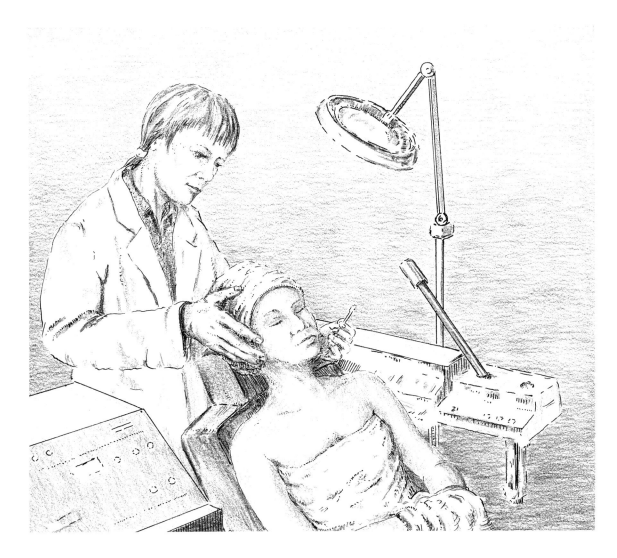

ments. With this focus the rest of the task was to select and present the material in a form that would be readable and useful.

Textbooks are of three types. There is the simple spoon feeding type of textbook that presents only the barest facts for an introduction to a subject. This I call a walking or flat plain book. Next, there is a hill book that requires some effort to read and digest while covering a great deal of the general material. Finally, there is the mountain book which is quite hard to read and is only for the highest level professional covering a great deal of minutiae. Advanced Professional Skin Care is designed as a hill book; you will need to expend some effort to learn from it.

## HOW TO USE THIS BOOK

This is a textbook designed for self education. (Later, a manual will be written which will provide a step by step instructional course with self evaluation tests included.) The chapters have been laid out to allow the reader to build a working knowledge of surface and skin anatomy, biochemistry, physiology, and skin pathology as a strong foundation. These subjects provide the basis for the next chapters on clinical skin care and the advanced chapters on nutrition and product design and use. What to include and what not to include has been tough. To keep this book from growing to a thousand pages and yet to provide an introduction to some important topics required constant compromise. References have been included to allow the reader to pursue those subjects which have particular personal appeal. In most cases textbooks are listed as reference materials.

### Concepts

Concepts are the key to learning most sciences and arts. If you are able to grasp the concept you can build onto it. It is a foundation, an anchor point on which to crystallize your thinking. Keep asking yourself "Have I learned the concept?" If you have, the rest will follow. Here is an example. Almost all skin diseases are characterized by the process of inflammation. To understand inflammation is to understand almost all of the reactions that occur in the skin, from a bug bite to complex immune disorders. Even cancers have an inflammatory component.

### Visualization

I have tried to make the material as visual as possible, though some concepts are very hard to visualize. Take each new concept and try to put it into your visual memory. Next, associate the new concept with a particular subject you have learned previously, or with which you are familiar. An example of this technique is product formulation. You can relate ingredient selection, following a recipe, measuring, and cooking to a similar process in formulation of a product. Similarly, skin care product appraisal is really no different from the appraisal of any other item that you will use on your body. You must know the ingredients and how they work in order to determine if the product will be effective.

### Repetition

Repetition is truly the secret to learning anything new, be it a language or a science. Go over the topics that you feel you have not grasped and read the chapter again, finding key words. Make sure you fully understand the key words. One of the greatest errors made by students of science is the failure to understand basic concepts. Students think the subject will clear up later when new topics are added but this is an error. Failure to master a basic concept is the same as building a house on sand; there is no solid foundation and in time the structure will fall.

### Patience

No one can eat one month's food in one day's time, nor can anyone digest a whole book at one sitting, or even in one week. It takes many years to master a subject and book learning is only a part of this process. You must work with clients and experienced skin care specialists to master this profession. Take heart, however, with the thought that the masters of today were the students of yesterday.

## AN INTRODUCTION TO TERMS AND CONCEPTS

You will be introduced to many new scientific terms in this book. It is the goal of science to measure things. The terminology of these measurements can be confusing to the beginner. We will cover some of these concepts now so that it will be easier for you in the later, more advanced chapters. First, let us look at physical measurements.

### The Metric System

The metric system is based on the meter (m) and the gram (g), whereas our system is based on the foot and the pound. One meter, when converted to inches, is 39.39 inches. We shall use the metric system in this book. From time to time I shall use some reference points to allow you a comparision to the inch/pound system. Linear measures, volume measures, and weight measures are looked at as separate topics.

<u>The Meter and Its Parts</u>

Since a **meter** is quite large it has been divided for convenience into units of one hundred parts and units of one thousand parts. A **centimeter (cm)** is one hundredth of a meter. A **millimeter (mm)** is one thousandth of a meter or one tenth of a centimeter. These measurements are great to measure a large item but when it comes to cells we need even smaller units. If we divide the millimeter by one thousand we have a **micron (µ)**. Hair diameter, for example, is measured in microns (about 150 microns for an average head hair). Again, we need a smaller measurement to study light rays so we divide the micron by a thousand and we have the **nanometer (nm)**. We speak of visible light ranging from 400 to 700 nanometers. Look at **Figure 1-1** to see these values in perspective.

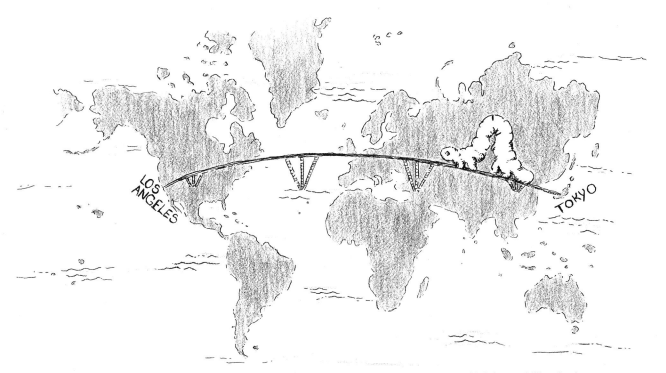

**FIGURE 1-1** Meter values. In order to visualize the relation of a meter to a nanometer, which is one billionth of a meter, we shall use a common measurement with which we are all familiar. Let us say , for the sake of description, that one nanometer equals one inch. (This is called a scale.) If one nanometer equals one inch then one micron would equal 1,000 inches or 83 feet. One millimeter would equal 1,000 x 83 feet or 16 miles. One centimeter would equal 160 miles and one meter would equal 16,000 miles, or the distance from Los Angeles east to Tokyo.

## Volume - A Three Dimensional Measurement

A cup of water is eight fluid ounces by our system. In metric terms it is about 240 milliliters. A milliliter (ml) is one thousandth of a liter, which is the volume contained in a vessel that measures 10 centimeters wide by 10 centimeters long by 10 centimeters high. Years ago we spoke of a milliliter as a cubic centimeter (cc). So a "cc" and a "ml" are the same thing. We shall speak of cubic millimeters of skin containing such and such hair follicles or nerves. This is a very small volume, not much bigger than a pin point.

## Weight - The Kilogram and the Gram

It is not easy to stop using pounds and ounces after a lifetime of use. Once you start with the metric system you will be captivated by the simple use of "tens" to change values. For instance, the **kilogram (kg)** is the weight, or mass, standard in the metric system. (For reference to our USA system it is about 2.2 lbs). If we deal in smaller amounts of material we need another unit, the **gram**, which is one thousandth of a kilogram. Even smaller units are obtained by dividing the gram by 1000 again to give us a **milligram (mg)**. Even this is large for some biological measurements so we divide again by 1000 and we have a **microgram (µg)**. We can go on and on, but for our purpose micrograms are about where we are in this text.

### Other Terms You Will Meet in This Text

## Rate

You will see phrases such as the "rate of penetration", "the rate of the reaction", and finally "the rate is a function". Rate means a certain amount of material and time are related in some manner. For example, the rate of water loss through the skin is measured at 0.5 mg/cm sq/hour. This means that one-half of gram of water is lost from every square centimeter of skin every hour. This is the rate of water loss. Using this number we can then calculate how much water is lost from an average person on an average day. All we need to know is how many square centimeters the average person has.

Surface area is a function of weight, so we

can work this out on a single square meter basis and then find the surface area and multiply our result for any particular person's surface area. One square meter has 100 cm x 100 cm = 10,000 sq centimeters. Next, we multiply 10,000 times 0.5 mg and we have 5000 mgs or 5 grams of water per hour for every meter of skin. In 24 hours a person will lose 5 gm x 24 hours or 120 grams of water/sq meter. Rates are important because they allow us not only to understand relationships but also help us to use these relationships for practical purposes. The little calculation I just did above is used to find water loss for hospitalized patients and to calculate the effectiveness of cosmetic moisturizers.

## CHEMICAL FORMULAE

You will recall from your early studies that all matter is composed of elements called atoms. Atoms, in turn, combine to form molecules of new materials; for example, water is hydrogen and oxygen, and salt is chlorine and sodium. We use chemical formulae to make the description of these reactions and compounds easier.

You will see many structural formulae in this text book. If you have no experience with this form of chemical shorthand the following may be helpful. The letter **C** stands for **carbon**, the most common element in the organic chemicals; **H** stands for **hydrogen**, the next most common element in biochemistry and **N** stands for **nitrogen**, an element seen in all proteins. Then we have **O** for **oxygen** and **P** for **phosphorus** and **S** for **sulfur**. These are the most important elements you will encounter in this textbook. In a structural formula the elements are put together according to chemical laws. We see them as only two dimensions on paper but there are actually three dimensions for every molecule. Remember that each formula stands for one molecule of that material. That is the beauty of chemical formulae. Here is an example for vinegar, known chemically as acetic acid:

$$
\begin{array}{c}
H \\
H\text{-}C\text{-}C\text{-}OOH \\
H
\end{array}
$$

This tells us the acetic acid is composed of two carbon atoms, two oxygen atoms, and four

hydrogen atoms arranged in a line.

Here is another example, a wax:

$$
\begin{array}{l}
H\,H\,H\,H\,H\,H\,H\,H\,H\,H\,H\,H\,H\,H\,H\,H\,H\,H\,H\,H\,H \\
H\text{-}C\text{-}C\text{-}C\text{-}C\text{-}C\text{-}C\text{-}C\text{-}C\text{-}C\text{-}C\text{-}C\text{-}C\text{-}C\text{-}C\text{-}C\text{-}C\text{-}C\text{-}C\text{-}C\text{-}C\text{-}C\text{-}COH \\
H\,H\,H\,H\,H\,H\,H\,H\,H\,H\,H\,H\,H\,H\,H\,H\,H\,H\,H\,H\,H
\end{array}
$$

This is called a $C_{22}$ wax because there are twenty two carbons, count them. This compound is also known as behenyl alcohol.

Just remember that the formulae are graphic descriptions of molecules that tell us both the composition and structure of the material. Chemists can get a great deal more information from the structural formula of a molecule, but for our purpose they are present so that the reader may be familiar with chemical families. In this way you will understand why certain groups of chemicals behave in a similar manner.

You will see terms, such as alcohols and aldehydes, used occasionally. **Alcohols** are compounds with C-OH groups, and **aldehydes** are compounds with

$$
\begin{array}{c}
\text{-C=O} \\
H
\end{array}
$$

which is much more reactive than an alcohol group. Notice the double bond in the oxygen molecule.

Just one more chemical item, valence. We use the term **valence** in chemistry for a number of things but for our purpose it means how many atoms of A may bind with atom B. Notice that carbon has a valence of 4, oxygen has a valence of 2, and hydrogen of 1. This means that carbon can bind four hydrogen atoms (that is, methane gas) or two oxygen atoms (that is, carbon dioxide or $CO_2$). When a double bond appears it means that the molecule is binding its atoms in a different way.

The term molecular weight refers to the total weight of all the atoms in a molecule. Let's take an example. Water is $H_2O$; hydrogen (H) has an atomic weight of 1 and oxygen (O) has an atomic weight of 16. The molecular weight of water is 2 + 16 = 18. Molecules may range in weight from 2 to many millions. We often speak of molecular weight in terms of daltons. Water is 18 daltons (d). A thousand daltons is a kilodalton (kd). Albumin, which is a common blood protein, is 40 kd in molecular weight.

## Ion

One of the most confusing terms to new students of chemistry is the word "ion". An ion is a charged chemical particle that represents an incomplete atom or molecule. Ions are usually found in solution but they may also occur in the atmosphere. Take, for example, salt which is sodium chloride, or NaCl. Sodium chloride is in crystal form when it is solid and dry. This is common table salt. When you add salt to water it will disappear as it dissolves and goes into solution. Now, we cannot see the salt but we know it is there for we can taste it, or if we let the water evaporate we see the salt again in crystalline form.

The salt in the water solution is said to be ionized. It is in the form of $Na^+$ and $Cl^-$ ions. Note that we must now write the Na with a + sign and the Cl with a - sign because they are now separated in solution as individual atomic particles or **ions.** There are three kinds of ions. The first is an **anion** which is a negative, the second is a **cation** which is postive, and the third is a **zwitterion** which can be both positive and negative.

Here is an easy way to remember which is which. The ions were named positive and negative because they will migrate in an electrical field. The negative electrode is called the cathode. That is the most important item to remember. The **negative electrode** is the cathode. Positively charged particles will migrate to the negative electrode, since opposite charges attract and like charges repel each other. A positively charged particle is called a cation since it moves to the cathode. Now it stands to reason that the anode is positive and the negative charge particle will migrate to the positive or anode electrode. It is just that simple. You need only remember one of the charges and the other then must be the opposite.

## Medical Terminology

For many readers this may be their first real brush with medical terminology. Most medical words are derived from Greek and Latin (used as universal languages among physicians). These words are composed of three parts: a stem or root word, a prefix, and a suffix. If you learn the major prefixes and suffixes you will have gone a long way to learning many of the medical words. The most common ones you will find in this book are explained and translated with the words. For example, in the word anaphylaxis: the prefix *ana* means "not", and the stem, *phylak* means "guard", so the word means "not guarded". Anaphylaxis is a serious allergic reaction to a food or drug. The suffix *axis* comes from the Greek *sis* which means "a condition or state". Anaphylaxis conveys a condition of danger, being unguarded or unprotected. Prophylactic, on the other hand, conveys a device that protects beforehand.

Here are some common prefixes.
*a-* not, or without, as in "aseptic"
*ab-* away from, as in "abnormal"
*ad-* towards, as in "adduct"
*ambi-* around, both sides, as in "ambidextrous"
*anit-* against, opposite
*ante-* before
*apo-* from, under, again
*bis-* two
*circa-* around, as in "circumcision"
*de-* from, away, down from
*dia-* through, in different directions, to the end
*dis-* opposite of
*dis-* asunder or apart, as in "dissect"
*dys-* ill or bad, as in "dysfunction"
*ektos-* outside, external
*endon-, ento-* within, inner
*eu-* well or true
*epi-* around, upon, on over, near, at, or before, as in "epidermis"
*ex-* out of, from, as in "excise"
*hemi-* half
*hyper-* over, as in "hyperplasia"
*hypo-* under, as in "hypoplasia", "hypodermic"
*infr-* below or underneath
*inter-* between
*intra-* inside
*kata-,* or*cata-* down from, against
*meta-* among, along with, afterwards
*ob-* before or against
*para-* besides, to the side of
*peri-* around, above, beyond
*prae-, pro-* before

*retro-* behind, back, backwards
*sub-* beneath, under
*syn-* with, together
*super-* above, as in "superficial"
*trans-* across, as in "transfer"
*ultra-* beyond, besides, over

Here are a few common suffixes.
*-itis-* inflammation of, as in "colitis"
*-ectomy-* to cut out of, as in "appendectomy"
*-otomy-* to cut, as in "episiotomy"
*-plasty-* to form, as in "mammoplasty"
*-orrhea-* to flow, as in "gonorrhea" (gona means seeds)
*-emia-* blood, as in "septicemia"
*-oma-* tumor, as in "fibroma"
*-osis-* a process or condition, as in "pediculosis"

Remember, do not be intimidated by words. After all, they have been created by a human mind just like yours.

### A NOTE ON PHYSICAL ATTRACTIVENESS

Since everything in this book is ultimately about physicial attractiveness, let us look at the importance of physical attractiveness.

It is common sense that attractive people are more easily accepted by other humans and are perceived to be happier than other people. Research on physical attractiveness, however, has shown many other benefits of being attractive that are not so obvious. In our society to-day it is believed by many that "what is beautiful is good". A recent study on the impact of physical attractiveness produced four generalizations.

1. Physically attractive people have more social power than physically unattractive people.
2. Individuals of higher physical attractiveness are accepted or liked more than individuals of lower physical attractiveness provided other characteristics are equal.
3. Physically attractive people are perceived to possess more positive personal and nonpersonal characteristics, such as intelligence, personality traits, and success in life, than physically unattractive people.
4. Physically attractive people have more positive effects on other people. They receive more positive responses from others, such as requests for work and requests for help, than do people of lower physical attractiveness.

The above summary is from The Physical Attractiveness Phenomenon, by Patzer, G.L., Plenum Press, 1985. This is an interesting study and is highly recommended reading if you wish to pursue this topic further.

Your aim is to make everyone healthy and attractive. To achieve this goal you shall use every means at your disposal, use every philosophy and science that relates to your skills, and through diligent pursuit of new knowledge and training, you shall keep those skills honed to a fine edge.

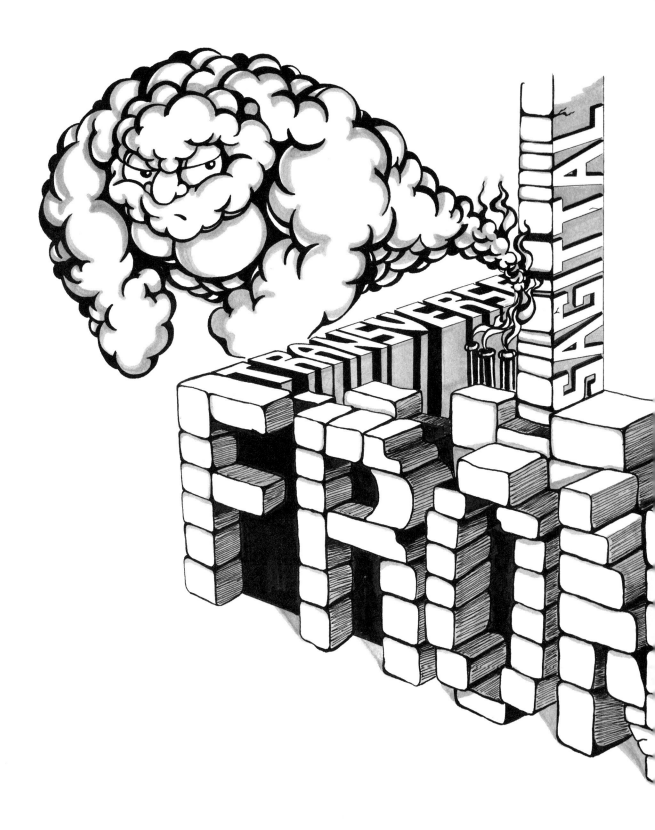

This place is incredible, but not invincible. No nook or cranny is insignificant to the whole operation. We're gonna stand back and get a bird's eye view of the place--look at the walls, the windows, and the landscape. We'll map out the territories and show you how to describe your location when you're calling in the allies to troubleshoot.

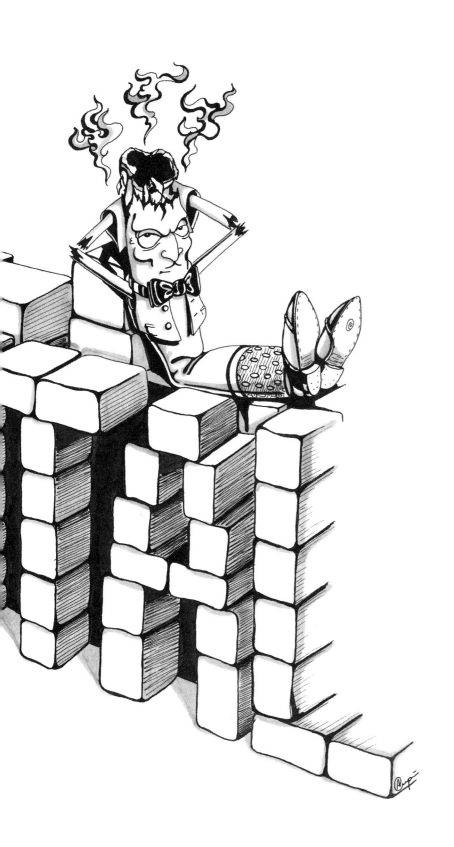

# Surface Anatomy

Anatomy is probably the oldest of the biological sciences. There was a vast accumulation of anatomical knowledge long before the practice of medicine was much more than hocus-pocus. The word "anatomy" comes from two Greek words, *ana* meaning "up" and temnein meaning "to cut". One learns anatomy by dissecting bodies. Fortunately for the skin care specialist this has already been done. As a science, anatomy studies the structure and the relation of body parts. Our study of anatomy will be the relation of the surface of the skin to the body parts below the skin. A detailed study of skin anatomy will be given in the next chapter. First, we need to learn the terms associated with the study of anatomy. This will allow us to find our way about the body as easily as following a road map. We shall look at planes and directions, for these are the basic starting points.

## ANATOMICAL PLANES AND DIRECTIONS OF THE BODY

"Divide and conquer" is the key phrase here. The body is divided into parts to help the student organize the accumulated knowledge into a workable system. This system permits accurate communication between all interested parties and prevents confusion. In essence, you will learn in sections and work each section into a complete system. Remember to take little bites, chew them well, and you will have no problem in digesting the whole thing.

### The Planes

Planes are nothing more than flat surfaces. In anatomy, they are imaginary and are used to divide the body into convenient parts. Let us consider, for example, a large sausage. It is round and has no flat surface to use as a reference point, therefore, it has no real front or back, no top or bottom. So we make a mark on the sausage and call the surface where we made the mark the front of the sausage. Now we have a reference point called a front. If we have a front, we also have a back. Since we have a front and back, we must also have two sides, a right and a left. We see that our sausage has two ends. Now we can change these terms into a more accurate description of our sausage. If we cut the sausage end to end, so that we have two long pieces, one being the front, the other being the back, this is then called a **frontal section**. If we cut the sausage end to end so that we have a right and a left side, this is called a **sagittal section**. These are the two main body planes that run from head to foot. Look at **Figure 2-1** and see these planes on the diagram. If we now decided to slice the sausage from side to side into little rings like the pepperoni on a pizza, we shall have made **transverse sections**. Here is the key to remembering the planes. Transverse planes are perpendicular to the long axis of the body, while frontal and sagittal planes are parallel to the long axis of the body. Remember that you always need a reference point when you describe a plane. Now let us look at the body directions to find the reference points.

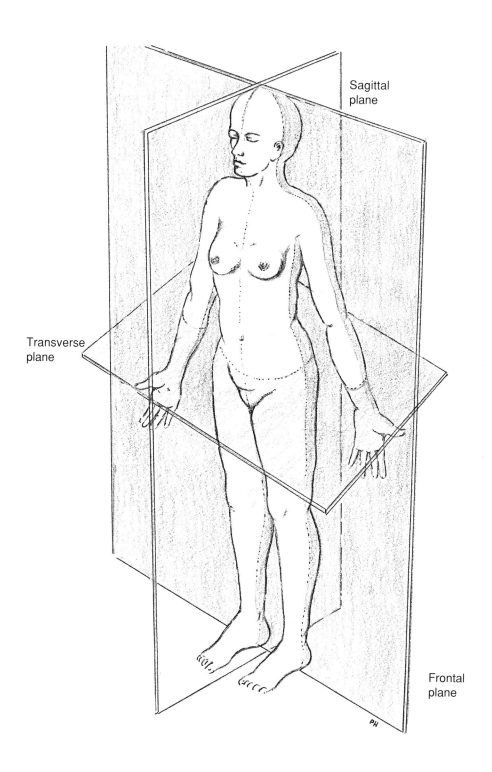

Sagittal
plane

Transverse
plane

Frontal
plane

PH

**FIGURE 2-1** The Planes. The planes are imaginary lines that divide the body into convenient sections for easy description.

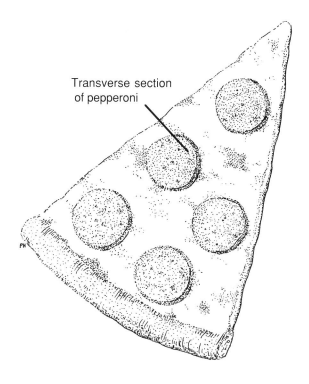

Transverse section of pepperoni

**Directions of the Body**

There are sixteen directions (see **Figure 2-2**), which seems like a lot, but none of them can easily be eliminated without resulting in confusion. We can break them up into four groups:

Group One:  Front and Back

**Anterior** - toward the front or face
**Posterior** - toward the back or behind the body
**Ventral** - toward the abdominal surface, or belly
**Dorsal** - toward the back
Example: The navel is an anterior or ventral structure lying in the frontal plane.

Group Two:  Sides and Ends

**Medial** - near or toward the midline
**Lateral** - to the side, away from the midline
**Superior** - above, toward the top
**Inferior** - below, toward the bottom
Example: The navel is a ventral midline structure inferior to the chest and superior

to the pubis.

Group Three:  Long and Short Distance Group

**Cranial** - cephalad, toward the head
**Caudal** - toward the tail or away from the head
**Distal** - away from the reference point
**Proximal** - near the reference point
Example: The navel is an anterior abdominal structure distal to the head and proximal to the pubis.

Group Four:  In and Out Group

**External** - outside, away from the center of the body
**Internal** - inside, near the center of the body
**Deep** - away from the surface of the body
**Superficial** - near or on the surface of the body
Example: The navel is a superficial midline structure on the ventral surface of the body halfway between the inferior border of the chest and the superior border of the pubis.

**A FEW MORE ESSENTIAL TERMS**

The joints of the body are moved by the muscles. Muscles can be attached to bone or tissue. The proximal end of the muscle is called the origin. The distal end is called the insertion. When a muscle contracts, movement is produced. These movements can be described in exact terms (see **Figure 2-3**). These are:
**Flexion** - to bend at an angle
**Extension** - to stretch out, or straighten out
**Abduct** - to draw away from the median plane
**Adduct** - to draw toward the median plan
**Circumduct** - to describe a cone in space, which combines the actions of flexion, abduction, extension, adduction and flexion again, or the motion of whirling a lasso
**Rotation** - to turn on a long axis, such as at the shoulder or hip
**Pronate** - to turn face down. This action refers mainly to the palm being turned down. When you are lying face down, you are prone.

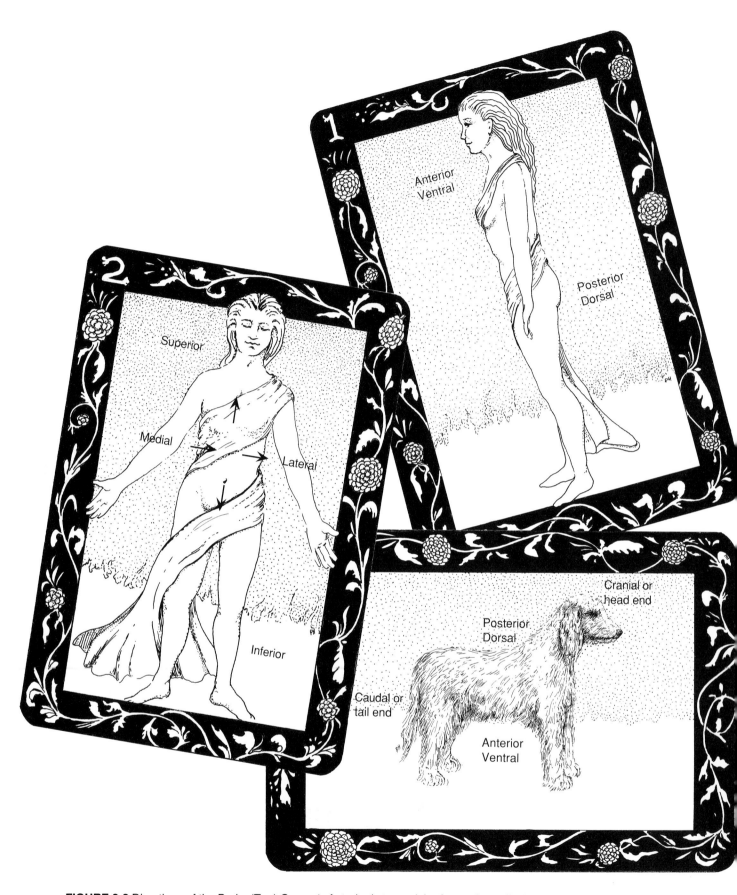

**FIGURE 2-2** Directions of the Body. (Top) Group 1. Anterior is toward the front, also called ventral or the abdominal side. Posterior is the back, also called the dorsal side. The relationship to a quadriped is seen in a dog. (Center) Group 2. Superior is top, and inferior is toward the bottom. Medial is toward the center of the body in the sagittal section. Lateral is away from the center of the body.

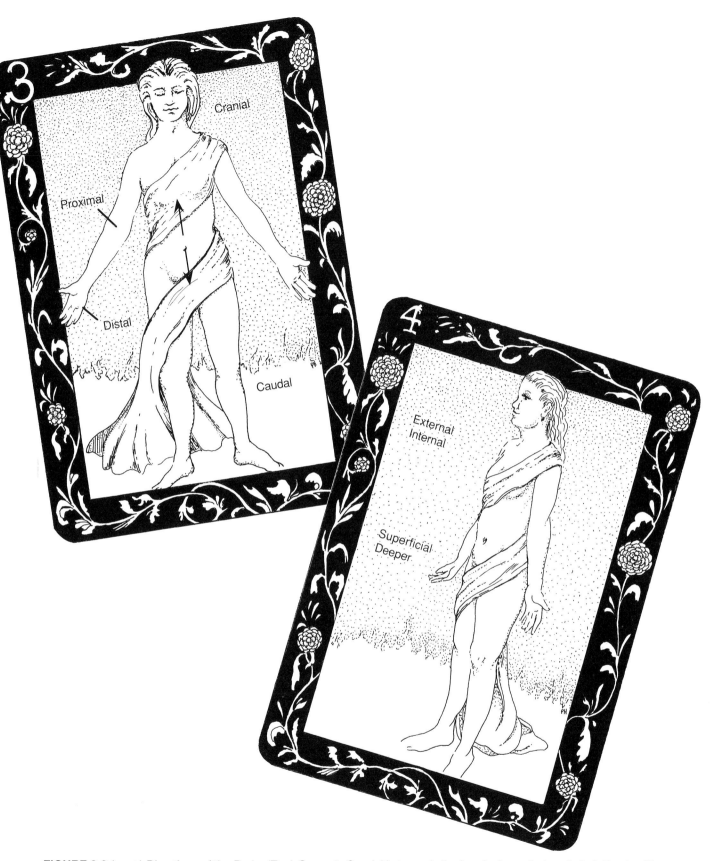

**FIGURE 2-2** (cont.) Directions of the Body. (Top) Group 3. Cranial is towards the head, also called cephalad. Proximal is close to the head or body. Distal means further from the head or body and caudal is away from the head, toward the tail. (Bottom) Group 4. External is outside of the body (nose), internal is inside the body (heart). Deep is towards the center of the body (cut or surgical wound) and superficial means surface or near the surface of the body.

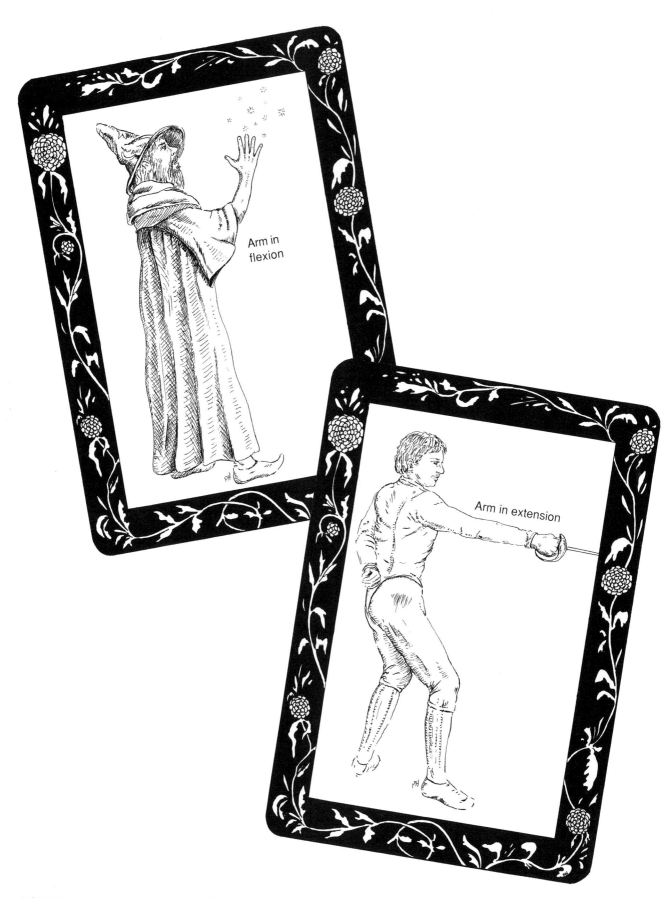

Arm in flexion

Arm in extension

**FIGURE 2-3** Essential Terms. (Top) Flexion. Arm bends or flexes at elbow. Leg bends at knee, as in sitting. (Bottom) Extension. In extension the arm and/or leg are straight.

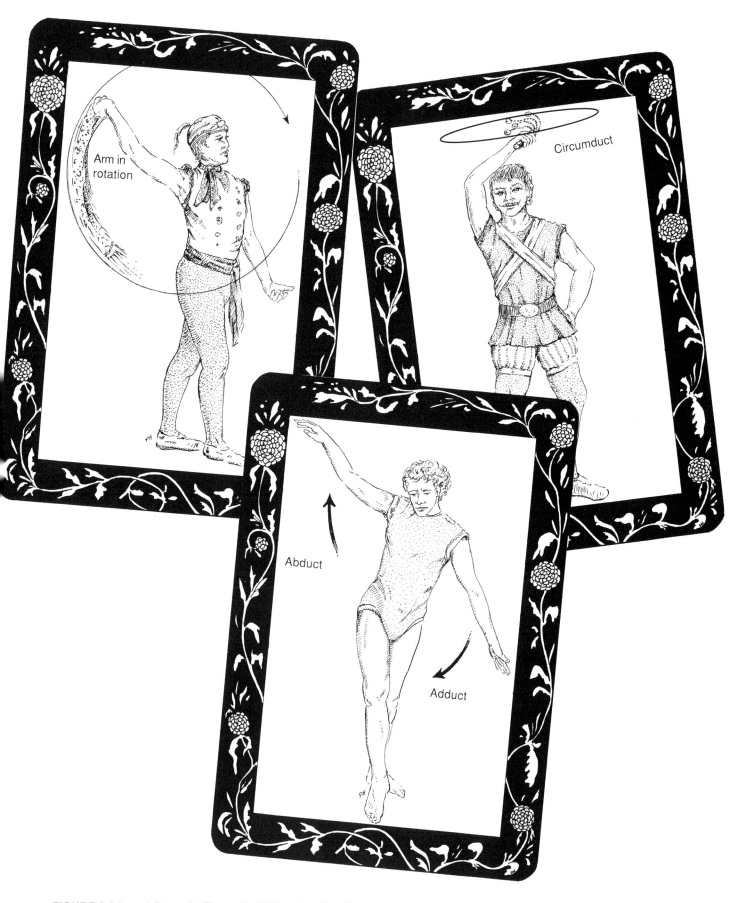

**FIGURE 2-3** (cont.) Essential Terms. (Left) Rotation. Rotation means to swing the arm at the joint in a **circular motion** but not in the **same plane**. (Right) Circumduct. Circumduct means to "lead around" or in circles. Think of drawing a circle with your finger on the ceiling, or floor. (Bottom) Abduct/Adduct. Abduction is moving away from the body while adduction is moving toward the body.

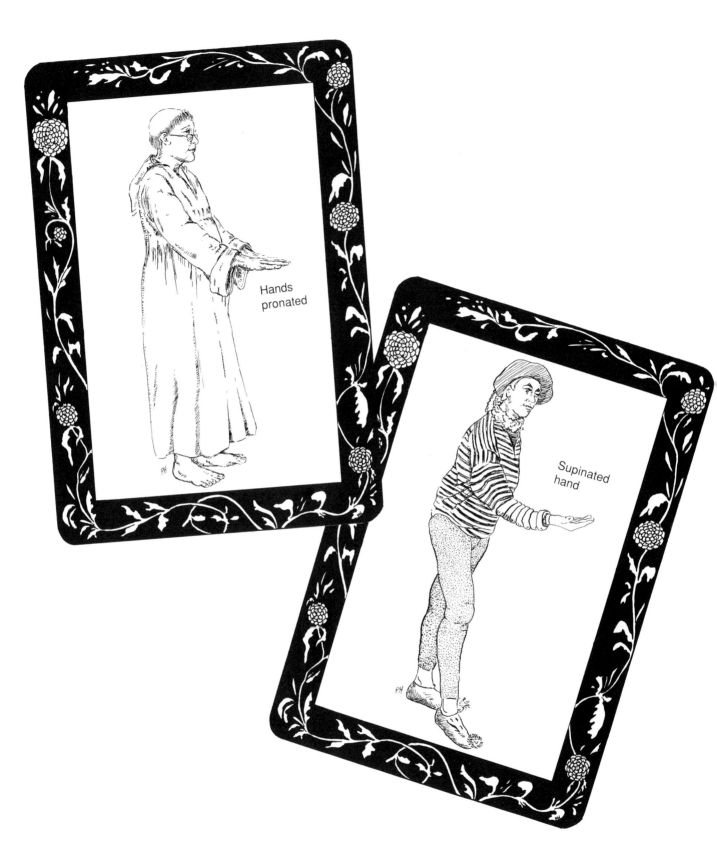

**FIGURE 2-3** (cont.) Essential Terms. (Top) Pronate. When you are prone you are flat on your abdomen and chest. Your hands are palms down in the prone position. (Bottom) Supine. Supine means "belly-up" or palms-up. A begger is a supplicant.

**Supinate** - to turn face up. When you rotate your hand so that the palm is up it is in the supine position. When you are lying on your back, you are supine.

## SURFACE ANATOMY OF THE HEAD

The head and the neck are the two most visible structures in man. Since you will spend most of your time as a skin care specialist working with these structures, it is a good starting point and one that we shall emphasize. We shall begin with surface markers and then examine the essential structures under the skin. Keep in mind that we need to know essentials which are different from details.

### Major Markers of the Head

Find the following markers:
The **nose** (see **Figure 2-4**) consists of thin

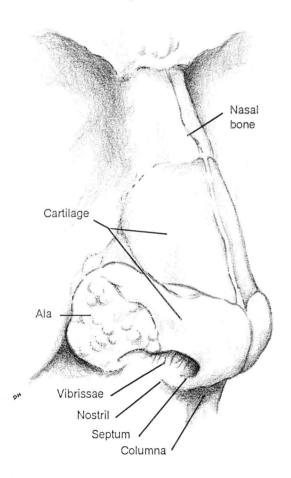

FIGURE 2-4 Structure of the Nose. Note the cartilage and bone locations. The nose is a thin and fragile structure. Not made for abuse.

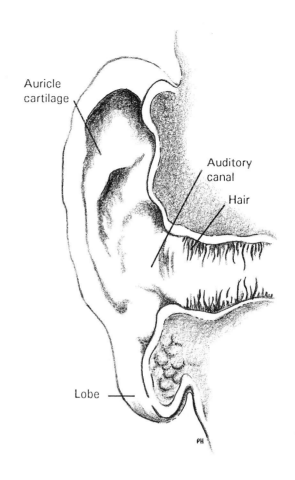

**FIGURE 2-5** Structure of the Ear. The ear contains a lot of cartilage and a fair amount of hair here and there. Note the ear canal contains hair follicles and wax glands (see text).

bone and cartilage. The tip is movable as are the alae or nostrils. These nostrils flare open by the action of small muscles on each side of the nose. The hairs in the nostrils are called vibrissae. Understand that the tip is composed of both cartilage and fibrous tissue and is divided by a septum, the lower border of which is called the columna.

The **ears** (see **Figure 2-5**), generally two, one on each side of the head, are placed at a level between the eyes and mouth when viewed from the side. The basic framework of the ear is a single piece of cartilage called the auricular cartilage to which is attached the ear lobe. This cartilage is part of the external auditory canal so that pulling on the ear also puts traction on the auditory canal. There is no fat under the thin skin that covers the ear cartilage, but there are numerous sebaceous glands and fine hairs over the ears. Coarse hairs are seen in the canal that guard the opening. The canal also contains wax glands that are activated at puberty.

The **eyes** (see **Figure 2-6**) are the most spectacular part of the face, which is the anterior part of the head. A line drawn through the eyes marks the center of the head in the average person. The eye is the most complex surface structure on the body. There are three major parts to learn - the orbit, the lids, and the eyeball itself. We need not concern ourselves with the eyeball as there are ample specialists who have devoted their lives and livings to this single organ. The orbit of the eye is a bony structure which has a prominent superior ridge called the supraorbital ridge. It is far more prominent in the human male (and gorillas) than in the human female. Surprisingly, the bones of the orbit are rather thin and weak. The eyelids are called palpebrae (Latin word *palpebra* meaning eyelid). Both upper and lower lids are separated by the palpebral fissure. At each corner of the eye are the angles called canthi. Each eye has a medial and lateral canthus. The space between the eyeball and the lids is the conjunctival sac. The membrane that lines this sac is called the conjunctiva.

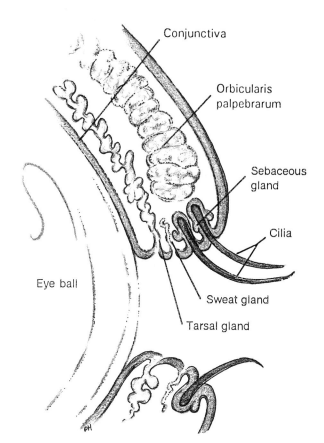

**FIGURE 2-7** Structure of the Eyelid. Look at the three types of glands in the lids. See text for explanation.

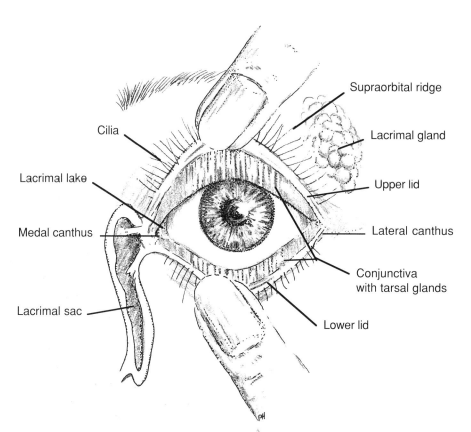

**FIGURE 2-6** Structure of the Eye. Notice the lacrimal gland is on one side of the eye (the lateral canthus) and the lacimal sac is on the other side. This allows tears to flow across the eye surface.

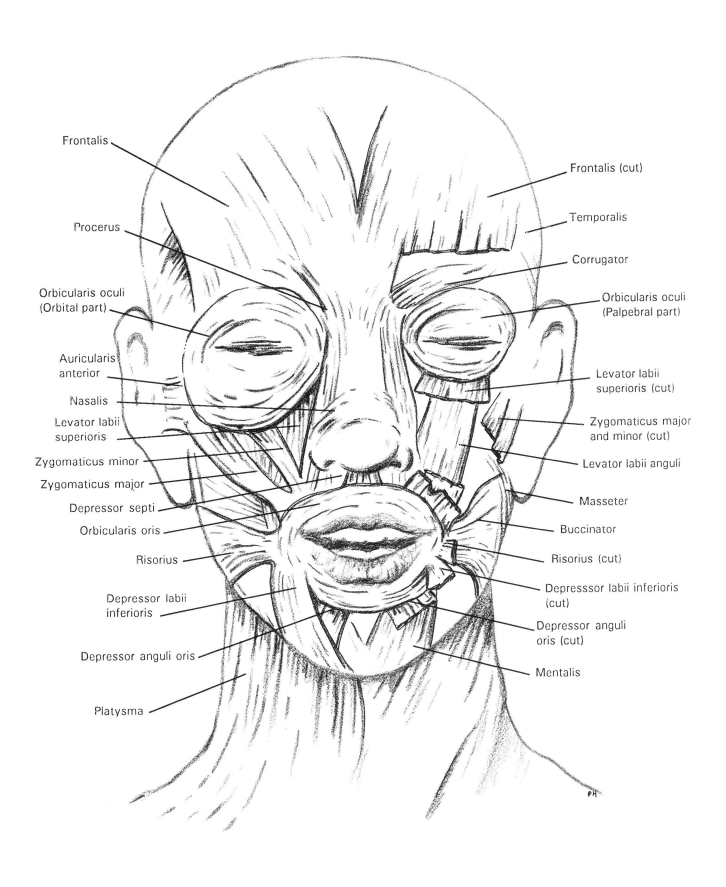

Frontalis

Procerus

Orbicularis oculi
(Orbital part)

Auricularis
anterior

Nasalis

Levator labii
superioris

Zygomaticus minor

Zygomaticus major

Depressor septi

Orbicularis oris

Risorius

Depressor labii
inferioris

Depressor anguli oris

Platysma

Frontalis (cut)

Temporalis

Corrugator

Orbicularis oculi
(Palpebral part)

Levator labii
superioris (cut)

Zygomaticus major
and minor (cut)

Levator labii anguli

Masseter

Buccinator

Risorius (cut)

Depresssor labii inferioris
(cut)

Depressor anguli
oris (cut)

Mentalis

**FIGURE 2-8** Muscles of the face. The buccinator keeps your food under your teeth for chewing while the masseter and temporalis are the main "power" chewing muscles.

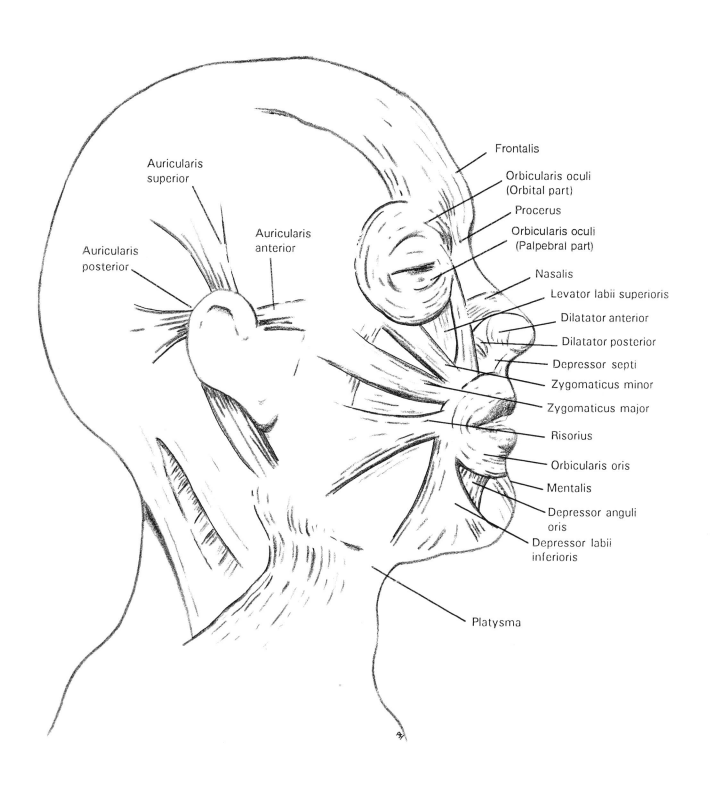

Auricularis
superior

Auricularis
anterior

Auricularis
posterior

Frontalis

Orbicularis oculi
(Orbital part)

Procerus

Orbicularis oculi
(Palpebral part)

Nasalis

Levator labii superioris

Dilatator anterior

Dilatator posterior

Depressor septi

Zygomaticus minor

Zygomaticus major

Risorius

Orbicularis oris

Mentalis

Depressor anguli
oris

Depressor labii
inferioris

Platysma

**FIGURE 2-8** (cont.) Muscles of the face. Superficial. These are the muscles of expression. Look at the **directions** of the muscles. Remember that wrinkles always form **across** these muscles (at right angles).

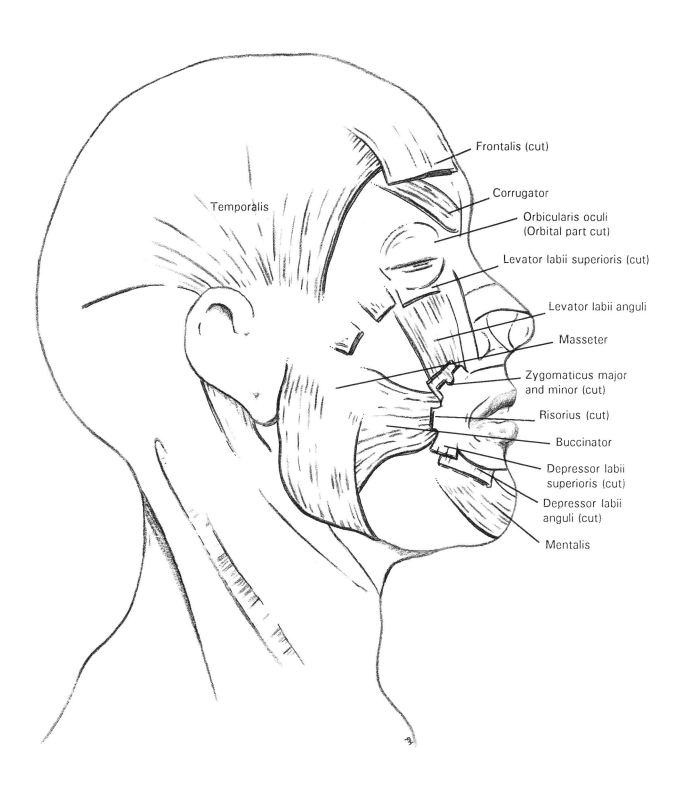

Frontalis (cut)

Corrugator

Orbicularis oculi
(Orbital part cut)

Levator labii superioris (cut)

Levator labii anguli

Masseter

Zygomaticus major
and minor (cut)

Risorius (cut)

Buccinator

Depressor labii
superioris (cut)

Depressor labii
anguli (cut)

Mentalis

Temporalis

**FIGURE 2-8** (cont.) Muscles of the face. Deeper. These are power muscles for chewing.

The **eyelids** are complex structures. Cilia (eyelashes) cover the outer five-sixth of the lids and are formed in two or three irregular rows (see **Figure 2-7**). These hairs are associated with both the sweat glands (the glands of Moll), and the sebaceous glands (the glands of Zeis), which open into the hair follicle. A third gland, the tarsal gland, is also known as the Meibomian gland. These glands are embedded in the tarsal plate behind the cilia and in front of the conjunctiva. The lacrimal apparatus or tear maker, consists of a gland under the lateral superior lid, a tear lake, and two small canals. The canals are located in the medial canthus and drain the tear lake into the nasal passage. This is why your nose runs when you cry.

The **mouth** is the most versatile movable structure in the body, and after the eye it is probably the most observed facial feature. It is a nearly oval oral cavity at the end of the digestive tube. It is bounded anteriorly by the lips and contains the tongue and teeth. The mouth is moved by the facial muscles, and this is where most students get hopelessly lost because of the apparent complexity of these muscles.

## THE MOUTH AND THE FACIAL MUSCLES

Following the "Divide and Conquer" principle, we shall separate these muscles into functional groups. Since you are going to be working on the surface of the skin only, you need not know all the details of the muscles in order to have a good working knowledge of facial anatomy.

The mouth (see **Figure 2-8**) itself is just muscles and skin and lies anterior to the maxilla, the upper immobile jaw, and the mandible, or lower movable jaw.

### The Deep Group, or Jaw Movers, or Chewing Muscles

The **temporalis** is a large muscle that pulls the jaw up and back. It is used to clench the teeth and close the mouth. You can easily feel the superior portion of this muscle on the head, but the part on the lower jaw is harder to feel. The **masseter** is a large powerful muscle with two parts. You can feel it on the angle of the mandible when you chew. It is the major muscle of

mastication or chewing. It is also used to clench the teeth and close the mouth.

The **buccinator** is a large, medium strength muscle that aids in mastication by pulling the cheeks against the teeth which keeps the food between the teeth. You can feel the buccinator on the inside of the mouth or on the external cheek.

The **pterygoids** are never seen and you cannot feel these muscles. They are the deep muscles used to move the mandible from side to side. Obviously, these muscles are important in mastication but of less importance to the skin care specialist.

### Mouth Movers or Muscles of Expression

Remember that muscles move things, usually bones, skin, or other muscles. When you move a body structure you must restore it to the original position so that it may be moved again. Muscles of expression (see **Figure 2-9**) are seen in pairs. It is best to learn them in pairs.

The **orbicularis oris**, or the kissing muscle, circles the opening of the mouth and functions to close the mouth and purse the lips. It is opposed by many muscles, chiefly the buccinator. This muscle is also important in chewing, but most of us use it far more often in the act of facial expression and speaking. Since the face is fairly symmetrical, the orbicularis oris is circular and equal on both sides of the face. It is the pulling and pushing of the mouth that changes the expression lines about the mouth.

The **depressor labii inferioris** pulls the corner of the mouth down. It originates at the mandible slightly to the midline on both sides. It is a deep muscle that lies above the mentalis and below the depressor anguli oris. The **mentalis** pulls the skin of the lower lip upward and outward, as in a pout.

The **depressor anguli oris** is attached to the corner of the mouth and the mandible. Its function is to pull the corners of the mouth downward. These muscles are opposed by the upper group of expression muscles.

The **levator labii superioris** pulls the corner of the mouth and part of the alae of the nose upward. It has three points of origin with the insertion in the skin and deep in the mucosa of the mouth. It is opposed by the lower group

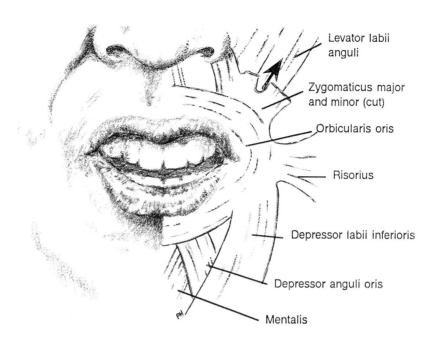

Levator labii
anguli

Zygomaticus major
and minor (cut)

Orbicularis oris

Risorius

Depressor labii inferioris

Depressor anguli oris

Mentalis

**FIGURE 2-9** Mouth muscles of expression. Growl. These muscles show the teeth. Teeth showing can be friendly, as in a smile, or a warning, as in a growl.

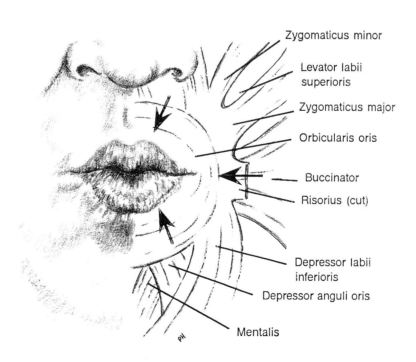

Zygomaticus minor

Levator labii
superioris

Zygomaticus major

Orbicularis oris

Buccinator

Risorius (cut)

Depressor labii
inferioris

Depressor anguli oris

Mentalis

**FIGURE 2-9** (cont.) Mouth muscles of expression. Kiss. The kiss is mainly produced by the orbicularis oris . (Think of a draw string on an old fashioned purse.

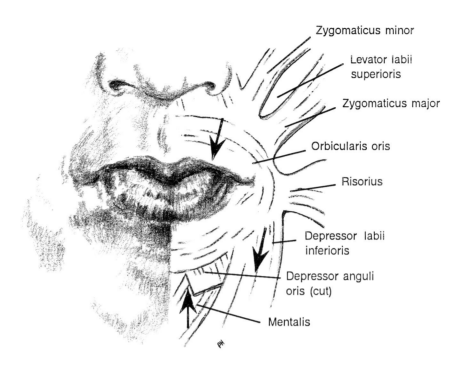

**FIGURE 2-9** (cont.) Mouth muscles of expression. Pout. A pout is a "pull down" muscle movement. It expresses quiet anger and frustration.

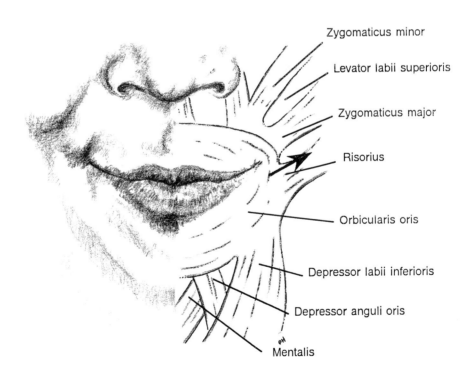

**FIGURE 2-9** (cont.) Mouth muscles of expression. Smile. Smiles are quantitative in nature, very subtle expressions of joy, surprise, anger, fear, etc. The risorius here is producing a "little smile".

member, the **levator labii inferioris**. This muscle works in conjunction with the zygomatic muscles of which there are two, a major and a minor. The **zygomaticus major and minor** arise from the zygoma and insert into the angle of the mouth from the corner to the base of the nares. They raise the angle of the mouth. The **risorius**, also known as the "smiling muscle" is a superficial muscle attached at the corner of the mouth and arising from the skin and fascia over the parotid gland (fascia is tough fibrous tissue that attaches muscle to skin and bone). Now, we are finished with the mouth group and we have to look at two more muscles of expression as we work our way up the face.

### The Eye and Forehead Group of Expression

The **orbicularis oculi** (see **Figure 2-10**) circle the eyes and oppose each other. This muscle pulls the eyelids down, closes the eyes, and compresses the tear ducts.

The **frontalis** arises from the front of the skull and inserts at the eyebrows, the skin and the nose. It is a big muscle and runs longitudinally over the forehead. Its function is to raise the eyebrows, and to draw the scalp forward, which causes wrinkles across the forehead. We shall learn more about the effect of the muscle fiber direction when we study the mechanism of aging. Let's move on to the nerves and blood vessels of the face which will be our final facial topic.

### THE BLOOD VESSELS AND NERVES OF THE FACE

Again, we shall stick to the essentials that relate to skin care technology. The muscles and skin of the face are supplied with nutrients and oxygen, mainly by the three arteries arising from the **external carotid artery** (see **Figure 2-11**) or branches of the external carotid. An essential point is at the angle of the neck formed by the mandible and the sternocleidomastoid muscle

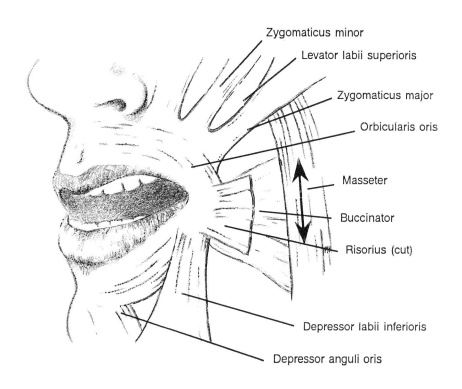

Zygomaticus minor
Levator labii superioris
Zygomaticus major
Orbicularis oris
Masseter
Buccinator
Risorius (cut)
Depressor labii inferioris
Depressor anguli oris

**FIGURE 2-9** (cont.) Muscles of chewing. Chewing is a powerful use of muscles, but it can be mild, controlled chewing as in chewing gum. (Gum chewing is a primative activity, much like thumb sucking, used to allay anxiety and insecurity).

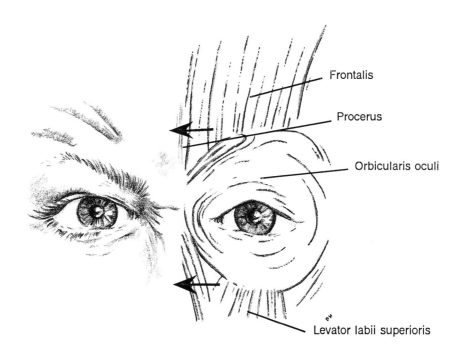

Frontalis

Procerus

Orbicularis oculi

Levator labii superioris

**FIGURE 2-10** Forehead muscles of expression. Anger. See the tension response. This is a brow knit, or "tight" movement, a squeezing of one's self.

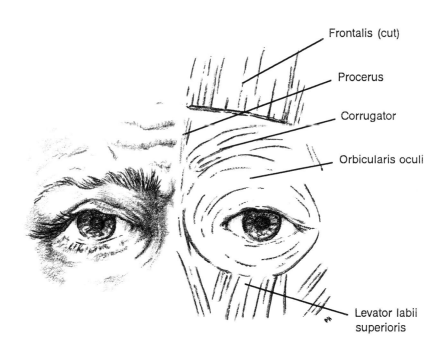

Frontalis (cut)

Procerus

Corrugator

Orbicularis oculi

Levator labii
superioris

**FIGURE 2-10** (cont.) Forehead muscles of expression. Crying. The crying face is a very complex face. Every muscle is used in both the upper and lower face.

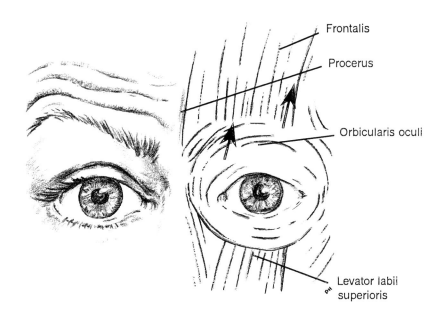

Frontalis

Procerus

Orbicularis oculi

Levator labii
superioris

**FIGURE 2-10** (cont.) Forehead muscles of expression. Surprise. Surprise is an "up-muscle" and an "eye muscle" movement. Notice the use again of the frontalis, a most versatile muscle.

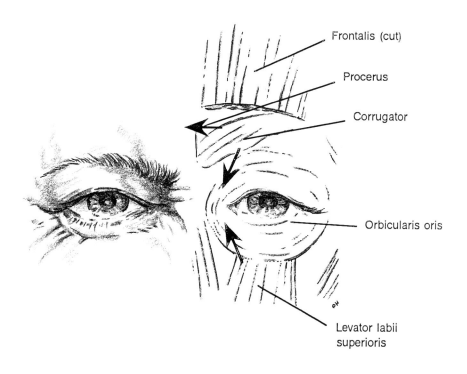

Frontalis (cut)

Procerus

Corrugator

Orbicularis oris

Levator labii
superioris

**FIGURE 2-10** (cont.) Forehead muscles of expression. Squint. Squinting is a very complex muscle activity. It is an attempt to improve the intake of light and focus of the eye. It expresses uncertainty, to take a closer look.

(SCM). (See Figure 2-16, structure of the neck.) There is a structure within the **internal carotid artery** called the carotid sinus body and it helps to control blood pressure. By turning the head sharply to the left or right and running your fingers up the SCM muscle, your fingers will strike the mandibular angle and you will feel the carotid pulsating beneath your fingers. You must be very careful in this area. Do not apply pressure as it can cause a sensitive individual to faint.

We need to recognize three main arteries.

The **facial artery** runs across the face from the top of the nose, between the eyes, down to about the middle of the mandible, and then goes deep. The **superficial temporal artery** at the top of the head supplies many branches for the scalp and forehead.

The **transverse artery** lies between the other two arteries of the face.

There are many branches, but the above three are the most important. Remember, the external carotid and its branches supply blood to most of the skin and muscles of the face. The internal carotid supplies the brain and other internal structures.

Now is a good time to reiterate the distinction between a vein and an artery. Veins take blood to the heart; arteries take blood away from the heart. The vein has only a thin muscular coat. The artery is heavier to expand and contract more quickly.

The major facial vein is the **anterior facial vein** (see **Figure 2-12**). It runs down across the face to join into the **external jugular vein** collecting many tributaries along the way. It collects blood from the **orbital vein**, the **frontal vein**, and the **superior labial veins**. Unfortunately, it also communicates with the cavernous sinus through the **opthamalic vein**. The **cavernous sinus** lies in the brain and connects to structures within the brain. There are no valves in these veins to prevent back flow and they are compressed by facial muscles. The area that drains has been called **the dangerous area of the face**. This is an extremely important aspect of the facial veins that must be known by every skin care specialist. **No infection, of any type, should be treated in this area, from the corners of the upper lip to the area between the eyes** as is seen in **Figure 2-13**. Any infection, such as a pimple, boil (furuncle), or cellulitis (red inflamed skin) seen in this area should be referred immediately to a physician for proper treatment.

## The Main Groups of Facial Nerves

There are both sensory nerves (see **Figure 2-14**) for feeling and motor nerves (see **Figure 2-15**) for moving the muscles of the face. Some nerves share both functions. When a sensory nerve is affected there can be either numbness in the face or an intense feeling. When motor nerves are impaired, it can result in muscle paralysis. A common temporary facial disorder is a paralysis of the facial nerve known as Bell's Palsy, manifested by drooping of the eye lid and mouth on one side of the face.

### Sensory Group

The major nerve for sensation of the face is the **trigeminal** nerve. It has three branches: the **opthalmic**, the **maxillary**, and the **mandibular** which are the first, second, and third branches of the Fifth Cranial nerve. Look at these nerves and see how they are distributed over the face. Most importantly, the trigeminal nerve emerges onto the face in front of the ear. Pressure in this area can cause damage to the trigeminal nerve. Individuals who hold a telephone to their ear with their shoulder, frequently produce damage to this nerve. The trigeminal nerve also supplies motor nerves to some of the muscles of mastication.

### The Motor Group

The **facial nerve** is the major motor nerve of the face. It also exits near the front of the ear and is easily damaged with excessive pressure. It supplies most of the muscles of expression of the face.

The facial nerve is the **seventh cranial nerve**. You do not need to learn all the branches but be familiar with the distribution.

## THE NECK

The **neck** is very often a neglected area in skin care. There are three major structures that we must look at in the neck. They are the muscles, the blood vessels, and the glands (see **Figure 2-16**).

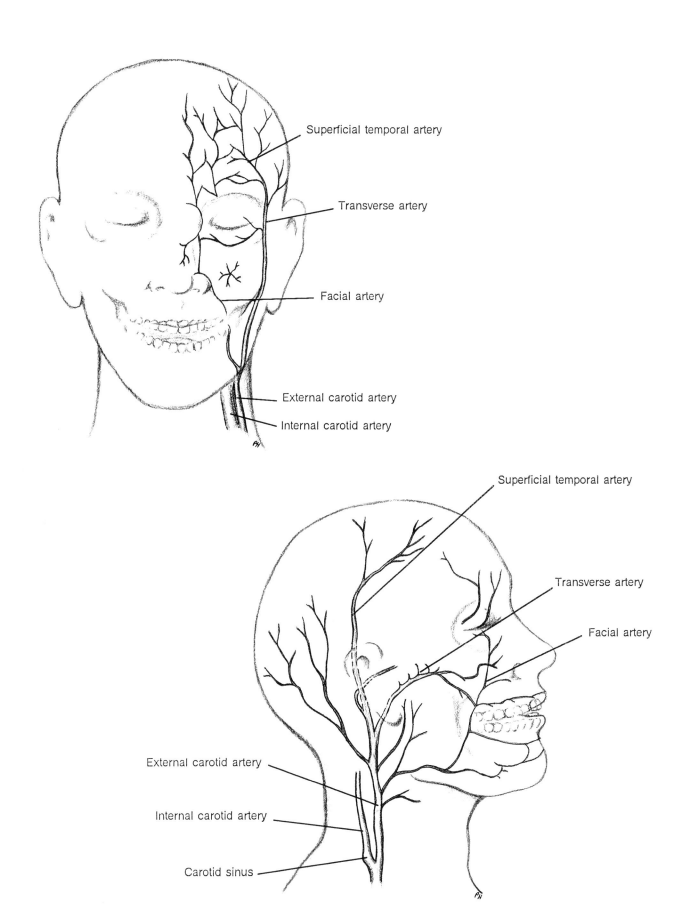

Superficial temporal artery

Transverse artery

Facial artery

External carotid artery

Internal carotid artery

Superficial temporal artery

Transverse artery

Facial artery

External carotid artery

Internal carotid artery

Carotid sinus

**FIGURE 2-11** Blood vessels of the face. Arteries. The external carotid supplies the skin of the face. The internal carotid supplies the brain.

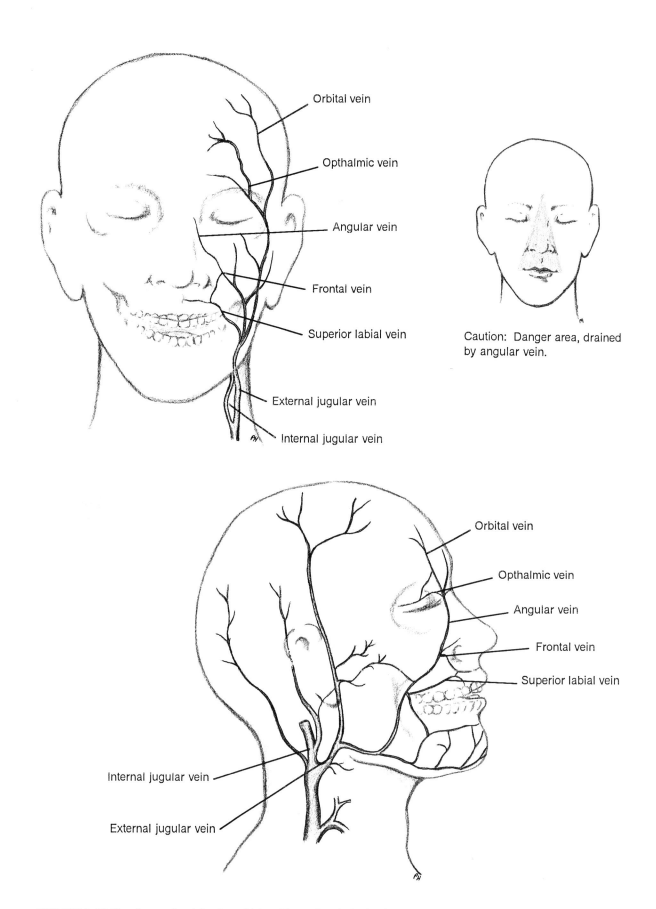

Orbital vein

Opthalmic vein

Angular vein

Frontal vein

Superior labial vein

External jugular vein

Internal jugular vein

Caution: Danger area, drained by angular vein.

Orbital vein

Opthalmic vein

Angular vein

Frontal vein

Superior labial vein

Internal jugular vein

External jugular vein

**FIGURE 2-12** Blood vessels of the face. Veins. The veins drain the face down to the external jugular vein, but the veins around the nose drain into the brain. **FIGURE 2-13** (Inset) Danger area of the face. Note the danger zone. It extends from the corners of the upper lip to the part between the eyes. Do not squeeze a pimple in this area.

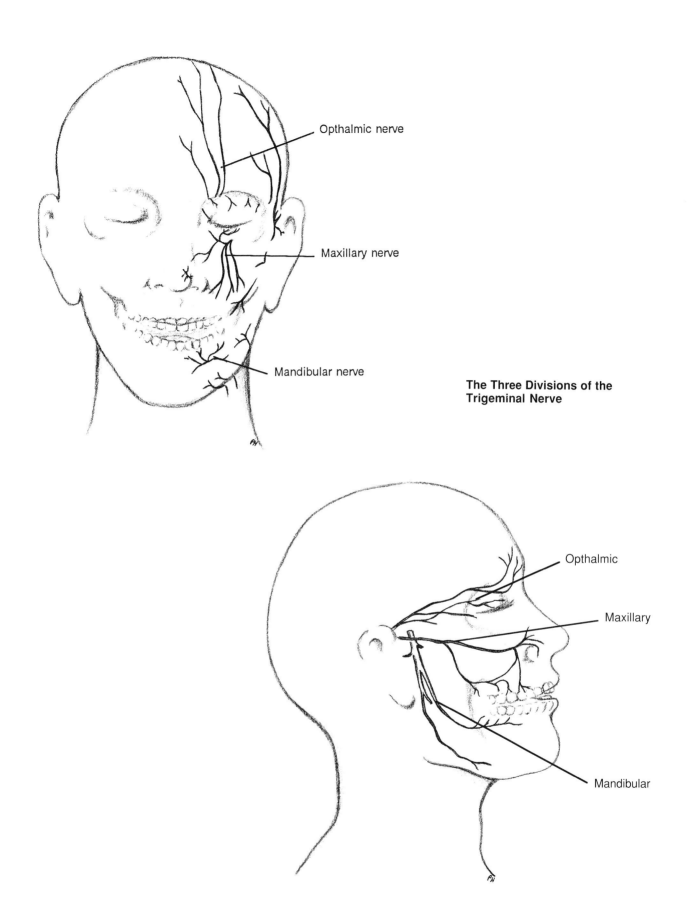

Opthalmic nerve

Maxillary nerve

Mandibular nerve

**The Three Divisions of the Trigeminal Nerve**

Opthalmic

Maxillary

Mandibular

**FIGURE 2-14** Nerves of the face. Sensory. Note the three facial nerve branches join inside the skull in the trigeminal ganglion, not shown in the illustration.

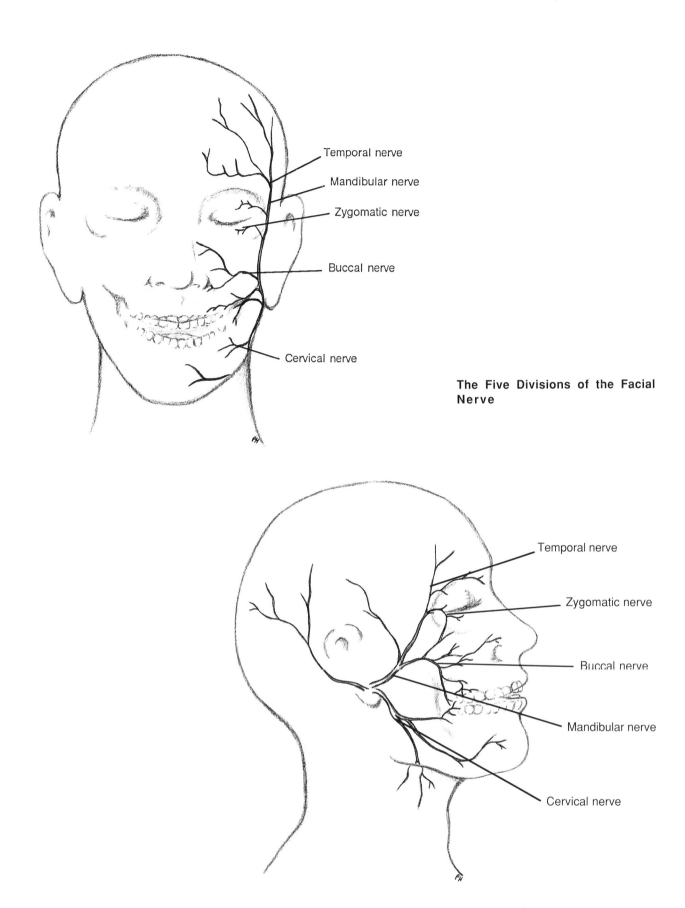

**The Five Divisions of the Facial Nerve**

Temporal nerve
Mandibular nerve
Zygomatic nerve
Buccal nerve
Cervical nerve

Temporal nerve
Zygomatic nerve
Buccal nerve
Mandibular nerve
Cervical nerve

**FIGURE 2-15** Nerves of the face. Motor. The facial nerve is a motor nerve that has five major branches, 1) the temporal, 2) the zygomatic, 3) the buccal, 4) the mandibular and 5) the cervical. Injury or infection of the facial nerve results in a condition called Bell's palsy.

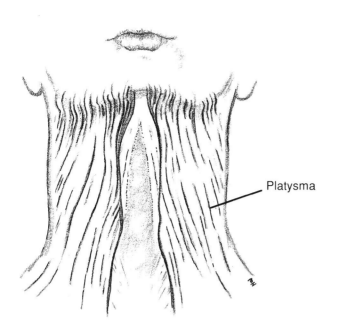

Platysma

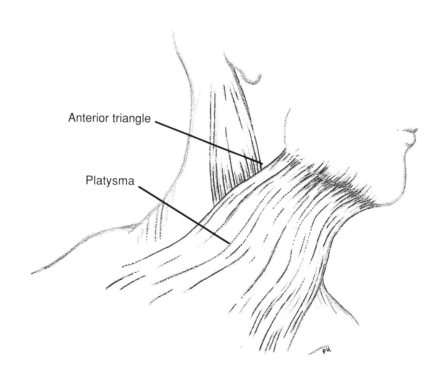

Anterior triangle

Platysma

**FIGURE 2-16** Structure of the neck. Superficial muscles. The platysma goes "bad" quickly and causes much distress to women and much delight to cosmetic surgeons.

### The Muscles

Only three muscles are important enough to warrant our attention. The **sternocleidomastoid (SCM)** is a very large muscle that runs from the manubrium in the chest to the mastoid process behind the ear on the skull. You can see it as rope-like cords when you turn your head sharply. The **platysma** muscle is a large, flat, thin muscle that is the bane of older men and women. It is the muscle responsible for "turkey neck". It arises from the skin and fascia of the upper chest

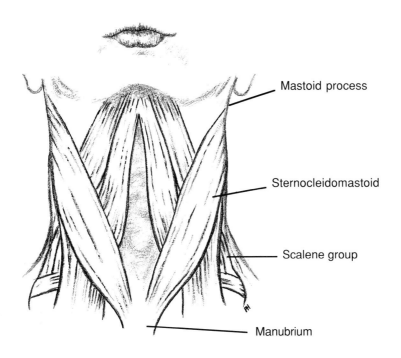

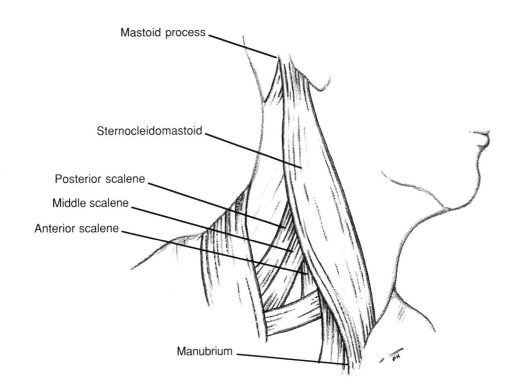

**FIGURE 2-16** (cont.) Structure of the neck. Deeper muscles. The main muscles are the sternocleidomastoid (SCM), and the scalene group. Use the SCM as an anatomical land mark.

and attaches to the skin over the cheeks, mouth, and under the chin. The **scalene group**, is a bundle of strap-like muscles in the lateral neck. They are deeper than the platysma and the SCM, and can be felt when the head is turned sharply. They are important because they can press on the nerves going to the arms (the brachial plexus nerves) causing pain and dysfunction.

**The Blood Vessels**

Only two major ones concern us: the **carotid**

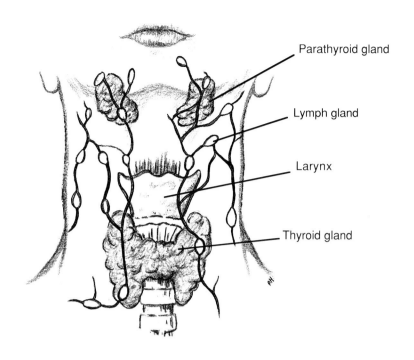

Parathyroid gland

Lymph gland

Larynx

Thyroid gland

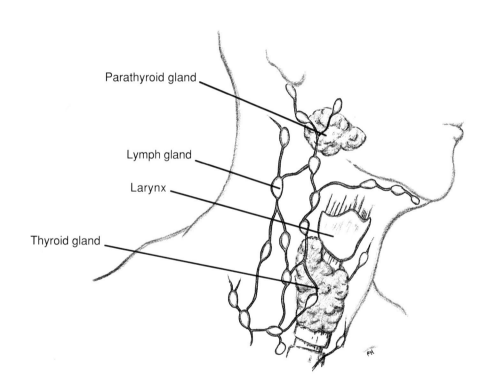

Parathyroid gland

Lymph gland

Larynx

Thyroid gland

**FIGURE 2-16** (cont.) Structure of the neck. Glands. The main glands are the thyroid and the parathyroids. In the presence of a sore throat the lymph nodes become enlarged and palpable.

**arteries** and corresponding **carotid sinus body**, and the **jugular veins**. The **common carotid artery** passes up the neck along the border of the SCM muscle, and is quite deep. It then splits into the internal and external carotid arteries. It can be felt in the anterior triangle of the neck, which is formed by the medial border of the SCM muscle, the inferior border of the mandible and the anterior platysma muscle. Divide this triangle into two parts by drawing an imaginary line from the middle of the SCM to the middle of the inferior border of the mandible.

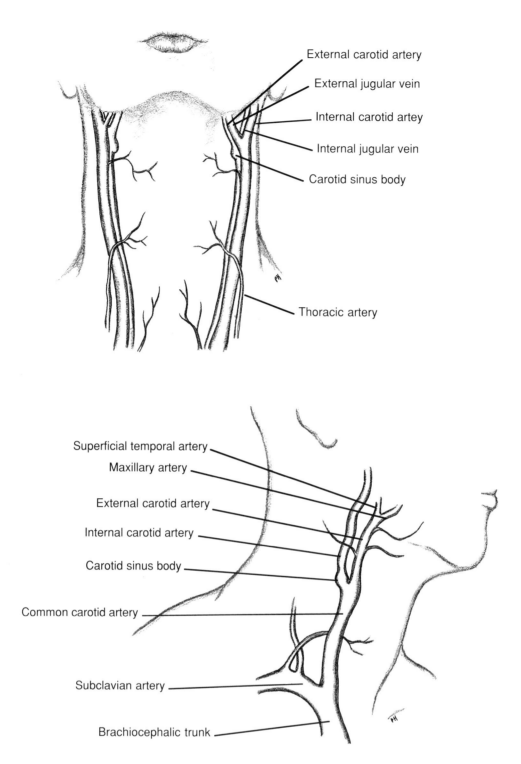

Labels in first diagram:
- External carotid artery
- External jugular vein
- Internal carotid artery
- Internal jugular vein
- Carotid sinus body
- Thoracic artery

Labels in second diagram:
- Superficial temporal artery
- Maxillary artery
- External carotid artery
- Internal carotid artery
- Carotid sinus body
- Common carotid artery
- Subclavian artery
- Brachiocephalic trunk

**FIGURE 2-16** (cont.) Structure of the neck. Blood vessels. The veins and arteries run close together. Stretching the neck as in looking up "or around" in older persons puts pressure on the carotid sinus and may cause dizziness.

You can then mark out the carotid triangle at the superior portion. In this triangle you can feel the carotid artery pulsating. Also passing through this triangle is the internal jugular vein. You cannot see it, but you can see the external jugular vein, which runs across the SCM into the lower neck.

### The Glands

There are two groups, the **thyroid-parathyroid group** and the **lymphatic group**. You can feel the thyroid if you turn your neck slightly and retract the SCM laterally. The thyroid sits in the notch above the manubrium and is below the voice box or larynx. The parathyroids are associated with the thyroid gland laterally. There are multiple lymph glands in the neck, chiefly in the anterior and posterior triangles. We can usually feel these if we extend the neck slightly for the anterior triangle and then flex the neck for the posterior triangle. They are important to us because they enlarge with certain diseases, such as infections of the skin, systemic infections, and other more serious diseases.

## THE CHEST OR THORAX

The **chest** is an anatomical site that is relatively easy, for the surface markings are few. The chest contains the heart, the lungs, the esophagus, and the diaphragm. The diaphragm separates the chest cavity from the abdominal cavity. Look at **Figure 2-17**, and identify these parts. Determine the relationship of the internal parts to the surface anatomy. This area is shown in the cross-sectional view of the chest (see **Figure 2-18**). While it is obvious, the examiner often forgets that these parts move as the body is turned from side to side, or as the

chest is flexed or extended. Keep in mind the comfort of your client, particularly your older client. Their bodies are no longer quite so resilient when you move or position them. There are areas of the chest that are relatively thin and cannot take much pressure. Make sure that you do not lean on the client's chest.

### Muscles of the Chest

There are only three groups on the anterior thorax that you need to know, the two **pectorales**, and the **intercostals**. (see **Figure 2-19**). The **pectoralis major** is a large muscle that flexes, adducts, and rotates the arm medially, e.g. pulls the arm across the chest as in folding the arms. It covers one half of the chest on each side, from the clavicle to the sternum, down to the muscles of the upper abdomen. (The **sternum** is a bony structure in the center or midline of the anterior chest. The sternum receives the ribs and the clavicles as an anchoring point). The breasts sit on top of this muscle. The **pectoralis minor** is deep or inferior to the pectoralis major. You cannot feel it. Its action is to pull the shoulder blade down, or to elevate the ribs. The ribs pull up and out in a flaring action when we take a deep breath. This is due to the action of

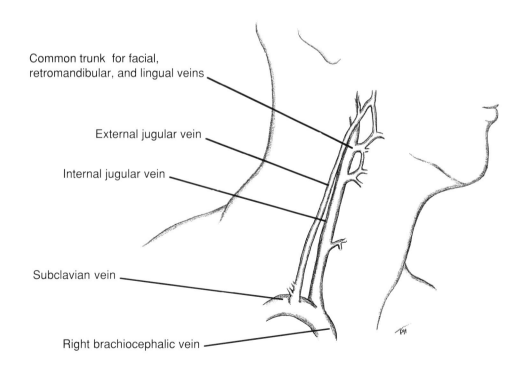

Common trunk for facial, retromandibular, and lingual veins

External jugular vein

Internal jugular vein

Subclavian vein

Right brachiocephalic vein

**FIGURE 2-16** (cont.) Structure of the neck. Blood vessels.

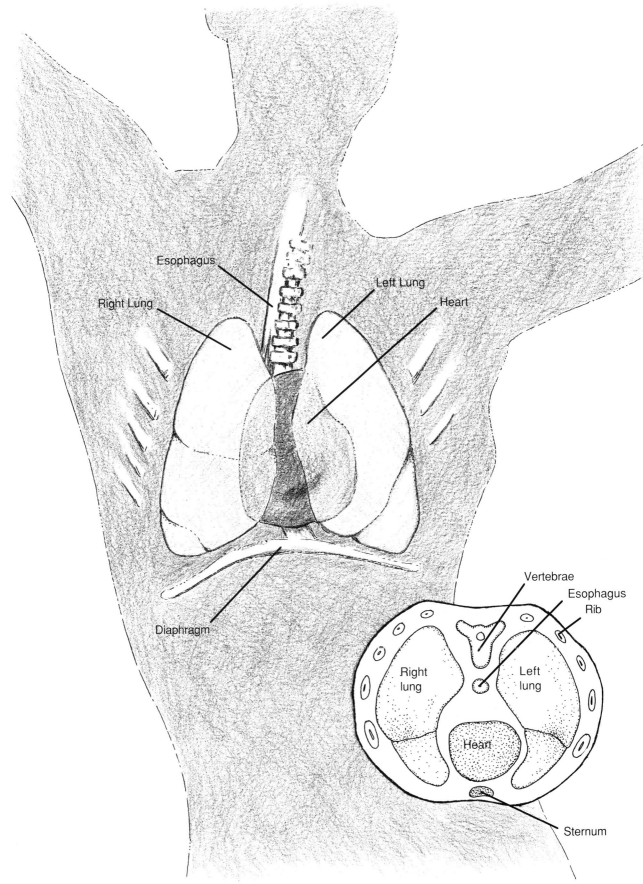

**FIGURE 2-17** Anatomy of the chest. Note the heart is near the center but off to the left side of the chest. **FIGURE 2-18** Cross-sectional view of the chest. The esophagus is directly behind the heart, and notice that the lungs are on either side of the esophagus.

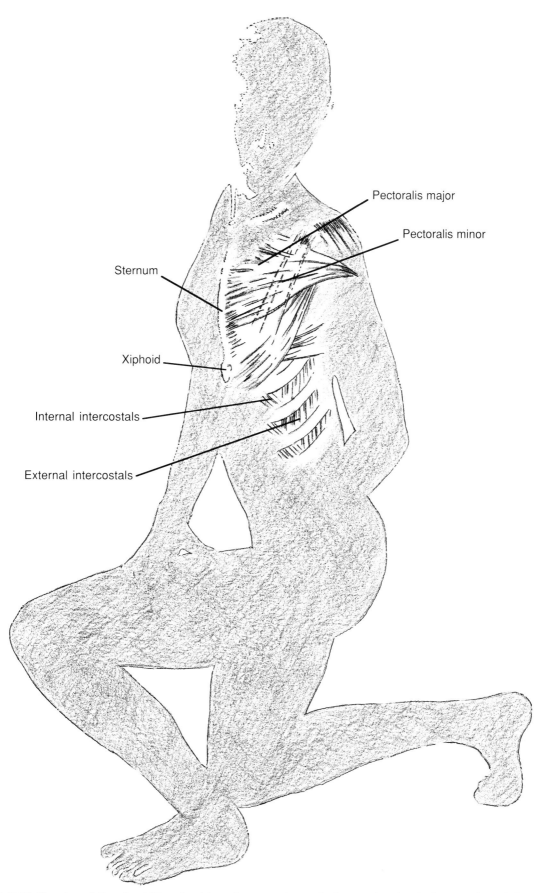

Pectoralis major

Pectoralis minor

Sternum

Xiphoid

Internal intercostals

External intercostals

**FIGURE 2-19** Muscles of the chest. The chest is quite muscular and often a site of pain from strain or inflammation. Breathing stretches these muscles and can aggravate any painful condition. Note the relationship of the large pectoral muscles **over** the ribs and extending to the sternum.

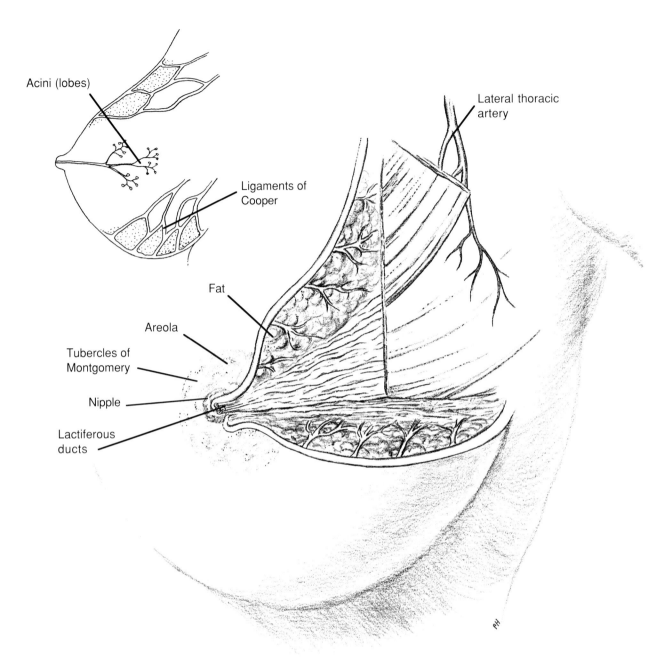

Acini (lobes)

Ligaments of Cooper

Fat

Areola

Tubercles of Montgomery

Nipple

Lactiferous ducts

Lateral thoracic artery

**FIGURE 2-20** Structure of the breast. The breast is a large apocrine gland consisting of mostly fat cells and ductile tissue. Note the ligaments that support the breast.

many muscles but is mainly due to the **inter-costals**. These muscles occur between the ribs as three separate muscles. They serve to draw the ribs together. Since the rib cage is "springy", none of the ribs are tightly fixed to the vertebral column or to the sternum. At the very bottom of the sternum is a projection called the xiphoid (a Greek word meaning "shaped like a sword"). The exact function of this structure is not known but it is important because it protrudes into the abdominal wall. You will become uncomfortable if this area is pushed or pressed too heavily.

## THE BREASTS

In the adult female the **breasts** (see **Figure 2-20**) are the most prominent structures. The breasts are derived from apocrine glands. They are superficial structures. The anatomy of the breasts is quite simple, but for many individuals understanding the limits of breast tissue is often difficult. This is most likely due to myths handed down through the ages, but also from limitless hope that the breasts may be altered at will. The breasts are located between the 2nd and the 6th ribs. They extend from the lateral border of the sternum to the mid-axillary line (the middle of the arm pit). The lower medial part of the breast actually rests on some of the superior parts of the abdominal muscles.

## Structure of the Breasts

The breasts are made up of five essential components: the acini, the ducts, the nipple, the ligaments, and the fat. Together, they comprise the structural and functional aspects of the breast. Bear in mind that the breast is a large, modified, apocrine-type gland that is a true skin derived organ. It reaches maturity only during pregnancy.

The **acini** are the smallest part of the gland. They are the true milk producers. They are arranged into lobules, which are then arranged into lobes, and finally are arranged radially (like spokes). They open into lactiferous ducts which convey the milk to the nipples. Each nipple has from 15 to 20 openings for milk secretion.

Immediately under the nipple the **lactiferous ducts** dilate, to form the lactiferous sinuses. They are tiny lakes that hold droplets of milk, which is expressed as the infant sucks.

The **nipple** is a raised structure. At its base is a circular pigmented area, known as the areola. The areola is composed of tiny, raised bumps called the tubercles of Montgomery or Morgagni (both men named these structures). They are enlarged sebaceous glands that protrude onto the surface of the skin.

The **Ligaments of Cooper** hold the breast to the muscle and fascial wall of the chest. They divide the various lobes of the breast. The ligaments of Cooper and the fat in the breast are responsible for the shape of the breast. In early puberty the breast will protrude outward in a small, conical form. This shape results from the lack of fatty tissue. Under the influence of female hormones and diet, the breasts will enlarge and fill with fat. This causes them to be round from the front view and assume a slightly pendulant, concave-convex shape from the side. In a mature female, the breast which protrudes sharply outwards in a conical shape, is an "assisted breast". The act of lying supine will cause the breast to assume a convex surface, with a flow laterally over the chest wall. The nipple will be in an outward position. Augmented or assisted breasts do not have this form and tend

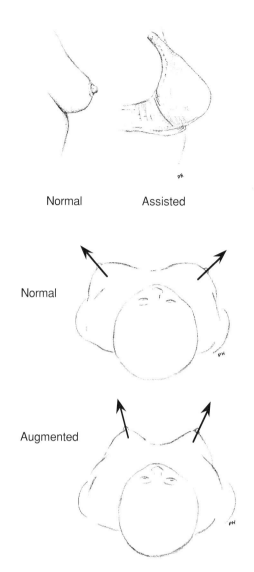

**FIGURE 2-21** (Top) Assisted breast. The use of breast supports do not necessarily prevent sagging with age. The prime purpose of the brassiere is to shape the breast. (Above) Augmented breasts. In the normal adult female the breast will be rolled to the sides of the chest in the supine position.

to be more upright, with a shorter radius of convexity. (See **Figure 2-21** to appreciate this phenomenon.)

The **fat** in the breast is behind the glandular portion and in front of the deep fascia. In the non-pregnant female, the greater part of the breast mass is fatty tissue.

The blood supply to the breast is from the **lateral thoracic artery** and the **internal mammary artery**. The nerve supply is from cutaneous branches of the intercostal nerves from 2-6. (The intercostal nerves run between the ribs.) There are also sympathetic nerves supplied to the mammary gland, which we will review in a later section.

One last comment on the breast. There is in mammals a "milk line" (see **Figure 2-22**). It runs from the axilla across the breast, down the lateral abdomen to the symphysis pubis (pubic hair region), and then down to the medial superior thigh. You may find little brown structures in this area that look like pigment moles, which in reality are accessory nipples.

## THE BACK OR POSTIOR THORAX

The **back** (see **Figure 2-23**) is another frequently neglected area for skin care because most of the time the client is in the supine position. Besides the universal muscle and bone problems of the back there is also a great deal of acne and other skin lesions associated with the back. It is best to consider the back as one unit, from the posterior neck to the buttocks. (While buttocks are frequent objects of ocular engagement, they too, have received little professional attention from any scientific group.)

We can divide the back into the chest portion or **posterior thorax** and the lower back or the **lumbosacral portion**. It is not necessary to know all the muscles of the back but you should be familiar with the larger ones. They run from the neck down to the sacrum:

The **trapezius**, which runs from the base of the skull superiorly to the last thoracic vertebrae inferiorly and to the apex of the scapula

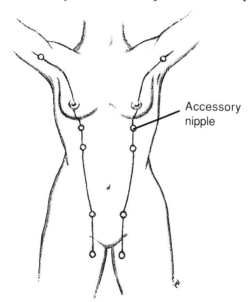

Accessory nipple

**FIGURE 2-22** Breast milkline. A vestigial structure that occasionally persists. Frequently are seen extra nipples in the lower chest in both males and females.

laterally, is the largest muscle in the back. The **latissimus dorsi** extends from the upper posterior humerus to the lower thoracic vertebrae, the lumbar vertebrae, and the iliac crest. It adducts, extends, and rotates the arm medially. The **deltoids** are partially on the back and that is why they should be mentioned here. The deltoids range from the lateral clavicle and scapula to the deltoid tuberosity of the humerus. It is an abductor muscle which aids in both extension and flexion.

The **nerves** of the back are many, but they are deep and most are not of our concern. However, the sciatic nerve should be learned. It is easily damaged with excessive pressure. It is located in the buttock area under the gluteus maximus and runs down the back of the thigh. It is the largest nerve of the body and it is the primary nerve of the leg.

## THE ABDOMEN

The **abdomen** is the major viscera-containing cavity of the body. The stomach, the liver, the spleen, the kidneys, the pancreas, and the intestines are located there. Look at **Figure 2-24** and locate the various organs. The abdomen is divided into four major quadrants. The right upper quadrant contains the liver, the gall bladder, and the top of the ascending colon. The left upper quadrant contains the spleen and the descending colon. In between these two quadrants is the epigastrium, which contains the stomach. The lower right quadrant contains the appendix and the cecum, while the lower left quadrant contains the sigmoid colon. None of these quadrants have sharp lines of demarcation. They serve mainly as general reference points to locate the internal organs.

The abdomen is covered with muscles that protect it from the outside forces. The major muscle that you need to learn is the **rectus abdominis**. This muscle runs down the midline from the lower chest to the symphysis pubis (pubic bone). It is a very large muscle that can be easily felt.

## THE EXTREMITIES

The anatomy of the extremities is quite complex when you consider all of the bones, the muscles, the ligaments, the blood vessels, and

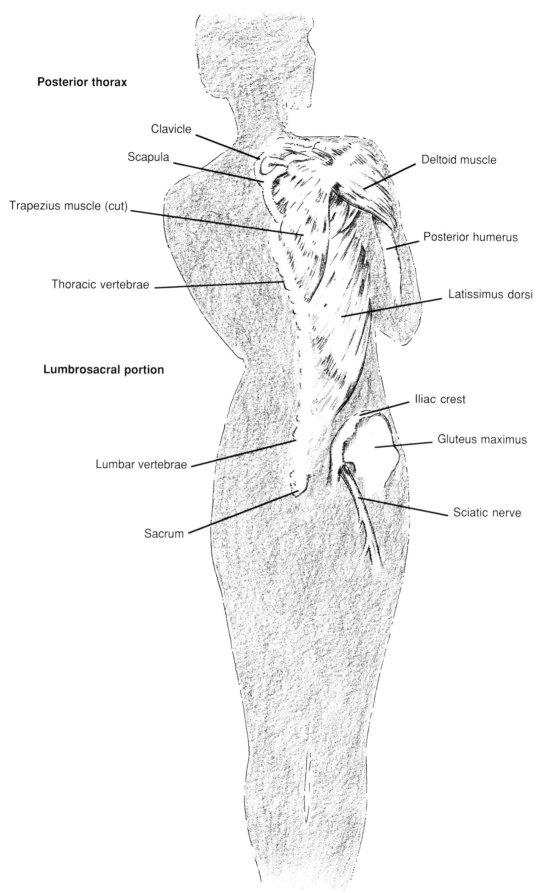

**Posterior thorax**

Clavicle

Scapula

Trapezius muscle (cut)

Thoracic vertebrae

Deltoid muscle

Posterior humerus

Latissimus dorsi

**Lumbrosacral portion**

Iliac crest

Gluteus maximus

Lumbar vertebrae

Sciatic nerve

Sacrum

**FIGURE 2-23** Structure of the back. The lumbrosacral area is the weakest part. Always bend the legs to pick up objects. These lower back muscles were not made for lifting.

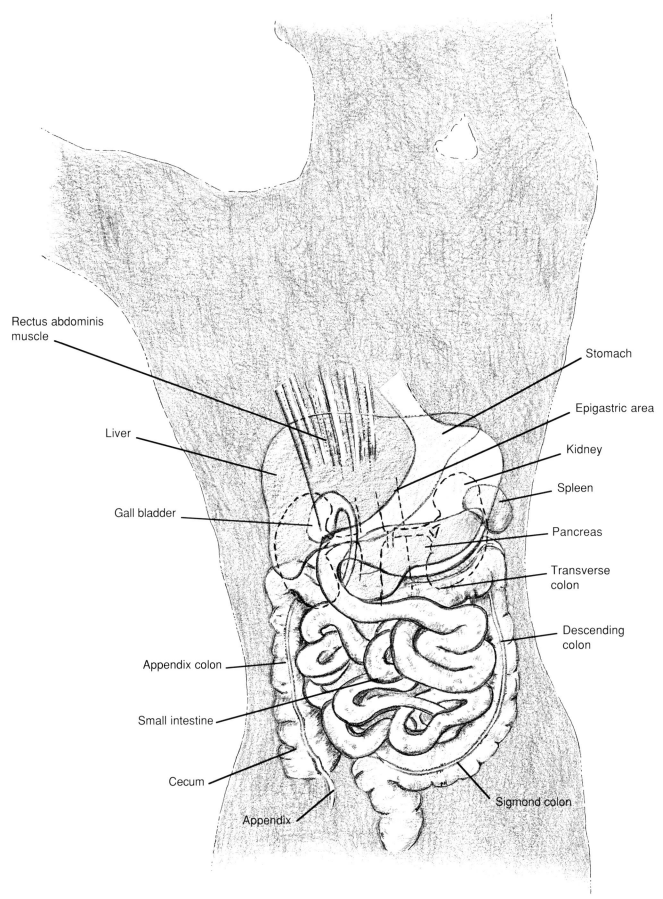

**FIGURE 2-24** Anatomy of the abdomen. Remember liver on right, spleen on left, stomach in the middle. Kidneys are on the back on either side, below the posterior chest.

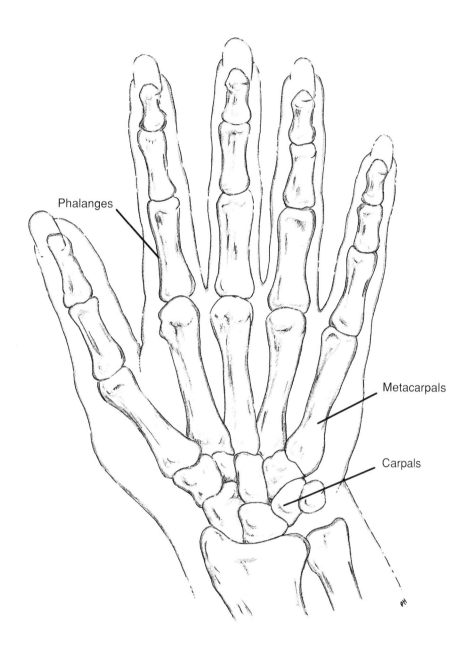

Phalanges

Metacarpals

Carpals

**FIGURE 2-25** (cont.) Structure of the hand. Bones of the dorsal hand.

the nerves. The skin care specialists focus is most likely to be the hands and the feet, even though the upper arms and the upper legs can be afflicted with so-called "cellulite". There are vascular problems with which we must also contend. But, I shall leave these subjects to later chapters and limit the coverage of the extremities to the hands and the feet.

## The Hands

The hands are one of the most expressive

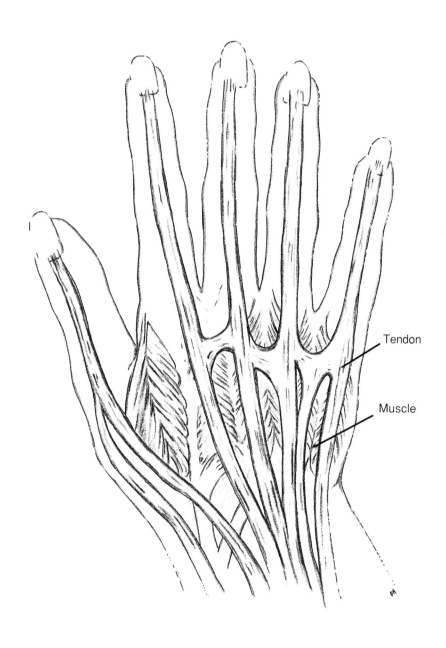

Tendon

Muscle

**FIGURE 2-25** (cont.) Structure of the hand. Muscles and tendons of the dorsal hand. Note the tendons extend to the tips of the fingers.

parts of the body. We shake hands, hold hands, and kiss hands. The hands are gentle or strong and can be used to stroke or strike. They are both tools and weapons. Above all, they are an extension of the self. One needs only to look at dirty, unkempt fingernails to learn a lot about the person on the other end. It is no joke that a rough, red hand is not a pleasure to see, or to feel. At the present time we have little to offer the older individual. Many problems are associated with aging hands. Dark pigmented spots, a thin dermis, and very prominent vessels do

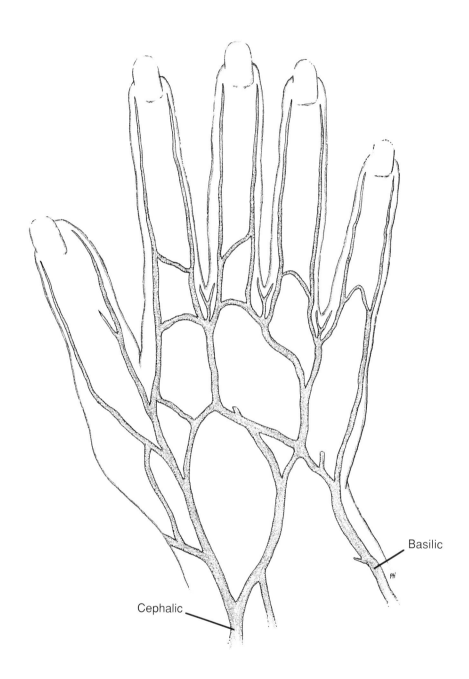

Basilic

Cephalic

**FIGURE 2-25** (cont.) Structure of the hand. Veins of the dorsal hand.

not make attractive hands. Look at the anatomy of the hand to see these areas.

The **hand** (see **Figure 2-25**) is composed of many bones and muscles along with nerves and blood vessels, all arranged to allow maximum versatility of action. The wrist joins the hand to the long bones of the lower arm, the **radius** and the **ulna**. There are eight **carpal bones** in the wrist which articulate with the **metacarpals** in the hand. The dorsal hand, between the fingers and the wrist, is the main area for skin defects. A cross section of the hand through the palm

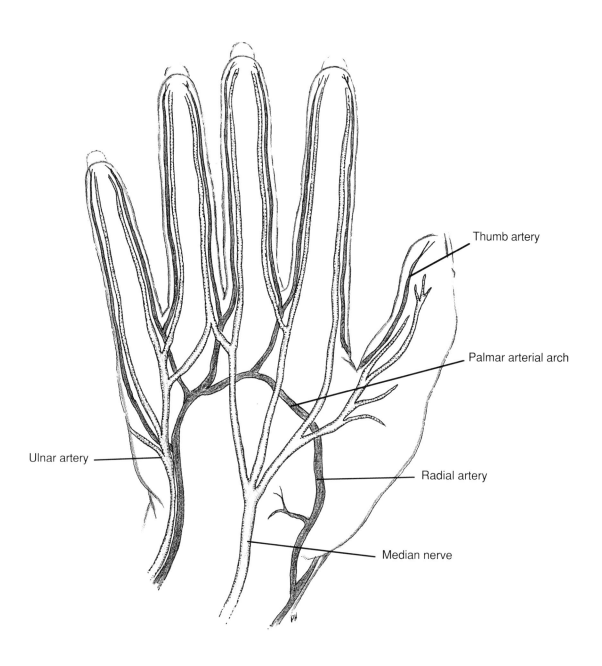

Thumb artery

Palmar arterial arch

Radial artery

Median nerve

Ulnar artery

**FIGURE 2-25** (cont.) Structure of the hand. Arteries and nerves of the palmer hand. Note the arc form of the blood supply and that both the ulnar artery and the radial artery are connected. Note also that the 4th finger is supplied both by the median nerve and the ulnar nerve.

shows the relation of the bones to the other structures. Notice that it is thin and devoid of fat, with prominent tendons and vessels. The palmar surface is not very different, except that there are no prominent veins.

The fingers contain three bones each, called

**phalanges**, which articulate with the metacarpals at the proximal end. There is a small amount of fat in the palmar side of the fingers which helps to ease the pressure of grasping and touching. The interphalangeal joints are frequently attacked by arthritis. This further disfigures the

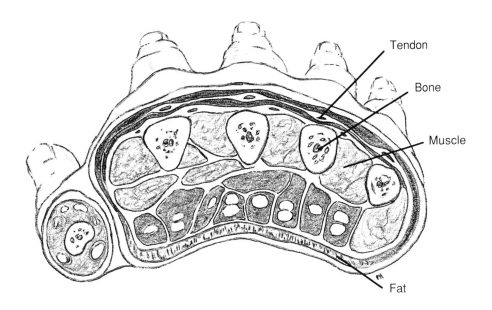

Tendon

Bone

Muscle

Fat

**FIGURE 2-25** Structure of the hand. Cross-sectional view. Note the relationship of bones, muscles and tendons.

hands.

The arteries of the hands are deep. You can easily feel the **radial artery** at the base of the thumb on the lateral volar wrist. The veins of the hands are the major cosmetic problem. If you hold your hand in your lap for about 3-5 minutes you can see that the veins begin to dilate. Now, raise your hand to the level of your eyes. You will see that the veins become flat and they almost disappear. Put the hand in your lap or on a table and watch the veins again dilate. Then, place your great finger on the vein with moderate pressure, just above the knuckle. Next with your index finger (the first finger) strip the vein cephalad, that is, up the wrist as far as your finger will go. You will see the vein disappear and it leaves a shallow depression. You can move your hands while still holding pressure on the vein and it will not fill up. Only when you release the pressure, will you see the vein fill rapidly. This experiment demonstrates the venous valves, which prevents back flow of the blood. It also shows us just how little pressure is required to stop the flow of blood, and how tight clothes can cause or contribute to the formation of varicose veins.

The basic landmarks on the hands are shown in **Figure 2-25**. For our purpose we need to know little else, unless you are involved in surgical aftercare of the hands. Being familiar with the fundamental structures and the major blood vessels and nerves is all that you need at the present. Because the hand is a prehensile or grasping tool, it requires muscles and nerves to activate this function. The **median nerve** and the **ulnar nerve** supply the muscle of flexion (to grasp) and the **radial nerve** the muscles of extension (grasp relaxation). The loss of any these nerves greatly impairs the function of the hand.

Notice that the webs of the fingers are only on the palmar side of the hand and not on the dorsum. Notice also, the finger print patterns with their ridges on which the sweat glands open. There are no sebaceous glands or hairs on the palms. Note that the middle digit is the most projecting finger with the ring finger being next. The index finger is the longest finger in one-third of white people and equal in length to the middle finger in one-fifth of the white people. In white females the number of individuals with a longer index finger is higher than in white males. This bit of information may not have any real value, but it is a good excuse to handle someone's hand at a party.

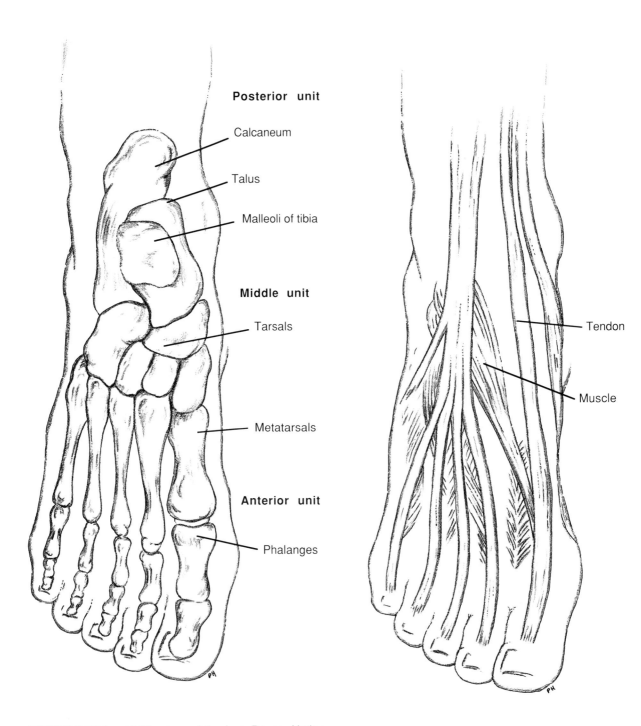

**Posterior unit**

Calcaneum

Talus

Malleoli of tibia

**Middle unit**

Tarsals

Metatarsals

**Anterior unit**

Phalanges

Tendon

Muscle

**FIGURE 2-26** (cont.) Structure of the foot. Bones. Notice that the bones must be aligned in a linear fashion. Tight shoes distort this structure giving rise to foot problems.

**FIGURE 2-26** (cont.) Structure of the foot. Muscles and tendons.

### The Foot

I am including the foot because I feel that in the future the skin care specialist will be working more closely with the elderly and that a specialist will need to offer foot-care. The feet are a

neglected area of the body, cramped into tiny, ill-fitting shoes or covered with sneakers that smell of indescribable ancient odors. Yet all one needs to do is to stub a toe to find out the utter importance of the feet. I do not profess to know or to even understand the origin of the foot fet-

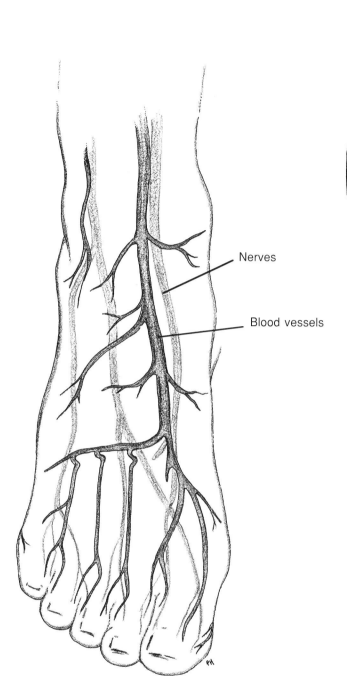

Nerves

Blood vessels

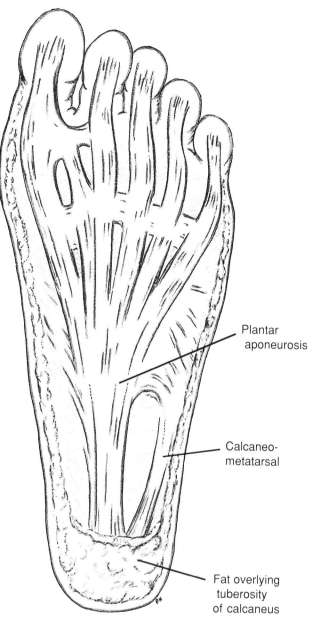

Plantar aponeurosis

Calcaneo-metatarsal

Fat overlying tuberosity of calcaneus

**FIGURE 2-26** (cont.) Structure of the foot. Blood vessels and nerves. Notice the fine circulation in the toes. They are adequately but not over-abundantly supplied with blood.

**FIGURE 2-26** (cont.) Structure of the foot. Ligaments of the sole of the foot. These are the main structures that support the arch. The calcaneus or heel bears much weight and can easily be injured by falls and poorly fitting shoes. Many nerves are seen in and about the ligaments. Reflexology is based on pressure stimulation of these nerves. Just plain walking accomplishes much of this stimulation, particularly if you are bare footed. (High heels negate most of the benefit of walking.)

ish fanatic, but somewhere there is a lesson here that tells us to take better care of our feet. I suppose that the skin care specialist who has spent so much time on the face will not be over-enthused about feet. Be that as it may, we shall nevertheless spend a little time on the anatomy of the foot.

The **foot** (see **Figure 2-26**) is divided into three units: the anterior, the middle, and the posterior foot.

The **anterior foot** is represented by the five metatarsals and the five phalanges (toes). The

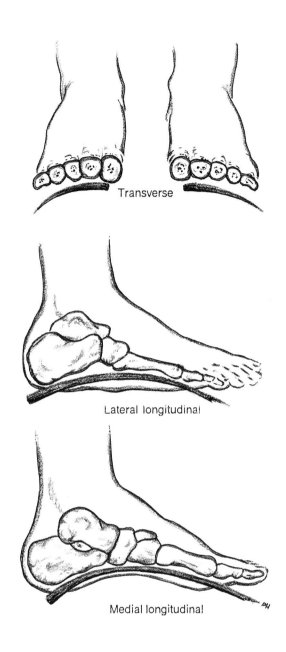

Transverse

Lateral longitudinal

Medial longitudinal

**FIGURE 2-26** Structure of the foot. The arches. Study the arches carefullly. Each foot provides half of the transverse arch. The longitudinal arch has both a medial and lateral aspect with the medial being higher.

toes are not weight-bearing (except in ballet dancers), but they are used for "spring action" in walking. In fact, the foot is not designed as a primary weight-bearing structure, but rather as a means of locomotion, as in walking. The **posterior foot** consists of the calcaneum or heel bone. Feel it as the big knob at the posterior part of your foot. Next is the talus which rests on the calcaneus. It receives the articulation of the tibia of the leg. Articulation means two bones coming together at a joint. You can feel the lateral and medial malleoli of the tibia as big projections on the outside and inside of the ankle. The middle foot consists of the five small tarsal bones, which roughly represents a wedge whose apex is lateral and base is medial.

In order to understand the foot you need to see the foot as a walking machine, based on the principle of the spring. The two arches, the medial longitudinal arch and the lateral longitudinal arch, are the main springs. The transverse arch forms only half an arch or spring but with your feet together you have a complete spring and arch.

The muscles and tendons of the plantar foot tie together the various bones in the arch structures. They supply the energy to the springs. Here again, you do not need to know all the details and names of the many muscles and tendons, but study the Figures to learn the general concepts.

Finally, the weight-bearing points on the foot are the median tubercle of the calcaneus, the heads of the five metatarsal bones, and the sesamoid bones.

And one last comment on the mystery of why some people are very ticklish on the feet and others enjoy a foot rub. Although there has been no scientific conclusion on this distinction one reference notes that people who are more sexually active are less ticklish.

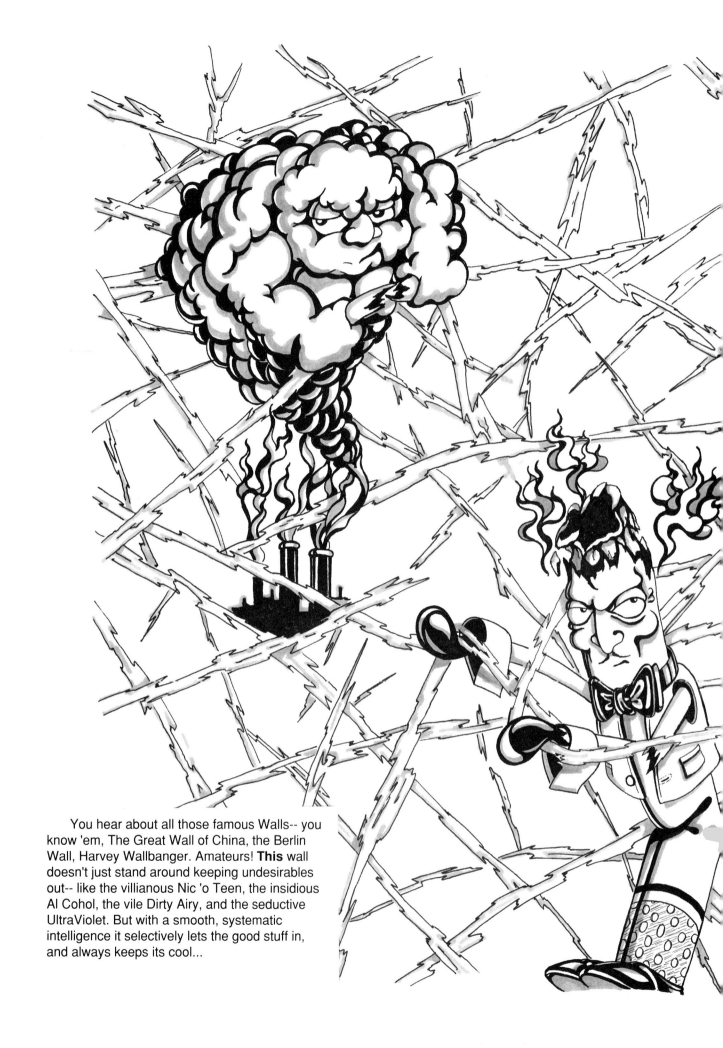

You hear about all those famous Walls-- you know 'em, The Great Wall of China, the Berlin Wall, Harvey Wallbanger. Amateurs! **This** wall doesn't just stand around keeping undesirables out-- like the villianous Nic 'o Teen, the insidious Al Cohol, the vile Dirty Airy, and the seductive UltraViolet. But with a smooth, systematic intelligence it selectively lets the good stuff in, and always keeps its cool...

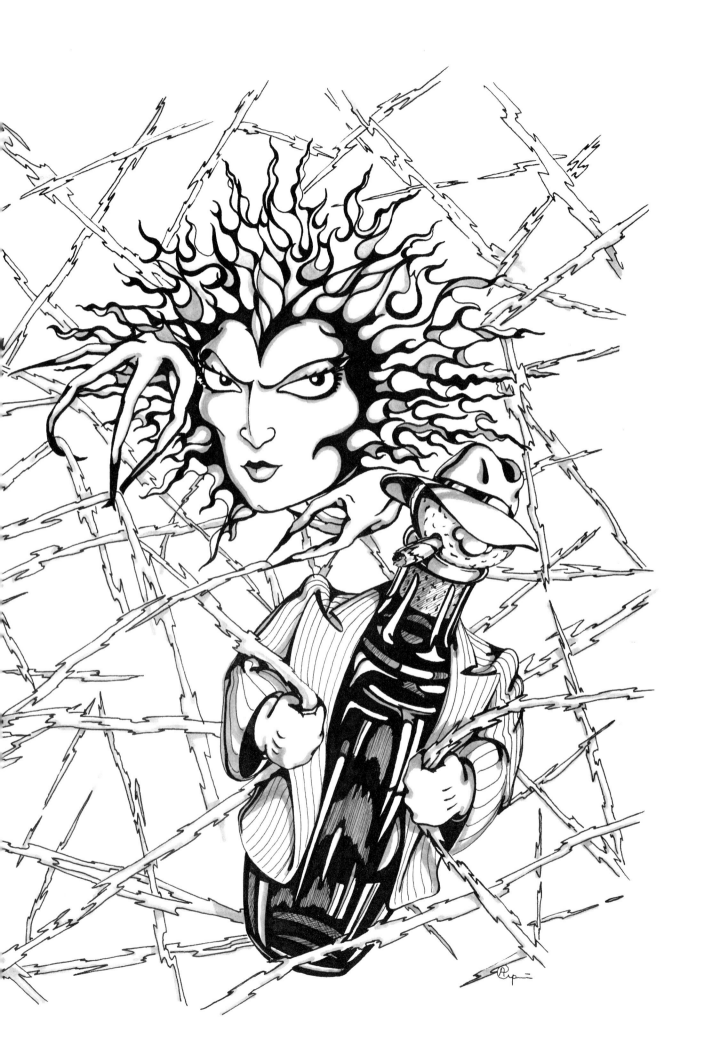

# Anatomy of the Skin

As skin care specialists, your main interest will be focused on the structure and function of the skin. Very little of the skin's structure is visible to the naked eye. This requires us to look at the microscopic anatomy to understand its real structure. At this point we shall leave the gross anatomy and get down to the cellular level. We shall need to look at the function of the skin in order to help us understand the structure. Some of what we learn now will be referenced in the Physiology chapter.

## ORIGIN OF THE SKIN

The skin structure developed over many millions of years to adapt to the environmental and internal needs of the animal. Look upon the skin as an active structure with two surfaces; an external surface and an internal surface. If you fail to grasp this fundamental concept you will have difficulty understanding the functional and structural aspects of the skin. Keep in mind the word dynamic. The skin is a very dynamic organ, meaning it is constantly renewing itself. The skin is also mosaic, meaning the cells don't always grow at the same rate. If this was not

the case, all cells would reproduce at once and we would molt like snakes.

Life appears to have started in the seas as a single cell formed over millions of years. It then developed into a more complex multicellular form after many more millions of years. The seas by this time were concentrated and a bit alkaline (pH 8.0). As the cell changed it had to protect itself from the changing sea environment. In other words, the cell made its own internal environment by separating itself from the sea with a living wall. This wall is the cell membrane. Like any wall, it is designed to keep things in and things out. But there must also be holes to let the free passage of needed things in, and things no longer needed out. All of this required many, many years and a great deal of biological experimentation, with more paths leading to extinction than preservation.

When the sea animals reached the land, the skin had to adjust to a new environment. No longer were there very large quantities of water to keep out. The animal needed to keep its water locked within its body. Actually, the animal was taking the primitive sea with it. Adjusting to dry land, heat, cold, wind, and sun helped produce many types of skin. All of these share essentially the same physiological principles. The fur on a polar bear and the feathers on a parrot are both special skin structures that developed to meet specific needs presented by the environment. The skin of man is no different in this regard. Now, let us add to the simple function of protection other needs of the animal such as body temperature regulation, sensory reception, recognition and sexual attraction, and other social interactions. We begin to see the complexity of the skin grow right before our eyes. The skin of man has no fur and is relatively hairless or glabrous; it also contains many heat-sensitive sweat glands that regulate body temperature. These two facts are the important differences between man and other mammals.

## SOME FACTS ON SKIN NUMBERS

The skin is the largest organ of the body with the liver next in line. It is slightly more than 3 kilograms in weight (6.6 pounds) and covers nearly two square meters of area. A meter is about 40 inches long, so picture an area 40 inches by 40 inches square and double it. This is

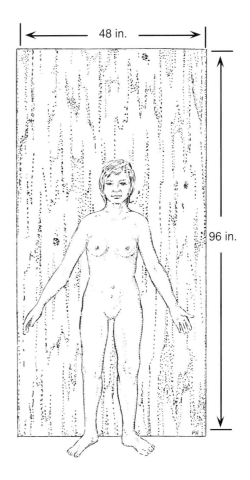

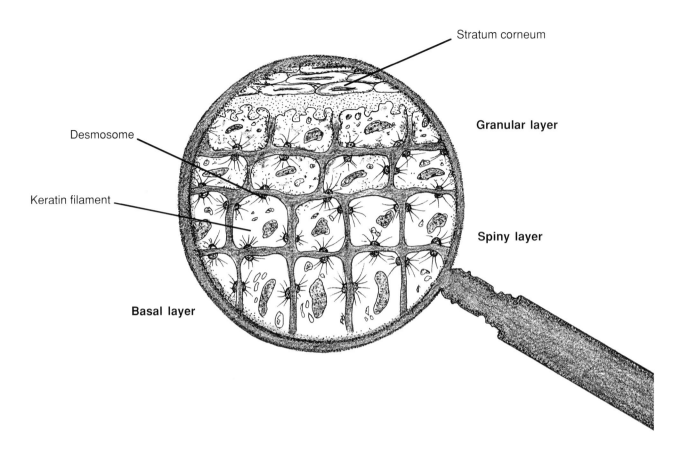

Stratum corneum

Granular layer

Spiny layer

Desmosome

Keratin filament

Basal layer

**FIGURE 3-2** The Epidermis. Keep in mind the four layers as a dynamic transitional process. The keratin fibers are formed in the lower layer to middle layer and increase in number as they move to the top.

roughly the area of a sheet of plywood, or an average sized wood panel. It would easily cover two regular kitchen table tops, or one large dining room table.

Skin is 1.5 to 4 millimeters (1 inch = 25.4 millimeters) thick depending on the location measured. It is thickest on the back and thinnest on the eyelids. The outer epidermal layer measures 75 to 150 microns. The soles and the palms may be 500 microns or 0.5 millimeters. This fact, that the outer skin layer (the epidermis) is the thinnest is truly startling. This tiny layer is our only real solid protection against the whole environmental world!

### STRUCTURE OF THE SKIN

As you look at **Figure 3-1**, please find the following: the epidermis, the papillary and reticular dermmis.

### The Epidermis

The **epidermis** (see **Figure 3-2**) is composed of four layers. Each layer consists of a specific type of cell. The outer layer is the stratum corneum. The inner three layers are the changing or differentiating layers. Starting at the inner most layer, we have the basal layer, the spiny layer, and the granular layer. We shall look at each one of these layers in detail.

The **basal layer** contains the living cells. They divide and differentiate to produce the upper layer cells. This layer is firmly anchored to the dermal layer beneath it by many fibrous bands. The basal cell forms two daughter cells upon division. The process of differentiation allows a cell capable of more than one function to go in only one biological direction. For example, the basal cell may divide to form two new basal cells each able to divide again. It may also form one basal cell and one end cell that will now differentiate into a stratum corneum cell. The basal cell is a basal keratinocyte. Ker-

**FIGURE 3-1** Structure of the skin. Note the relationship of the various dermal structure to the epidermis. The hair follicle is really part of the epidermis but it goes deep into the dermis. Note also that the nerve endings without receptor organs are high up in the dermis, while sense receptors range superficial to deep.

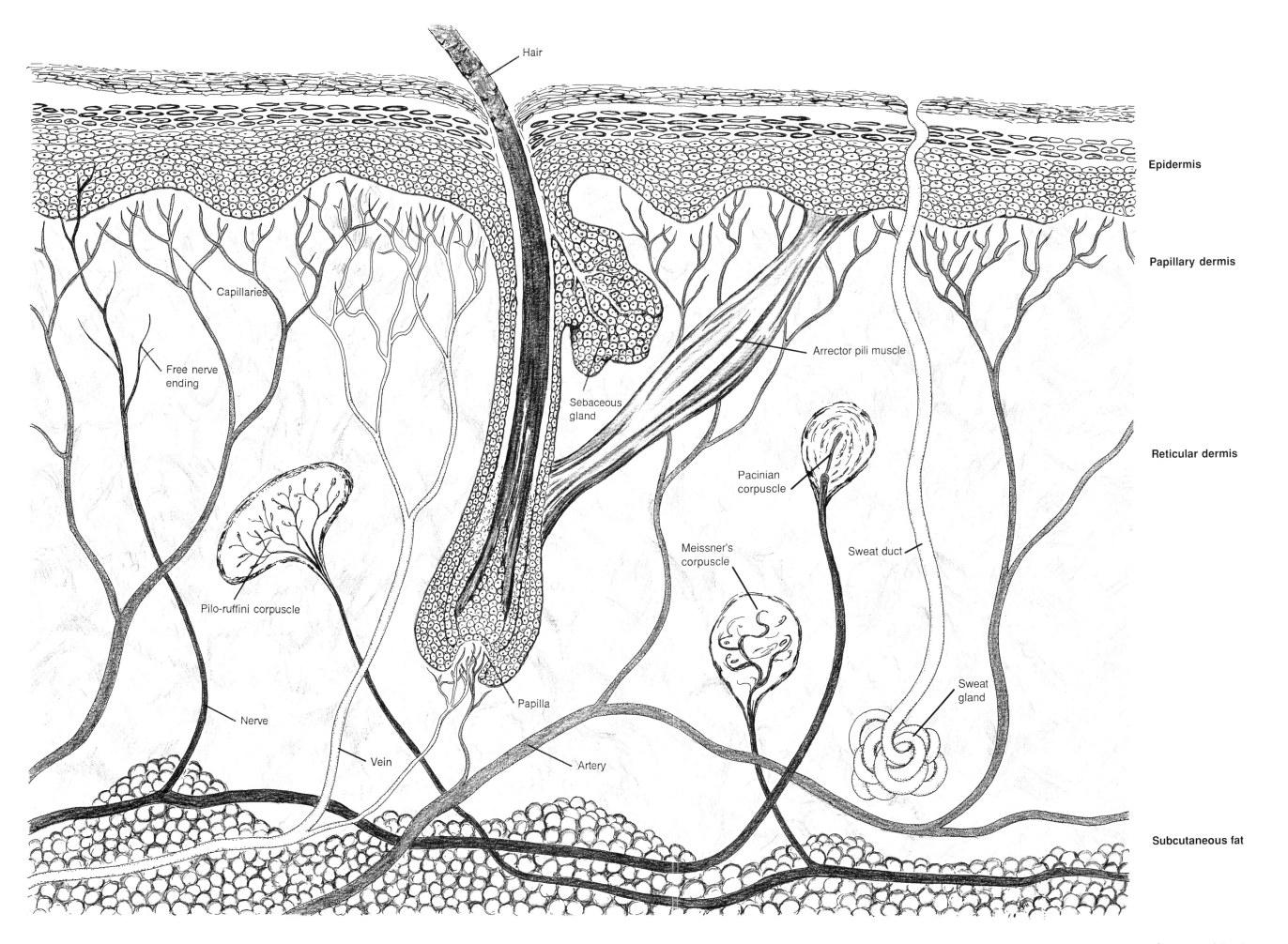

Hair

Epidermis

Papillary dermis

Capillaries

Free nerve
ending

Arrector pili muscle

Sebaceous
gland

Reticular dermis

Pacinian
corpuscle

Pilo-ruffini corpuscle

Meissner's
corpuscle

Sweat duct

Sweat
gland

Papilla

Nerve

Vein

Artery

Subcutaneous fat

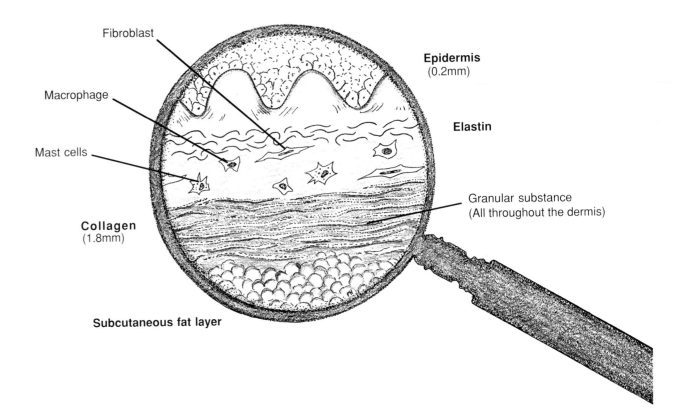

Fibroblast

Epidermis
(0.2mm)

Macrophage

Elastin

Mast cells

Granular substance
(All throughout the dermis)

Collagen
(1.8mm)

Subcutaneous fat layer

**FIGURE 3-3** The dermis. Collagen fibers are much thicker than elastin fibers. They provide strength to the skin to resist tears, while elastin fibers provide "snap-back" or elasticity to the skin. Note also the cellular components, the fibroblast, the mast cell and the macrophage. We shall study these cells in detail later.

atinocytes produce a protein called keratin. About 90 to 95% of the epidermal cells are keratinocytes with the rest being melanocytes, mast cells, or Langerhans cells all of which we shall study later.

The **spiny layer** consists of a differentiating keratinocyte which is immediately above the basal cell. The cell's shape is more ovoid than the basal cell and it possesses keratin fibers in early form. The spiny name comes from the little bridge-like hairs that join the cells in this layer. These are in fact the desmosomes which are complex attachment sites between the cells. As the cells move upward these attachments become less and less until at the stratum corneum they disappear. This allows the cells to flake off.

The **granular layer** is composed of cells that have undergone greater differentiation and now consists mostly of keratin fibers, a degenerated nucleus, and many lamellar bodies. The lamellar bodies are key structures in the skin for they are the origin of the lipid barrier of the stratum corneum. More of this structure will be discussed later.

The **stratum corneum layer** is composed of flat, hard, and mostly "dried cells" that form the outer layer of the skin. These cells are renewed every day. Within a period of two weeks all the stratum corneum may be replaced by new cells. This process is called cellular proliferation and is highly controlled by many unknown mechanisms. There may be 10 layers of cells in the stratum corneum or more than 50. The eyelid is the thinnest and the palms and soles are the thickest.

### The Dermis

Beneath the epidermis is the **dermis** (see **Figure 3-3**) which is the support layer of the skin. There is only one layer between the epidermis and the fat or adipose layer and we call that the dermis. Within the dermis are the nerves, blood vessels, and the organs of the skin appendages (the glands and hairs). These structures are unique and we shall discuss them separately. Consider the dermis as a tough but highly resilient structure that allows the skin to move, take shocks, cool and warm the body, and permits the passages of nutrients to the epidermis. At the same time it interacts with both the inside and outside changes which constantly take place.

This is a good time to look at a few more facts on skin numbers. The dermis is thickest on the back, being about 4 millimeters thick, and thinnest on the eyes and scrotum. The skin of the scalp, forehead, wrist, and palm are all less than two millimeters thick while the abdomen and thigh are between two and three millimeters thick.

The dermis and the epidermis are joined by an undulating membrane which forms ridges and grooves known as the **papillae**. These papillae are a subject of much discussion. The current belief is that the dermis actually forms these ridge structures, like mountain ranges, and the epidermis fits into the valleys between the ridges. This process is lost as we age. Now the presence of this particular structure allows us to further functionally divide the dermis into the papillary dermis and the reticular dermis. This is not done to confuse you but you will see these terms in other texts and you need to know them.

The **papillary dermis** is under the epidermis. It undulates, and contains smaller, widely spaced collagen and elastin fibers. It contains large amounts of interfibrillar "gel substance" (the ground substance of the dermis), chemically known as the mucopolysaccharides. More on this later, keep relaxed. Also in the papillary dermis are the capillary vessels, the small nerves, and the lymphatic vessels. The papillary dermis accounts for about 10 - 20 percent of the dermis.

The **reticular dermis** is beneath the papillary dermis and makes up the bulk of the dermis. It is relatively devoid of cells and blood vessels. It contains heavy, closely packed collagen and coarse elastin. The major support of the skin is derived from this layer. The structure of collagen resembles woven strands that in some manner relates to the surface pattern on the skin.

### Components of the Dermis

The connective tissue consists of three types of fibers, known as collagen, elastin, and reticulin. Each of these are chemically distinct from the other and have separate physical properties and functions.

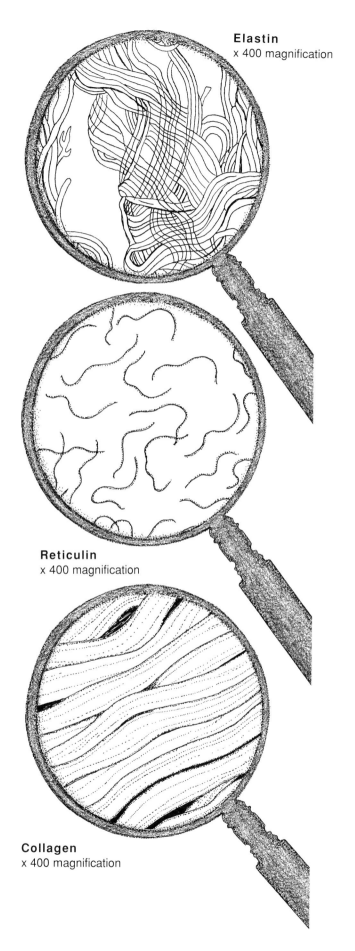

**Elastin**
x 400 magnification

**Reticulin**
x 400 magnification

**Collagen**
x 400 magnification

**Collagen** is composed of complex fibers made up of protein and arranged in long chains. It is tough and does not stretch easily. Collagen makes up 10 - 30% of the wet weight of the dermis. **Elastin** is composed of a highly resilient material that chemically is vastly different from collagen. Only about 1 - 3% of the dermis is elastin. Reticulin is probably a subdivision of collagen chemically. It is composed of small fibers which mainly appear in the papillary dermis.

### The Blood Vessels of the Skin

The human skin is unique in that the skin serves also as a thermo-regulatory organ, that is, as a heat control organ. The sweat glands and the blood supply to the skin are the chief players in this system along with heat receptors and the central and sympathetic nervous system. At this point our interest is mainly in the blood vessels of the skin. Study this intricate structure in fine detail (see **Figure 3-4**).

The **peripheral blood vessel system** is a three dimensional maze of both large and small arterial and venous vessels. Starting with the cutaneous arteries, a number of smaller arterioles are given off to form the subcutaneous vascular bed. At the top of this system the fine capillaries of the papillary dermis serve to nourish the epidermis. The vertical vessels connecting the capillary loop are the major vessels employed in thermo-regulation. The capillary is a key structure in the skin and we need to understand this small vessel in detail.

**Capillaries** arise from mesenchymal tissue about the fourth month of gestation. By the fifth month new vessels form from existing vessels by budding. At this stage of fetal development, the skin is very thin, only a few cells thick, but it now increases rapidly. There is active and rapid blood vessel proliferation. The tiny capillaries now form into arterioles and venules, developing muscular coats and spreading through the underlying tissue. These vessels will be the adult subcutaneous blood vessels. The ability of skin to repair itself after injury lies in this primitive ability to grow new vessels from capillaries.

The **capillary loop** is characteristic of adult skin while the infant's capillary structure is less organized, yielding a more vascular skin. The capillary loop begins as a 100 μ diameter artery in the lower dermis, then branches to 50 μ arterioles with fine walls and few muscle fibers. The vessels get thinner on their way to the epidermis finally becoming only 15 μ in diameter as they form into capillaries. Arising from these fine vessels are the loops. They are vertical, sharply looped as a hair pin, and supply the papillary structures. On the down side of the loop they enter the venous vessel and drain into the horizontal sub-papillary venous vessel. These vessels, of 40 - 60 μ, are very numerous in the skin. As they enter into the lower dermis they may be 100 - 400 μ in diameter, and gradually add more muscle cells to their wall.

Visualize the capillary network as a series of loops. They arise from arteries which become smaller and smaller until they form tiny vessels of a few microns. After exchanging certain substances they become tiny venules that reverse the direction and grow larger as they return to the dermis.

The inner lining of both veins and arteries is called the **endothelium**. It is a thin layer of living, ameboid cells that respond to many stimuli to produce various sizes and shapes of blood vessels. The best picture analogy ever given for these cells is that of Dr. Terrance Ryan of England. He describes the cells as "lightly fried eggs rolled over to form a tube. The yolk represents the nucleus and shows only variation between the disk-shaped and the round, whereas the white of the egg represents the cytoplasm and can be spread out, or closely circumscribed, smooth, or irregular at the periphery, homogeneous in texture, or full of bubbles." Consider these cells as the key to the blood vessels, always active and constantly ready for a change in the environment.

The **internal elastic lamina** is present in arteries but not in veins. It is an elastic circle of tissue that helps the artery to change diameter. Moving outward, the next layer is the muscle layer which is larger in arteries and smaller in veins. Remember that these structures change as the vessels get larger or smaller. Only endothelial cells with a few support muscle cells are found at the capillary loop.

Some Statistics on the Capillary

The length of a capillary loop is 0.2 to 0.4

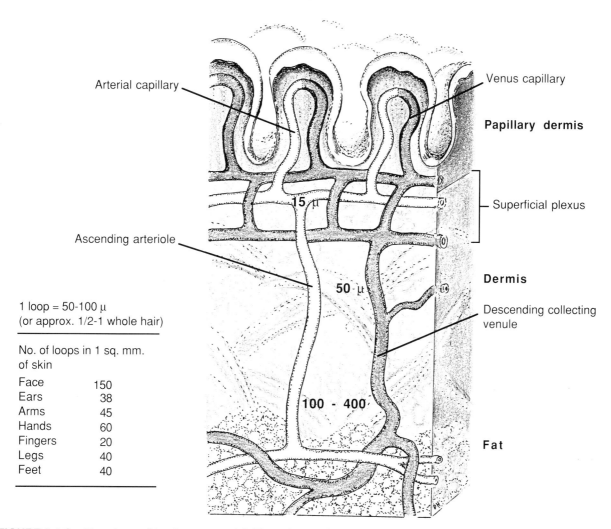

**FIGURE 3-4** Capillary loop. (Not drawn to scale). These loops of capillaries supply the epidermis with everything it needs to survive. There is no blood in the epidermis, so it is fed is by passive diffusion from the blood vessels to the cells.

Labels in figure:
- Arterial capillary
- Venus capillary
- **Papillary dermis**
- Ascending arteriole
- **Superficial plexus**
- **Dermis**
- Descending collecting venule
- **Fat**
- 15 μ
- 50 μ
- 100 - 400

1 loop = 50-100 μ
(or approx. 1/2-1 whole hair)

No. of loops in 1 sq. mm. of skin

| | |
|---|---|
| Face | 150 |
| Ears | 38 |
| Arms | 45 |
| Hands | 60 |
| Fingers | 20 |
| Legs | 40 |
| Feet | 40 |

mm. The diameter of an arterial capillary arm is about 10 u with the venous side being 13 - 20 μ. One capillary loop supplies 0.04 - 0.27 square mm of skin. The average distance between one loop and the next loop is 50 - 100 μ. In one square mm of skin there is an average of 150 loops on the face, 38 on the ears, 100+ on the neck, 45 on the arms, 60 on the hands, 20 on the fingers and 40 on the legs and the feet.

**The Cutaneous Nerves**

The skin is the largest sensory organ in the body. It must be able to detect many sensations such as pain, pressure (touch), itch, heat, cold, and tickle. This is an area in which more than one book has been written and even more could be written. At present we do not have an adequate understanding of the nervous system of the skin, but there is a great deal known. We

shall start with the sensory nervous system and then discuss the motor nerves of the skin.

**The Sensory Nerves of the Skin**

The sensory nerves all arise from the spinal nerve branches. In the face, the sensory nerve is the **trigeminal nerve**. These nerve branches are arranged in a pattern on the surface of the skin so that one branch serves an area which is called a dermatome. Look at **Figure 3-5** and you will see this pattern. It is very important to know this concept in order to understand the distribution system. Notice that on the trunk the dermatomes are horizontal while on the arms and legs they are more vertical and irregularly distributed. It is of interest that there is a very sharp line of demarcation of the nerves between the right and left sides of the body (the midaxial line), but between adjacent nerves on each side there is

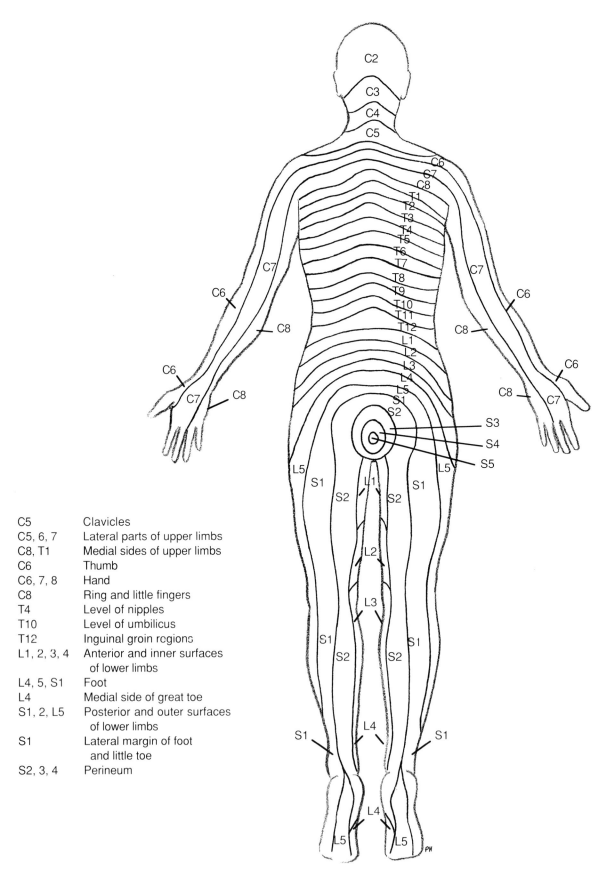

| C5 | Clavicles |
| C5, 6, 7 | Lateral parts of upper limbs |
| C8, T1 | Medial sides of upper limbs |
| C6 | Thumb |
| C6, 7, 8 | Hand |
| C8 | Ring and little fingers |
| T4 | Level of nipples |
| T10 | Level of umbilicus |
| T12 | Inguinal groin regions |
| L1, 2, 3, 4 | Anterior and inner surfaces of lower limbs |
| L4, 5, S1 | Foot |
| L4 | Medial side of great toe |
| S1, 2, L5 | Posterior and outer surfaces of lower limbs |
| S1 | Lateral margin of foot and little toe |
| S2, 3, 4 | Perineum |

**FIGURE 3-5** Dermatomes of the body. Back. Note here the different areas of the body surface are supplied by different nerve roots; the letter C corresponds to the regions of the spine. C=cervical or neck, T=thoracic or chest, L=lumbar or lower back, and S=sacrum or lower posterior pelvis. The arrangement is similar in animals who walk on four legs, quadripeds.

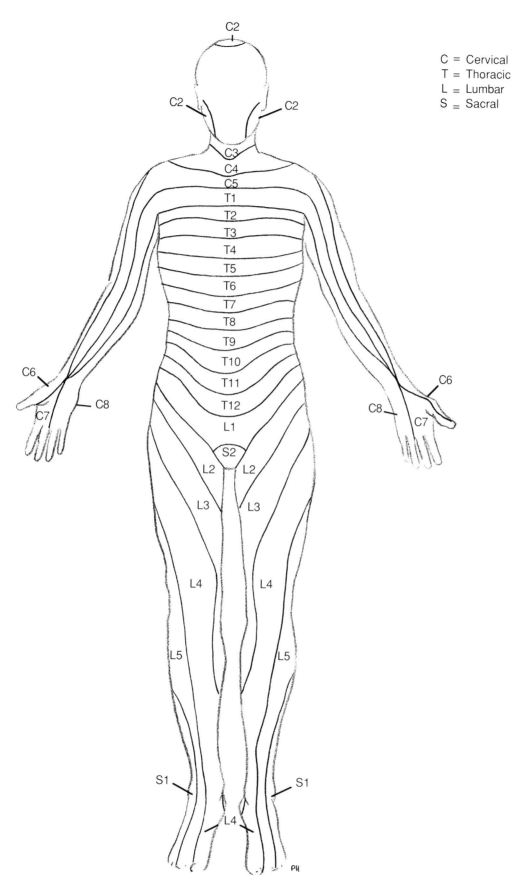

C = Cervical
T = Thoracic
L = Lumbar
S = Sacral

**FIGURE 3-5** (cont.) Dermatomes of the body. Front. Notice that the dermatomes cover specific areas that represent distribution of spinal nerves.

considerable overlap. We are not dealing with a static system here, these nerves are constantly changing according to the body's needs.

A **single nerve fiber** (see **Figure 3-6**) arises from the spinal cord, or from the trigeminal nerve. It is a single neuron with the cell body in the central nervous system and the dendrites pushing to the periphery. The dendrites receive impulses and carry them to the nerve cell body. Once in the cell body, this impulse is carried away by the axon, and transmitted to other nerve cells. The nerves are covered with a complex sheath which is multilayered. On the outside of some nerves are the glial (Schwann) cells that wrap around the fiber to protect it. Under the Schwann cell is a white substance called myelin. Myelin is mainly a lipid material. Nerves lacking this substance are called unmyelinated nerves. Unmyelinated nerves are more sensitive and can operate without receptors. The outside of the Schwann cell is further covered with the endoneurium. Bundles of nerves are in turn covered with the perineurium. It is impressive that for every cubic millimeter of nerve there are about 12,000 myelinated nerve fibers and about 45,000 unmyelinated nerve fibers! These nerve fibers join to sensors in the skin and relay messages to the brain.

The Sensors

1. Free Nerve Terminals

The sensory system has a variety of receptors in the skin to detect and sort out sensations of heat, cold, pressure, pain and itch (see **Fig-**

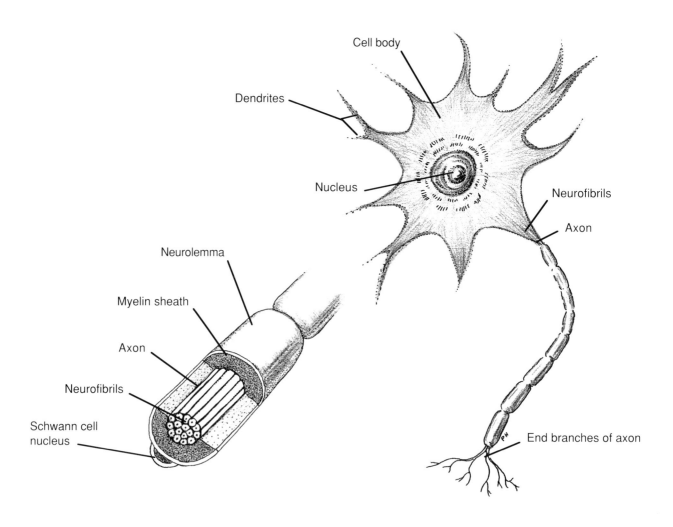

**FIGURE 3-6** A single nerve fiber. The nerve fiber must be insulated by fat, a poor conductor, to allow flow of current with a short-circuit. The flow is in one direction.

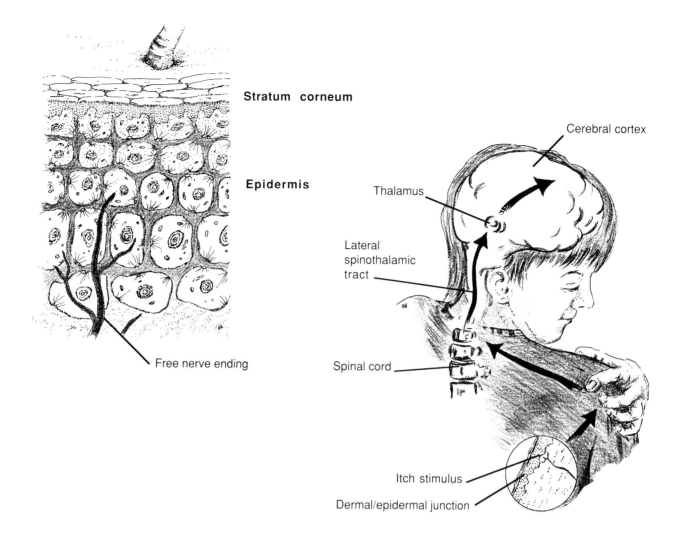

Stratum corneum

Epidermis

Free nerve ending

Cerebral cortex

Thalamus

Lateral
spinothalamic
tract

Spinal cord

Itch stimulus

Dermal/epidermal junction

**FIGURE 3-7** The sensors. The free nerve endings carry pain, temperature, and itch sensation. These are tiny unmyelinated nerves. Most end in the papillary dermis and surround hair follicles. It was suggested that itching sensation is a variety of pain since itch and pain travel similar nerval paths, but today itching is believed to be a distinct and separate sensation from pain.

ure 3-7). The vast majority of these endings are free nerve terminals which do not have a specialized ending. They are associated with pain and itch sensations and their endings are closely applied to the epidermal tissue in the hairy areas of the skin.

### 2. Hair Follicle Endings

Single nerve fibers join at the hair bulb and wrap around the end of the hair in fine body hair, but in other hairs the nerve is above the hair bulb encircling the external root sheath.

### 3. Hederiform Endings

**Hederiform** means "ivy shaped" and re-

fers to a nerve that occurs in glabrous, or hairless skin. They are also called **Merkel's discs** by some anatomists since they were first described by Merkel. As the nerve ending approaches the base of the epidermis it expands into flattened leaves which lie close to specialized cells in the epidermal rete pegs. Each of the receptors consists of a modified epidermal cell (the Merkel cell) and its disc-shaped terminal. They are attached to the local keratinocytes by desmosomes. These receptors are thought to be mechanoreceptors for touch and other internal functions.

### 4. Meissner Corpuscle

The **Meissner corpuscle** is found in frictional areas of the skin, that is, the hands, fingers, soles

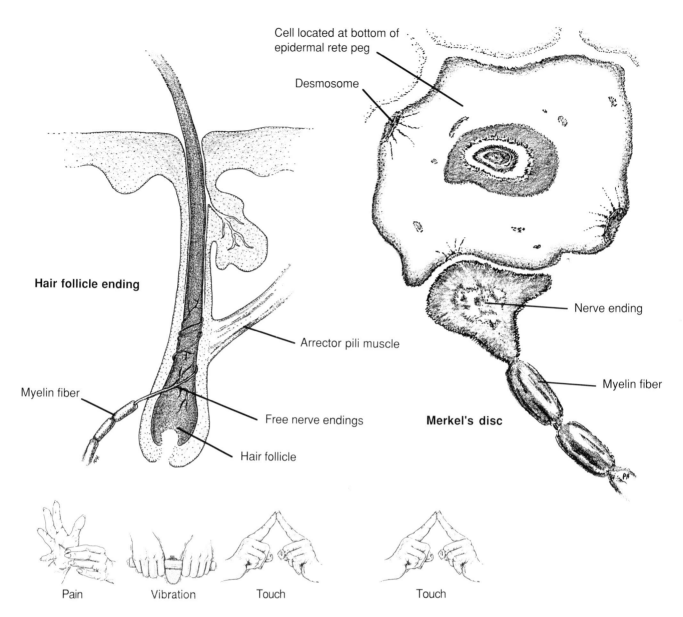

Cell located at bottom of epidermal rete peg

Desmosome

Hair follicle ending

Arrector pili muscle

Myelin fiber

Free nerve endings

Hair follicle

Nerve ending

Myelin fiber

Merkel's disc

Pain    Vibration    Touch

Touch

**FIGURE 3-7** (cont.) The sensors. Hair follicle endings. These free nerve endings surround the hair follicle and transmit pain, vibration and touch. They are very numerous.

**FIGURE 3-7** (cont.) The sensors. Merkel's disc. (F. Merkel, German anatomist, 1845-1919.) Merkel's discs are actually transmittors that relay signals which may be associated with other skin sensory receptors in free nerve endings. The last word on Merkel's disc has not been written.

of the feet, and on the glabrous skin of the toes. They are circular or ovoid structures with a distinct connective tissue capsule. They are supplied by myelinated nerves, and are fairly large, 20 - 40 x 150 microns in size. They transmit touch, pressure, and cold.

5. Pacinian Corpuscle

The **Pacinian corpuscles** are very large, 0.5 to 3 - 4 mm in size. They occur in the deep part of the dermis of the palms and fingers near the bones. They are also found in the external geni-

talia and the breast. Many internal organs also contain these corpuscles. The ovoid capsule is layered around an unmyelinated nerve, which arises from a myelinated nerve at the base of the corpuscle. This Pacinian corpuscle is called a multilamellar structure. They are believed to transmit vibration and pressure.

6. Mucocutaneous Corpuscle

This type of ending was previously called a Krause's end-bulb and occurs in the dermis in transitional zones between the skin and mucous

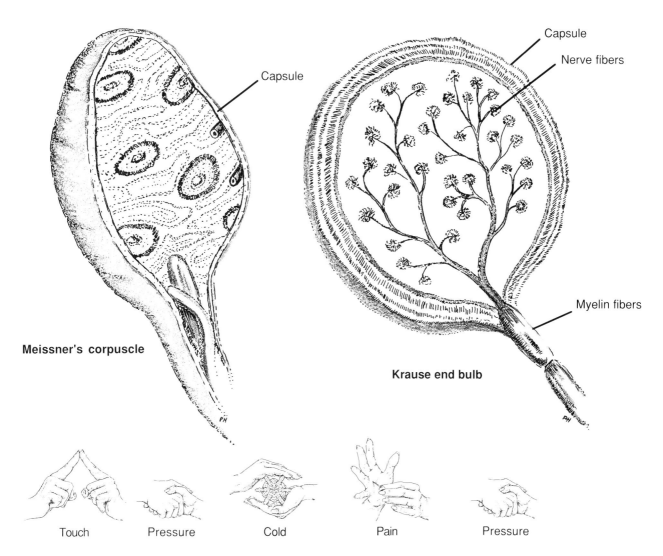

Capsule

Capsule

Nerve fibers

Myelin fibers

**Meissner's corpuscle**

**Krause end bulb**

Touch        Pressure        Cold

Pain        Pressure

**FIGURE 3-7** (cont.) The sensors. Meissner's corpuscles. (G. Meissner, German physiologist, 1829-1905.) Meissner's corpuscles are located in the papillary dermis on palms and soles. They are encapsulated nerve endings that detect pressure, touch, and cold. Temperature sensation is a very sensitive mechanism in the skin. Heat is a positive quantity that is detected by the skin's sensor with as small a rise as 0.001 degree centigrade per second. Cold is detected as a fall in temperature; the skin can detect a fall in temperature as small as 0.004 degrees centigrade.

**FIGURE 3-7** (cont.) The sensors. Krause end bulbs. Krause end bulbs (F. Krause, German anatomist, 1833-1910) detect pain and pressure. They are encapsulated endings of myelinated nerves. Pain sensors are spread all through the body. They are able to detect mechanical, electrical, chemical and extremes of temperature as stimuli causing pain. At 44.5 degrees centigrade the skin senses temperature as pain.

membranes such as the penis, clitoris, lips, tongue, and the eyelids. It does not occur in the hairy or frictional skin areas. They are not universally accepted as distinct entities. They resemble hair bulb endings and are probably pressure receptors. Their endings are unmyelinated nerves arising from myelin fibers.

7. Pilo-ruffini corpuscle

These are cylindrical encapsulated nerve endings encircling hair follicles just below the sebaceous duct. They are very complex struc-

tures consisting of branching terminal nerve fibers enclosed in a unique connective tissue compartment that consists of bundles of collagen and elastin fibers and some connective tissue cells called "septal cells". These receptors are believed to function as transmitters of slow mechanoreceptors, such as pressure.

The Nerve Reflex Circuit

**Figure 3-8** is a representation of a **nerve reflex circuit** (or arc). The nerve from the skin to the spinal cord forms a synapse or junction

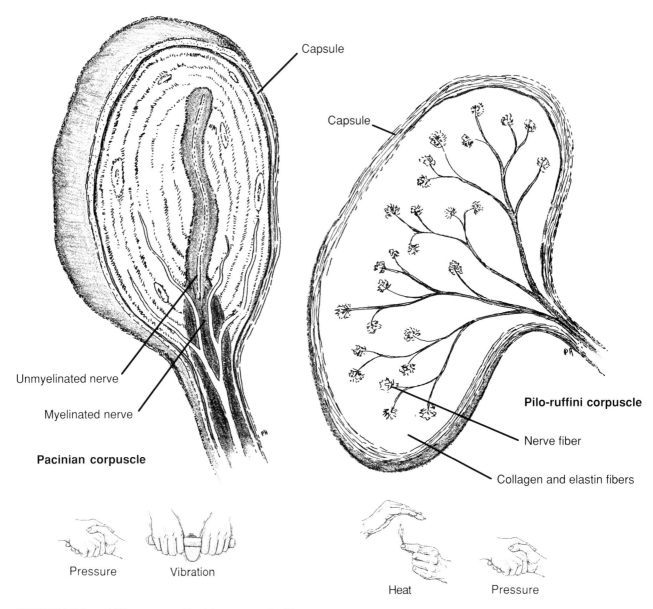

Capsule

Capsule

**Pilo-ruffini corpuscle**

Nerve fiber

Unmyelinated nerve

Myelinated nerve

Collagen and elastin fibers

**Pacinian corpuscle**

Pressure          Vibration

Heat          Pressure

FIGURE 3-7 (cont.) The sensors. Pacinian corpuscle. The Pacinian corpuscle (after F. Pacini, Italian anatomist,1812-1883) is a pressure and vibration sensor. They are located in the deep dermis and subcutaneous fat and are found mainly in weight-bearing areas.

FIGURE 3-7 (cont.) The sensors. Pilo-ruffini corpuscle. Ruffini corpuscle ( A. Ruffini, Italian anatomist 1864-1929) or end organ is a touch sensor that detects pressure and heat. They are located in hairy skin.

with a motor nerve that effects the response. The nerves in the spinal cord that run to the brain also synapse with the incoming nerve so that the brain is aware of what is happening.

bers. The fibers are running along with the myelinated sensory nerves. We shall pursue this in the Physiology Chapter.

Motor Nerves of the Skin

The **motor nerves** (see **Figure 3-9**) of the skin supply the sweat glands, the pilomotor apparatus and the muscle, and the adventitia of the microvasculature. It consists of postganglionic sympathetic fibers (more on this later, don't worry now) without parasympathetic fi-

**The Skin Appendages**

There are three skin appendages that we need to learn. They are the hair follicle, the sweat glands, and the apocrine glands. Each of these structures could command an entire book and indeed books have been written on each of these appendages. At this stage we shall only look at the basic anatomy of these structures and leave

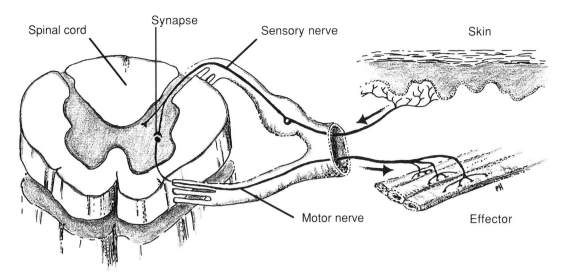

**FIGURE 3-8** Path of the nerve impulse. This is a complete "circuit". Notice that the sensing nerve must connect or "synapse" with the effector, a motor nerve.

their physiology for Chapter Four.

### The Hair Follicle

The **hair follicle** is also termed "the pilosebaceous apparatus" for it consists of the hair shaft, hair bulb, sebaceous gland, and the apocrine gland. You could use either term and be correct though the hair follicle is used at times to express only the hair bulb and shaft.

You will find hair follicles all over the body except on the palms and the soles. They are present at birth but do not develop into the mature form until puberty. Some parts of the body such as the breast and the ear canals have only

the apocrine glands without the rest of the apparatus. You must remember that the hair follicle develops from the epidermis at about 9 weeks of fetal life, with the sebaceous gland appearing at 13 weeks and the apocrine gland at 17 weeks. The entire apparatus can be found in the axilla, in the pubic area, on the face, and on the chest and back.

### 1. The Hair Structure

Each **hair** (see **Figure 3-10**) begins as a bud, or peg and grows by the division of cells from the hair bulb located in the dermis. Only the lower growing end is alive, the rest of the hair is

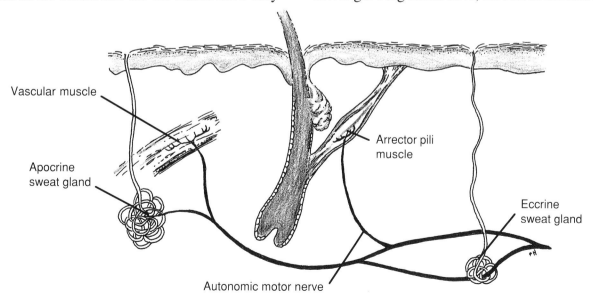

**FIGURE 3-9** Motor nerve action. The autonomic system is an involuntary, or automatic system. When you are cold or frightened the hair will stand-on-end by action of the arrector pili muscle.

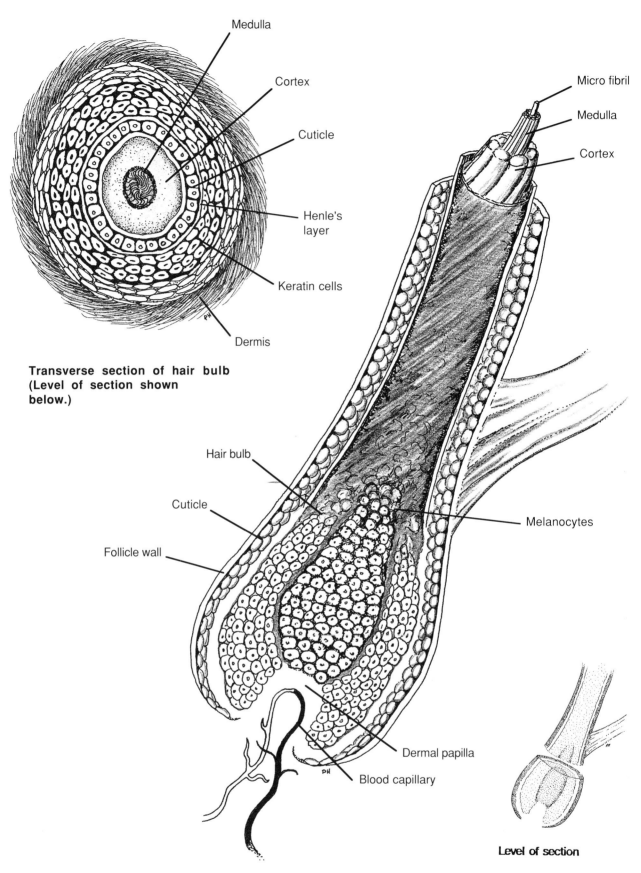

Medulla

Cortex

Cuticle

Henle's layer

Keratin cells

Dermis

**Transverse section of hair bulb (Level of section shown below.)**

Micro fibril

Medulla

Cortex

Hair bulb

Cuticle

Follicle wall

Melanocytes

Dermal papilla

Blood capillary

**Level of section**

FIGURE 3-10 Structure of the hair. (Top) Cross section of a hair above the papilla. (Center) Only the bottom of the follicle is actually growing. Note that the melanocytes, the pigment-making cells, provide color to the hair (see Chapter 4). Note also the fibril character of the cortex. It is the structure that allows you to comb your hair without breaking it.

a compact mass of keratin cells. The three parts of the hair when examined in cross section are the cuticle, the cortex, and the medulla. Each hair has a nerve plexus and a blood vessel plexus. We must study the hair growth cycle to understand the hair.

## 2. The Hair Growth Cycle

Hair grows in three phases. **Telogen** is the resting stage or club stage. **Anagen** is the growth stage. **Catagen** is the regression stage. During telogen the club hair is high in the follicle and the lower hair bulb is inactive. When anagen is started there is a great increase in mitotic activity and a downward growth of the hair bulb. The hair shaft grows upward and dislodges the club hair. When this stage is over the hair bulb ceases mitosis and moves up in the dermis and the hair shaft becomes a club hair again. See **Figure 3-11** for this cycle.

## 3. Types of Hair

We classify hair as vellus hair when it is soft and fine, very short, and unpigmented. You see vellus hairs on the non-hairy parts of the body as fine "down". These hairs have a short anagen and a long telogen. Terminal hairs are the heavy, coarse, long, and pigmented hairs seen in the hairy areas of the body, scalp, beard, pubic areas, eyebrow, eyelash, and in the axilla. The intermediate hair is seen between the size and shape of the vellus and terminal hair. They are found frequently on the arms and legs of adults.

Hair follicles may also be classified as non-sexual and sexual depending on how they respond to hormones. Ambosexual hair follicles are found in both sexes and respond to androgens. They are converted from vellus to terminal hairs at puberty and are found in the pubis and in the axilla. Male sexual hair responds only to androgens and is seen in the beard area, the ears, nasal tip, chest, and pubic area.

## The Sebaceous Gland

**Sebaceous glands** are widely distributed over the body. They are on the face, scalp, back and chest in profusion. They are absent on the soles, palms and lower lip. Every hair is associated with a sebaceous gland but not all sebaceous glands are associated with hair follicles. They are then called sebaceous follicles and can

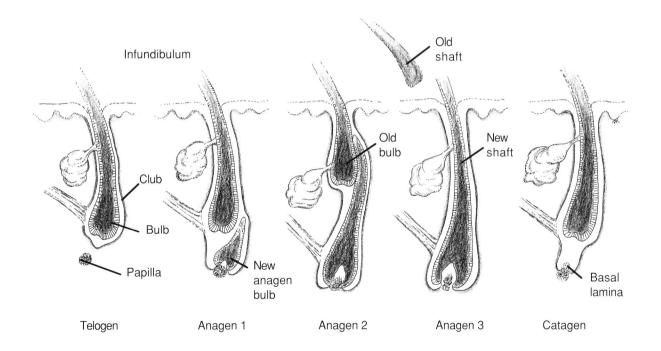

FIGURE 3-11 The hair growth cycle. Essentially there are three periods - anagen or growth stage, telogen or resting stage, and catagen or dying stage. Keep in mind the three letters A.T.C.

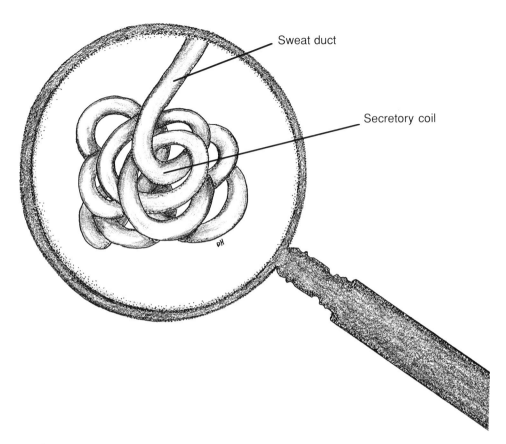

FIGURE 3-12 The sweat gland. Sweat is secreted and the water concentration adjusted carefully. The lumen carries the sweat up to the surface.

be found on the face, back, chest, buccal mucosa, nipples, upper lip, prepuce, and the glans penis.

Sebaceous glands are numerous. About 100 glands can be found per square centimeter on most areas, but on the face and scalp there may be as many as 400 - 900 per sq cm. These glands are holocrine glands "*holo* = entire", that is, glands that secrete cells along with the material they produce. The fatty substance secreted by the gland is called sebum. There is no known function of sebum. The gland secretes at the level of the infundibulum (hair pore) of the hair shaft. When not associated with a hair, it secretes directly on the skin surface, as in the upper lip.

### The Sweat Gland

Two entire industries have arisen around this gland, the antiperspirant and air conditioning. The sweat gland or sudoriferous gland (*sudor* - "sweat") is employed to regulate body heat. The underlying principle of this system is evaporation of water. The heat required to change water from a liquid to a gas or vapor is taken from the

body and used up in this conversion. As a result the body cools down as the sweat evaporates. We shall learn more about the physiology of sweat in Chapter Four, but for the present time you need to know only the basic principle of heat control.

There are two to three million sweat glands in the human body with varying distribution in different regions of the body. The soles of the feet have the most (600 per square centimeter) and the legs have the least (150 per square centimeter). These glands are widely distributed in man, but very limited in other animals. Monkeys and apes have the same sweat glands as humans but of a much lower density (fewer glands per square cm).

### The Apocrine Gland

These are the real mystery glands of the skin and much has been written about their purpose. It is believed that they are vestigial glands in the human without any true function at this stage of our evolution. They are found in the axilla, the pubic area, the anal area, the mammary areolae, and the face and scalp, developing at puberty. In the ear, they are the glands that produce ear wax (cerumen). In the eyelids they are called the glands of Moll. They are about as numerous as the sweat glands in the axilla. Otherwise, they are believed to occur at about 1 apocrine gland to every 10 sweat glands.

These glands are located in the lower dermis, and are complex tubular structures with compound secretory coils. Their ducts run parallel to the hair follicle and they empty above the sebaceous gland. Their secretion is thicker and more complex than true sweat glands, which we shall consider later.

## Eccrine Gland

Sweat is composed mainly of water (99%) and minute quantities of dissolved substances including sodium chloride, urea, sulfates, and phosphates. Sweat is odorless until bacteria act upon it, producing body odor.

The sweat gland (see **Figure 3-12**) consists of two components, a secretory coil and a duct.

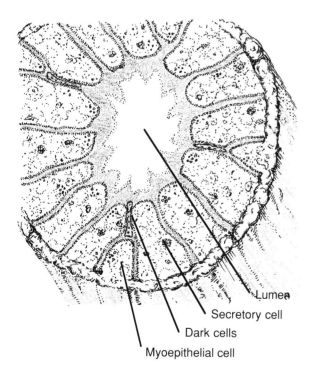

FIGURE 3-13 Transverse section of a secretory coil loop. The coil at the bottom of the sweat duct provides a large area for sweat production. The coil carries the sweat to the surface. Activation of sweat secretion is by the autonomic nervous system.

There are three cell types in the secretory part of the gland, 1. secretory (clear), 2. mucoid (dark), 3. myoepithelial.

The **secretory coil** rests directly in the basement membrane and is an irregularly coiled tube. The tube is lined with a single layer of epithelial cells which surround an open space called the lumen. Within the duct are the clear and the dark cells. The function of the dark cells remains unknown. They contain a granular substance which is "a muco-protein" but the composition is not fully known. The clear cells are believed to be the true secretory cells of the sweat gland, in that, the secretions of the gland on the skin comes from these cells. They contain many mitochondria. There is an intricate infolding of the cell membrane which forms the basal labyrinth. (See **Figure 3-13**). Where two or more clear cells join, there are structures called intercellular canniculi, which connect the cells with delicate passageways that drain eventually into the lumen of the tube.

The **sweat duct** starts abruptly after the secretory portion. It is characterized by having two to three layers of cells rather than a single layer, but it is more narrow than the secretory duct. As the duct rises, it becomes wider and in the epidermis it starts to form a spiral. At the surface it is quite wide when compared to the lower part. Just before the tube opens onto the surface, the body absorbs key salts in order to maintain a healthy balance. This is the basis for a skin condition called miliaria (prickly heat).

Nerves and blood are plentiful in sweat glands. An unmyelinated nerve from the sympathetic system supplies the gland. However, they function as if they were a part of the parasympathetic system.

The **myoepithelial** cells are located in the basal lamina of the gland, between the lamina and the clear cells. These cells act like smooth muscle cells and contract in response to stimuli, but they appear to be independent of some secretory functions.

The **basal lamina** surrounds the secretory portion of the gland. It is contiguous with the basement membrane of the epidermis but it is immunologically distinct.

We shall discuss more aspects of the sweat gland in both the biochemistry of the skin and the physiology of the skin chapters.

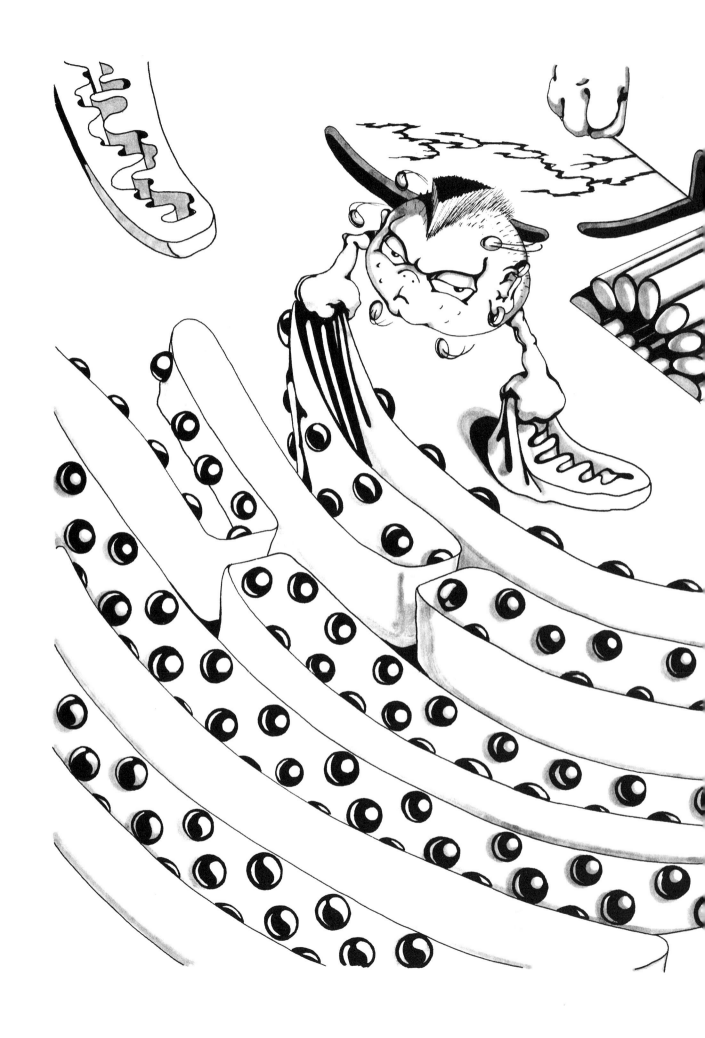

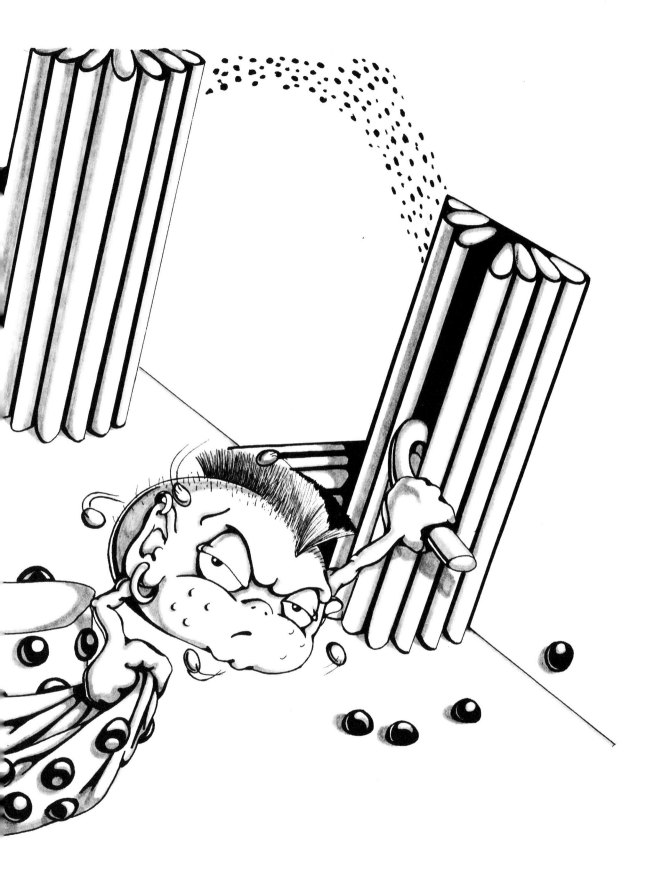

You're going to meet a rotten little group of troublemakers now. The Free Radicals. These punks thrive around Playgrounds-- you know, places where there's "fun" going on with our villians Al Cohol, Nic o'Teen, Dirty Airy  and UltraViolet. Together they spread their influence so powerfully that once they get inside, the very pillars of the community start to crumble! In this town, man, these characters are the Main Dog.

# The Essential Physiology and Biochemistry of the Skin

Biochemistry is the study of life at the level of the molecules. At this point we go deeper into the cell and try to find out how the cell works. We shall enter a world of extreme complexity and endless fascination. For the purpose of the skin care specialist only the bare essentials of this field are needed in order to understand the functioning of the skin.

The growth and repair, nourishment and appearance, health and disease, and aging of the skin are all related to biochemistry. The study of biochemistry is also essential to understand the physiology of the skin. In the study of skin physiology, we shall combine our knowledge of anatomy and biochemistry to learn about the functions of the skin.

The primary functions of the skin are protection, sensory perception, and acting as a barrier to the passage of water, chemicals, and microbes. The secondary functions, which developed later in evolution, are thermoregulation, endocrine functions (such as sex hormone and vitamin D3 production), and communication.

After reading this chapter, you may be motivated to learn more about these topics by reading some of the general references and original articles listed at the end of this book.

I shall start with a basic review of cellular structure and components. The terms and definitions given in this chapter will be used throughout the book. We shall study three major areas of biochemistry which are classified according to the three basic types of biological compounds: proteins, lipids, and carbohydrates. Each of these basic compounds comprises substances that are essential for life and the proper functioning of the body. As you read and follow the text remember that the first time you are introduced to a new subject is very similar to the first time you are introduced to a stranger. It is a little awkward and confusing until you are more familiar with the new person... so it is with biochemistry. Hang in there and you will find an exciting friend for life.

## THE CELL - THE BASIC UNIT OF LIFE

Biologists have tracked the cell's origin to the oceans. The primitive environment of the ocean is imitated in the living cells of today as a microenvironment enclosed by the cell membrane. Most cells are characterized by some or all of the following functions:

1. Nutrition - the process of food and oxygen intak, its conversion to energy, and the elimination of waste
2. Response to the environment
3. Growth and repair
4. Reproduction
5. Differentiation

We shall discuss each of these points, but first let us look at **Figure 4-1** and find the main features which are described below.

## Cell Membrane

The **cell membrane** (see **Figure 4-2**) is composed of lipids and proteins arranged in a bilayer. Picture a two layer structure, the top layer appearing much like a lot of plastic balls floating tightly together on water. Now imagine each ball with a stick a little longer than the ball (much like a caramel apple on a stick) pointing downward into the water. Next picture a second identical layer below this, with the sticks pointing upward, toward the top layer, and the whole thing floating in water in an organized manner.

Throw into this structure some very large watermelons, cucumbers, and cantalopes so that they extend through the bilayer and you will then have a fairly good idea of what a cell membrane looks like. The watermelons, cucumbers, and cantalopes represent the protein receptors and other membrane components. The whole cell membrane (also called the plasma membrane) is held together by both chemical and physical forces into a unified functional whole. All material which passes into or out of the cell must do so by one of the established pathways. Some of these pathways require energy input and others do not. Each is specific to the functioning of the cell. There is much about the cell membrane and the transportation of materials across it that remains unknown.

## The Nucleus

The **nucleus** of the cell is the major director of biochemical activity. Around the nucleus is a second membrane, the **nuclear membrane**. This membrane separates the nucleus from the rest of the cellular materials. It is the presence or absence of this nuclear membrane that forms the

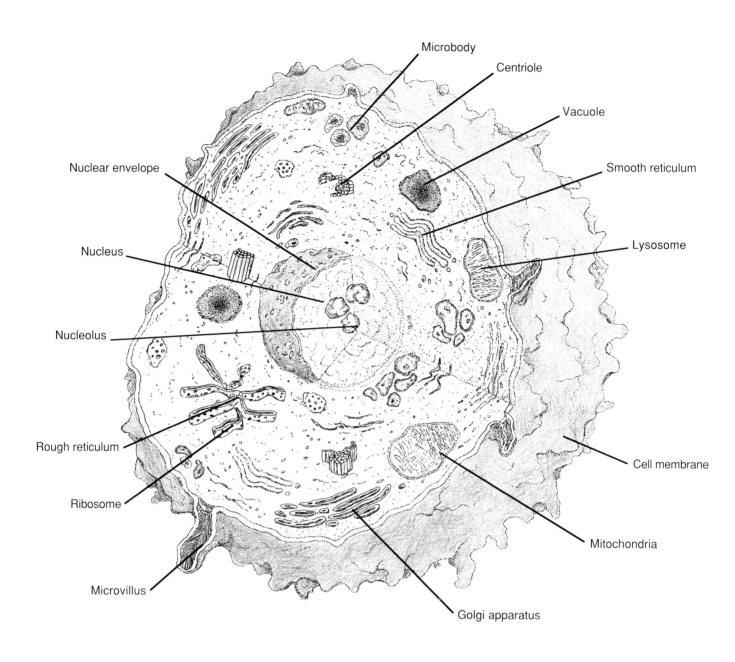

Microbody

Centriole

Vacuole

Smooth reticulum

Nuclear envelope

Nucleus

Lysosome

Nucleolus

Cell membrane

Rough reticulum

Ribosome

Mitochondria

Microvillus

Golgi apparatus

**FIGURE 4-1** Structure of the cell. This is a three dimensional view of the cell. Note all of the organelles. Try to visualize the cell as a virtual powerhouse of incessant activity that must always be alert to respond to external stress as well as internal regulation.

basis for classification of all cells into two types, prokaryocytes and eukaryocytes.

The term prokaryocyte (*pro* = before + *karyon* = nucleus) is used for all simple bacteria and blue-green algae. Eukaryocyte (*eu* = true + *karyon* = nucleus) is used for all cells with a

nuclear membrane and a complex organization of cell organelles. All mammalian cells are eukaryocytes.

The nucleus contains the genetic material **DNA (deoxyribonucleic acid)**. The DNA acts as the storehouse of genetic information and as

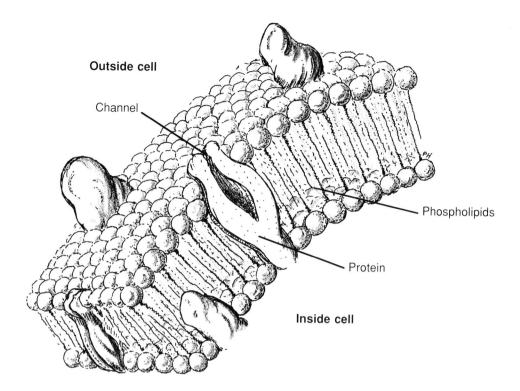

Outside cell

Channel

Phospholipids

Protein

Inside cell

**FIGURE 4-2** The cell membrane. The cell membrane is fluid, yet is very selective in passage of materials. Note that the large proteins go all the way through the cell membrane. See them as special passageways or channels allowing only those substances to pass that have the "key".

the master template for protein synthesis. The nucleus controls the potential scope of the cell's activity. The cell's environment determines what action will be taken. For instance, damage to a tissue releases substances that will cause the nucleus to initiate cellular repair and cellular division.

The **chromosomes** (*chromo* = color + *soma* = body) are in the nucleus of the cell. There are 46 chromosomes or 23 pairs in normal human cells. These cells are called diploid. When only one chromosome of each pair is present, as in the ovaries or sperm cells, they are called haploid. The chromosomes contain the DNA and generally are not visible unless the cell is dividing.

The **nucleolus** is a dark area within the nucleus. There may be more than one. It contains fibers or granules that may synthesize **RNA (ribonucleic acid)**.

### Cell Cytoplasm

The **cytoplasm** is the fluid part of the cell. It is an aqueous, colloidal material containing many fibrillar particles, lipid globules, and cel-

lular organelles. Organelles are membrane bound structures which perform specialized functions. Some of the more important components are the following:

**Ribosomes** - tiny (20 nanometer) spherical structures that synthesize proteins. The proteins carry out the complex functions of the cell such as building and repair, digestion, and energy production.

**Endoplasmic reticulum** (ER) - a membranous system containing ribosomes that manufacture proteins which are used outside of the cell (such as collagen). Both smooth and rough endoplasmic reticulum are seen. The smooth ER has no apparent ribosomes attached while the rough ER contains attached ribosomes.

**Golgi complex** (named after Camillo Golgi, 1898) - consists of vesicles, vacuoles, and flattened cisternae (bags or sacs that store proteins). The proximal face of the Golgi complex faces the nucleus. The distal face is oriented away from the nucleus. There is still a large amount of controversy about the Golgi complex. We believe it is involved in the secretion activity of the cell as well as in certain synthesis processes, such as melanin formation.

**Lysosomes** - membranous sacs that contain many digestive enzymes. The process of autolysis (self-digestion) occurs when the lysosomes rupture and literally digest the cell.

**Mitochondria** (*mito* = thread + *chondrios* = granule) - easily seen in cells though they are only 0.5 μ to 3 μ long and 0.1 μ to 0.5 μ wide. They contain all the enzymes (cytochrome system) and components to produce adenosine triphosphate (ATP) which is the major energy source of the body. The energy needed for cellular transport, movement, contraction, biosynthesis, and digestion is completely supplied by the ATP of the mitochondria. The unraveling of the mystery of the mitochondria is one of the most fascinating and exciting stories in all of biology and chemistry. Names such as Hans Krebs, Albert Lenninger, and Britton Chance will always be associated with the mitochondria and ATP generation. The presence of DNA in the mitochondria was a remarkable discovery. The mitochondria are capable of a separate replication system. It is important for you to know that energy is mainly produced in the mitochondria and that the entire process of food and oxygen utilization eventually ends up in the mitochondria. We shall discuss more of this later.

There are a few other organelles shown in Figure 4-1, but we have covered the essential ones. Remember that cell anatomy and physiology are dynamic sciences that are expanding day by day. No one person can keep up with all the new information. Don't despair. New information will appear in condensed form by some reviewer. Let us now look at the basic building blocks of proteins and protein structure.

## PROTEINS

Proteins are the most plentiful compounds in the body, other than water. They are involved in nearly all body functions. Here are some of the roles they play:
1. Mechanical support - fibrous proteins such as collagen and elastin
2. Motion and mobility - muscle proteins
3. Transmission of messages - nerves and specific receptors
4. Control of growth and differentiation - mediated by DNA
5. Enzymatic reactions - needed to build other proteins and to drive many chemical reactions
6. Transport and storage
7. Immunological functions - antibody production.

All of these functions require some type of specific protein which is made up of units called amino acids.

### The Amino Acids

The building blocks of the proteins are the amino acids. All amino acids contain four components.

Amino Group - ($-NH_2$)
Carboxyl Group - ($-COOH$)
Hydrogen Atom - ($-H$)
R Group - R is a variable group. It is this group which gives each separate amino acid its

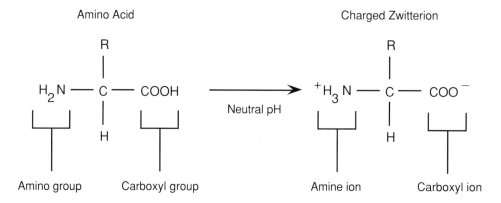

FIGURE 4-3 Structure of amino acids. This is an important concept which relates to pH. The zwitterions can swing back and forth between a negative anionic molecule and a positive cationic molecule. The implications for biological functions is obvious. For example, if the pH of the blood would change from a slightly alkaline (7.4) to a more neutral range, there would be an adverse effect on protein structure and function.

## CLASSIFICATION OF AMINO ACIDS

SINGLE AMINO, SINGLE CARBOXYLIC
STRAIGHT SIDE CHAIN GROUP
1. Glycine (Gly)- the most common and most simple.
2. Alanine (Ala)
3. Valine (Val)
4. Leucine (Leu)
5. Isoleucine (Ile)

AROMATIC SIDE CHAIN (SIX CARBON RING SIDE GROUP)
6. Phenylalanine (Phe)
7. Tyrosine (Tyr)
8. Tryptophan (Trp)

HYDROXYAMINO GROUP
9. Serine (Ser)
10. Threonine (Thr)

DICARBOXYLIC GROUP (2 CARBOXYL GROUPS)
11. Aspartic Acid (Asp)
12. Glutamic Acid (Glu)

ACID AMIDE GROUP (HAS A CO.NH2 GROUP)
13. Asparagine (Asn)
14. Glutamine (Gln)

BASIC GROUP (TWO OR MORE AMINO GROUPS, ONE CARBOXYL GROUP)
15. Lysine (Lsy)
16. Arginine (Arg)
17. Histidine (His)

SULFUR-CONTAINING GROUP
18. Methionine (Met)
19. Cysteine (Cys)
19a. Cystine

SECONDARY AMINO GROUP
20. Proline (Pro)
20a. Hydroxyproline (Hyp)

**TABLE 4-1**

unique structure and function. The R Group is also called a side chain.

We shall list the amino acids in a convenient classification by structure. You need not memorize them but study the essential differences in structure and make-up among the various groups. This will help you to appreciate and understand protein function more easily.

One bit of chemical knowledge you need to know about amino acids is that they are very sensitive to pH. Changes in pH cause them to change their net electrical charge, so that at a neutral pH they are zwitterions. This means that the carboxyl group is dissociated (ionized) into a carboxyl ion ($-COO^-$). The amino group gains a proton ($H^+$) and is protonated to become an amine ion ($-NH_3^+$). While at first, this seems hard to understand, look at the diagram in **Figure 4-3** and you will see these changes.

When the amino acids are in an acid solution that is below pH 7 the carboxyl group remains as -COOH and the amino group becomes ionized to $NH_3^+$. In an alkaline solution the carboxyl group becomes ionized to $-COO^-$, while the amine group remains $-NH_2$. We have not discussed pH so just keep these concepts in the back of your mind until we cover pH in more detail. These little bits of information are needed now to go on with our presentation of proteins.

The most important amino acids are shown in **Table 4-1**. You will find other amino acids listed in text books, but at this time, you need not be concerned with them.

### The Peptide Bond

Amino acids form proteins by combining with each other in several ways, the most important of which is the peptide bond. This is a chemical structure that is very strong and results when the carboxyl group of one amino acid joins with the amino group of another amino acid (see **Figure 4-4**). Water is eliminated as a result. When two amino acids join we have a **dipeptide** and when many amino acids are joined we have a **polypeptide**. Proteins are nothing more than large groups of polypeptides joined in a highly specific configuration to serve a particular purpose.

### The Making of Cellular Proteins

I have included this section mainly as a refresher. We shall use terms later in the chapter that are perhaps new to the reader. Many of these terms are related to the synthesis of proteins in the cell, starting with the nuclear DNA and proceeding to the finished protein.

DNA is a double stranded molecule consisting of a backbone of alternating sugar and phos-

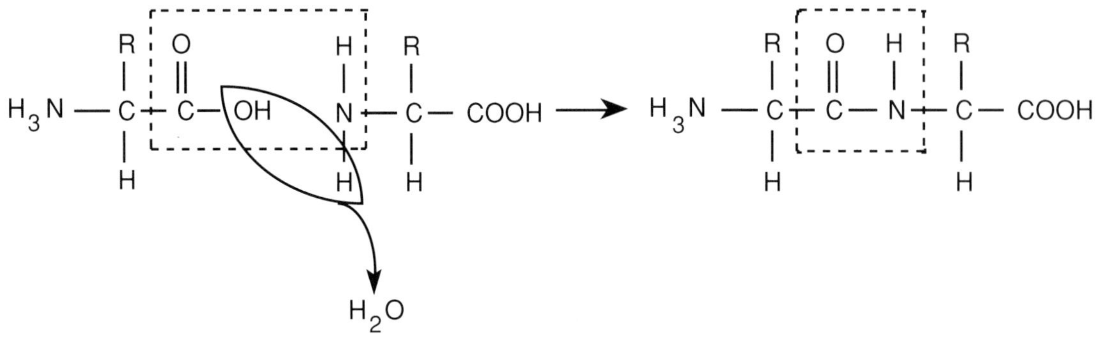

**FIGURE 4-4** The peptide bond. The peptide bond unites amino acids. It can also bind proteins together. Most amino acids are linked by peptide bonds to form large proteins.

phate molecules, each of which contains one of four bases: adenine, cytosine, guanine, thymine. The two strands are held together by the union of the bases, adenine to thymine, cytosine to guanine. The process of protein synthesis starts with the DNA molecule opening to allow an RNA molecule to be synthesized. The RNA makes a reverse copy of the DNA (that is, of the four bases of RNA: adenine, cytosine, guanine, and uracil instead of thymine) link with the bases on the DNA molecule. The linkage is always as is depicted in **Figure 4-5**. This process is called transcription. Once the RNA is formed, it separates from the DNA template and is termed messenger RNA (mRNA), a coded molecule carrying the information for a specific protein. Moving to the cytoplasm the mRNA joins with the protein synthesis area of the ribosomes in the endoplasmic reticulum. Here amino acids are added to the specific sequence of base units to form a small polypeptide or a complete protein. This process is called translation. This process is described in detail in "The Science of Molecular Biology" (see references). These terms will come up again when we explore the pathology of skin disorders.

## THE FOUR HORSEMEN OF THE SKIN. THE KERATINOCYTE, THE MELANOCYTE, THE LANGERHANS CELL, AND THE FIBROBLAST.

I have chosen to divide the biochemistry and physiology of the skin into an explanation of cell types and function. These four cell types account for most of the biochemical activity of the skin. We shall start with the keratinocyte

since it is the most versatile of skin cells.

### The Keratinocyte

I believe the keratinocyte and its complex of proteins will be future markers for determining the state of health of the skin. Changes in the keratins within the stratum corneum cells have been observed in psoriasis and may soon be used to show the response of this disorder to treatment.

Keratin is a protein that belongs to a class of structural proteins called intermediate filaments which make up the structural components of the cell (also called the cytoskeleton). Much remains to be known about this group of proteins as a class. Keratin is found in the cells of many tissues including the epidermis, sweat ducts, hair follicle, breast, vaginal and anal mucosa, bile and pancreatic ducts, intestinal mucosa, trachea and bronchial epithelium, ovarian and uterine structures, and the renal collecting ducts. These keratins all share certain characteristics but we shall confine our discussion to only the keratins of the epidermis and related structures. Keratin is formed initially in the cells of the basal layer and as these cells move up, the keratin is modified. The synthesis starts with DNA, then proceeds through RNA to prekeratin, tonofilaments, prekeratin filaments, tropokeratin filaments, and results in keratin filaments. We have a very heterogeneous group of keratin proteins in the skin as determined by the molecular weights of the polypeptides resulting from hydrolysis of the keratin proteins. The molecular weight analysis of the polypeptides serves as the basis for keratin identification. Let us look now at the struc-

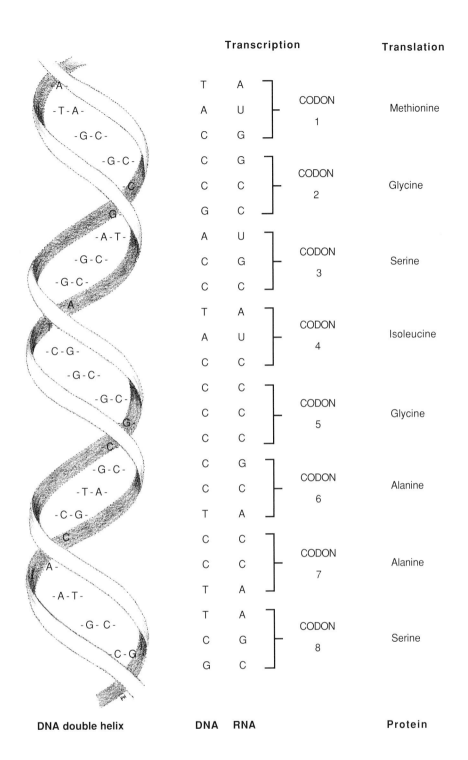

| | | | | Transcription | | | Translation |
|---|---|---|---|---|---|---|---|

| DNA | RNA | | |
|---|---|---|---|
| T | A | | |
| A | U | CODON 1 | Methionine |
| C | G | | |
| C | G | | |
| C | C | CODON 2 | Glycine |
| G | C | | |
| A | U | | |
| C | G | CODON 3 | Serine |
| C | C | | |
| T | A | | |
| A | U | CODON 4 | Isoleucine |
| C | C | | |
| C | C | | |
| C | C | CODON 5 | Glycine |
| C | C | | |
| C | G | | |
| C | C | CODON 6 | Alanine |
| T | A | | |
| C | C | | |
| C | C | CODON 7 | Alanine |
| T | A | | |
| T | A | | |
| C | G | CODON 8 | Serine |
| G | C | | |

**DNA double helix**          **DNA   RNA**                          **Protein**

**FIGURE 4-5** The transcription process. The only way the DNA strands can combine is by linkage of thymine (T) to adenine (A) and cytosine (C) to guanine (G). This is why animals of different groups (Genus) can not reproduce. The sequence of DNA bases is quite different among various animals; this prevents exact matching of the base sequence.

ture of keratin protein.

The basic structure of the keratin protein is the alpha helix (or coil) composed of polypeptide subunits. These subunits are arranged into a strand of alternating subunits with four strands to a protofilament and nine protofilaments to a keratin protein filament. The subunits are composed of segments 47 nm long. In each segment there are two helical proteins each 18 nm long separated by a non-helical protein of 4 nm. At each end there are additional non-helical structures of 4 nm. Now, this appears quite complex and indeed it is for the exact structure has not been completely determined. We do know that these subunits make up the various polypeptides seen in different layers of the skin, and in various regions of the body. What is important to understand is that there are several different forms and they have different functional properties. The molecular weights of the polypeptides that make up the keratin segments identify particular keratin proteins in the cells. There are many references to this subject, a few of them are listed in the bibliography.

Another protein linked with keratin is filaggrin, or "stratum corneum basic protein". This protein is aggregated with keratin filaments to form keratin macrofibrils which are highly insoluble. Filaggrin is derived from a large precursor molecule, profilaggrin (between 450 - 600 kd). This protein is seen in the keratohyaline granules in the lower epidermis. At the very top of the epidermis the keratinocyte hardens into a cornified cell. This requires the action of two additional proteins, involucrin and keratolinin, which are components of the rigid crossed-linked insoluble envelope of the corneocyte. Involucrin (Latin -*involucrin* = envelope) is not a keratin protein and is not synthesized in the basal layer but rather in cells further up, when the cells no longer can divide. Thus, the cells can serve as markers of advanced differentiation.

To review the above, let us follow a keratinocyte from the basal layer to the corneocyte.

1. Keratin is formed in the basal layer as tonofilaments.
2. The keratin filaments are formed.
3. The cell moves towards the surface and keratohyaline granules are formed.
4. The cell moves into the upper granular layer (lower layers of the stratum corneum) where the keratin fibrils are formed and the involucrin is produced.
5. The cell now consists of packed keratin fibrils inside and a tough crossed-linked envelope outside.

There are three other proteins that we shall look at briefly that occur in the basement membrane. They have considerable importance in some skin disorders so the skin care specialist must be aware of them. At first these are confusing and not easy to remember, but we shall encounter them again and they will seem more

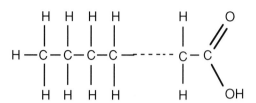

**FIGURE 4-6** Structure of fatty acid. A fatty acid has a long carbohydrate chain. The dotted line represents more of the H-C-H groups. The short chained fatty acids and the fatty acids with double bonds tend to be liquids at room temperature. The longer the chain, that is, the more H-C-H groups, the more solid the material. Fatty acids above 20 carbons form waxes.

friendly. These proteins belong to a large group known as glycoproteins or sugar containing proteins. Here are three in the basement membrane:

**Fibronectin** - not a glycoprotein specific to the basement membrane. It is also found in and about other cells and in the serum. It has strong surface attachment properties and strong binding affinities. It plays a role in the cellular attachment to the basal lamina.

**Laminin** - a very large glycoprotein (950 kd) that is believed to be a structural component of the basement membranes, possibly of the basal lamina.

**Entactin** - a newly discovered glycoprotein whose function is unknown. There is some evidence that it is a separate basement membrane component. It is important to us now only as a distinct protein of the skin that may have future impact on skin health.

Lipids and the Barrier Function

The two most important chemical substances in the skin are the keratins and the lipids since they provide the materials for mechanical protection and the permeability barrier of the skin. Lipids are water insoluble compounds that are soluble in organic compounds such as ether and chloroform. They have many forms, but for our purpose we will look at phospholipids, glycolipids, and cholesterol. The fatty acids are basic structures in lipids so we need to look at this structure first. Fatty acids are usually straight chained hydrocarbons, that is, many carbon and hydrogen molecules linked together in a line (see **Figure 4-6**). At one end there is a carboxyl group. (Sometimes there is one on each end and that is called a dicarboxylic fatty acid). We talked about lipids when we discussed the cell membrane. Many of these membrane lipids are phospholipids. Phospholipids are composed of a glycerol backbone or a complex alcohol called sphingosine, two fatty acids usually with 14 to 24 carbons, and a phosphorylated alcohol. The 16 carbon fatty acid is called palmitic acid and the 18 carbon fatty acid is called stearic acid. Together they are the most common fatty acids in the body.

Glycolipids are sugar-containing lipids composed of a sphingosine backbone, a fatty acid, and one or more sugars. They are important in many ways which we shall touch on later.

Cholesterol is an extremely important lipid in the cell membrane and in the stratum corneum. The structure of cholesterol is shown in **Figure 4-7**. The basic structure of cholesterol is seen in many hormones such as cortisone, estrogen, and testosterone. You need to be familiar with this molecule as it will come up time and again.

For many years the barrier of the skin was believed to be protein and the sebaceous secretion. This myth has been dispelled and the new findings provide an elegant explanation of the barrier make-up. First, the barrier layer is only in the stratum corneum. Strip that away and the water will come forth! The work of Elias has shown that the intercellular space is the key to barrier function. He pictures the stratum corneum as bricks (the corneocytes) and mortar (the lipid-containing intercellular spaces). To understand this concept refer to **Figure 4-8** as you read the text and find all the components in the diagram.

The **lamellar body** is the major player in the two compartment model of the lipid barrier. Lamellar bodies are very small granules of 0.2 to 0.3 microns in diameter which are synthesized in the granular layer. These secretory granules which are found in the upper granular layer fuse with the plasma membrane and secrete their contents into the intercellular space. The intercellular space then expands to a point where it comprises 10 to 40% of the total volume of the stratum corneum. How this occurs, what triggers the process, and what controls the process is unknown. The lipids in the intercellular space are arranged in laminar fashion and contain free fatty acids, sterols (both free and esterified), and sphingolipids. There are no phospholipids in the stratum corneum, but there are some very long fatty acids, such as waxes.

One other observation by Dr. Elias is important for the skin care specialist. The ability of the skin to resist permeation is not related to the thickness of the skin but rather to the amount of lipids present in the skin. It is known that the eyelid and skin of the human scrotum are ten

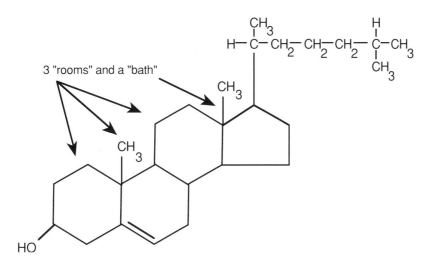

**FIGURE 4-7** Structure of cholesterol. This is the basic molecule for many hormones. Visualize the benzene symbol as six carbons linked in a circle. All cortisone hormones and male and female hormones have this basic structure. It is easy to remember if you consider the three six-carbon molecules as "rooms" and the five-carbon molecule as the "bath".

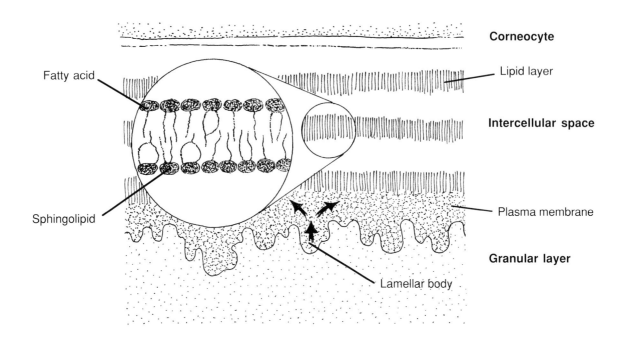

Corneocyte

Lipid layer

Intercellular space

Plasma membrane

Granular layer

Fatty acid

Sphingolipid

Lamellar body

**FIGURE 4-8** The barrier function. While (fatty) lipid materials pass easily into the stratum corneum, water soluble materials also penetrate but at a slower rate.

times more permeable to lipid material than other body areas. It is not only that these areas are thinner but that the lipid content is much less than other body areas.

### Carbohydrate Metabolism, the Keratinocyte and Energy

We have discussed the role of proteins and lipids mainly as building components of the body cells and tissue. We have also discussed sugars as components of both glycolipids and glycoproteins. Sugars belong to a group of compounds known as carbohydrates. Carbohydrates are chemical compounds composed of carbon, hydrogen, and oxygen. The hydrogen and oxygen are present in a ratio of two to one, the same ratio that is in water ($H_2O$). Many carbohydrates are saccharides (sugars and starches). Glucose is the most common sugar in the body. It is also the simplest sugar (six carbons) and is called a monosaccharide. Two monosaccharides linked together form a disaccharide such as sucrose (common table sugar) which is composed of glucose plus fructose. When many sugars are linked together we have a polysaccharide, such

as starch and glycogen. These carbohydrates are very important because they are the major source of energy for the body.

When a carbohydrate is broken down by the body the energy used to hold the carbohydrate together is released and used immediately or stored in the body. This process is called metabolism. Metabolism is divided into two major functions: anabolism (synthesis functions) and catabolism (decomposition functions). Most of these reactions would be extremely slow unless they were helped along by special proteins called enzymes. Enzymes are protein catalysts which greatly increase the rate of reaction of many metabolic functions.

The reader must understand the importance of enzymes in the body, otherwise the whole concept of metabolic function will be lost. Enzymes function by joining to the substrate (reactant) to form an enzyme-substrate complex and then produce the products of the reaction. The enzyme is not used up in this reaction, but is released to be used over and over again. See **Figure 4-9**, which illustrates this reaction. Enzymes can only react with specific substrates under certain conditions. Certain compounds called coenzymes are required for some reactions (eg. - vitamins are coenzymes in some reactions).

When I was a small child I was curious about many things and it was inevitable that the ticking clock would fall victim to this curiosity. I discovered two things when I dismantled the family clock - one was that it was very complicated and the second was that taking a clock apart produced a spanking. Now this certainly was an unplanned and unexpected reaction to a simple process. Only later in life did I learn that there is no such thing as a simple action. One little act sets into motion many events that must be balanced by other events. In the body this whole process is called **homeostasis,** that is, maintaining a constant internal environment. All of the metabolic processes are geared to keep this environment stable. If a clock is broken, the cause must be found and dealt with, and the clock repaired or replaced. All of this requires energy and expense and produces heat (in more places then one). We shall discuss this process and see how the skin gets its energy to do work.

As we have described above, the source of energy for the body is a chemical called adenosine triphosphate or **ATP** (see **Figure 4-10**).

Let us take a simple glucose molecule and see how this is broken down to produce energy. While this will seem complex to you at first, you will see later why a basic understanding of this process is necessary for anyone dealing with the skin.

Glucose must first be taken out of the blood stream, and then is linked with a phosphate group to become glucose-6-phosphate. It is then converted to fructose-6-phosphate and another phosphate group is added. Next, it is split into two three carbon compounds and each of these two compounds is metabolized via the Krebs cycle into carbon dioxide and water with the production of energy. This Krebs cycle is diagrammed for you in **Figure 4-11**. You need not learn all the steps, but observe that ATP is ultimately produced at several places in this cycle. Most of the ATP is produced in the electron transport system (cytochrome system). This system requires oxygen which combines with the electrons produced in the citric acid cycle (Krebs cycle) to produce water. This process is called oxidative phosphorylation. Think about this a minute. If you are choking on food, your oxy-

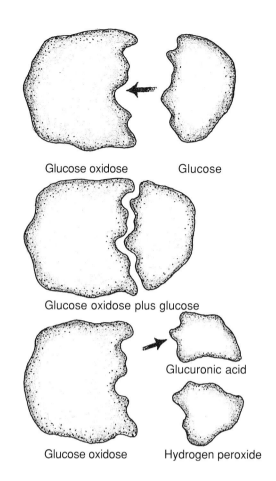

Glucose oxidose          Glucose

Glucose oxidose plus glucose

Glucose oxidose          Hydrogen peroxide

Glucuronic acid

**FIGURE 4-9** Enzyme reaction. Enzymes are not used up in a reaction. Just remember the three steps. 1. Enzyme + substrate 2. Enzyme-substrate complex (the intermediate compound) and 3. Enzyme + product. Now the enzyme can be used again.

gen supply is being cut off and your cellular electron transport system stops. You lose all energy and if not supplied with oxygen, you will become unconscious and then die. So oxygen is vital to this metabolic pathway.

The skin, however, can get by without oxygen for a time. The first part of the glucose metabolic pathway needs no oxygen and is called anaerobic and produces very little ATP. For some reason the skin does not use glucose as its main energy source but uses lipids instead.

Lipid metabolism is more complex and proceeds by way of a process called fatty acid oxidation (beta oxidation). Again, you need not learn all the pathways but remember that the end product of fatty acid metabolism is a compound called acetyl-CoA (see **Figure 4-12**), which is an important component of glucose metabolism. If there is no glucose present to produce oxalo-

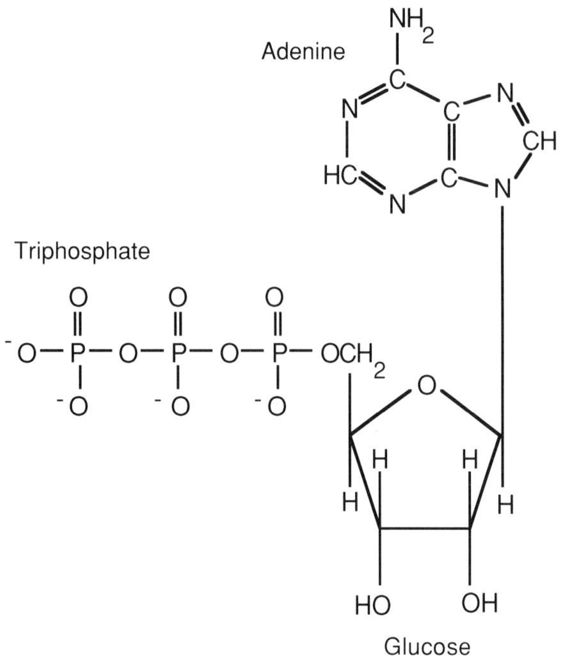


**FIGURE 4-10** Structure of ATP. ATP is the energy source for most body reactions. Remember that there are three parts to the molecule. Adenine, glucose and the triple phosphate. As energy is lost phosphate is lost and we end up with adenosine diphosphate (ADP) and adenosine monophosphate (AMP). The whole process of food metabolism is used to regenerate ATP.

acetate then the fatty acids will produce acetoacetate and other compounds known as ketone bodies. This occurs in individuals with diabetes. I have outlined this pathway in **Figure 4-13**. The key concept to remember is that the skin uses fatty acids as its major source of energy and that glucose is needed to help metabolize the fatty acids. The generated ATP is used by the body whenever an energy requiring reaction takes place. All living things need energy to move, to transport molecules, to build molecules, and to perform cellular movements. One thing more, all energy for life on earth comes from the sun. It is through the food chain that we use most of this energy, not through our skin.

## Epidermal Kinetics or How the Skin Maintains Itself

We have stated that one of the main functions of the skin is to provide a protective barrier. This barrier must be both effective and efficient to be of real value. We have seen that the biochemistry of the individual keratinocyte is beautifully developed to enable the cell to perform well as a barrier. We have, however, many millions of cells in small areas of the skin that must be organized in a physical manner or structural pattern that will actually form the barrier against the outside world. The study of this structure and how it is maintained is our next topic.

As an early student of the skin you must have seen many drawings of the epidermis depicted as neatly structured in four layers. When you see the epidermis removed from the body, stained and examined with a microscope it does not have this very neat, well organized appearance. In fact, in the beginning you will have trouble distinguishing one layer from the next. There is order in this system, though, and you must understand this mechanism to appreciate the functionality of the stratum corneum. The epidermal cells are aligned in a columnar fashion depending on where they are located. This arrangement probably represents the need to establish short pathways to the surface for cell replacement, or for the effective inhibition of penetrants, or to prevent frictional forces from shearing the cells from the surface. Many of these questions remain to be answered. We do know some facts about the rate of cell growth and the transport of cells to the surface. This process of renewing cells is called epidermal cell kinetics. There are four types of cell growth based on the rate of mitosis or cell division. These populations are:

1. The static cell - the brain.
2. The expanding cell - the liver, kidney, and muscles which reach a maximum of mitosis at maturity and then decrease.
3. The renewing cell - the epithelial tissues (which includes the skin) and the blood cells.
4. The neoplastic cell - includes benign and malignant tumors, characterized by a net over production of cells. We are concerned herewith the renewing cell population of the epidermis.

The epidermis may be divided into three basic compartments, for the purpose of studying cell kinetics. These are the germinative, the differentiated, and the cornified compartments. The basal layer and the layer immediately above it (the suprabasal layer) form the germinative compartment. Above the germinative compart-

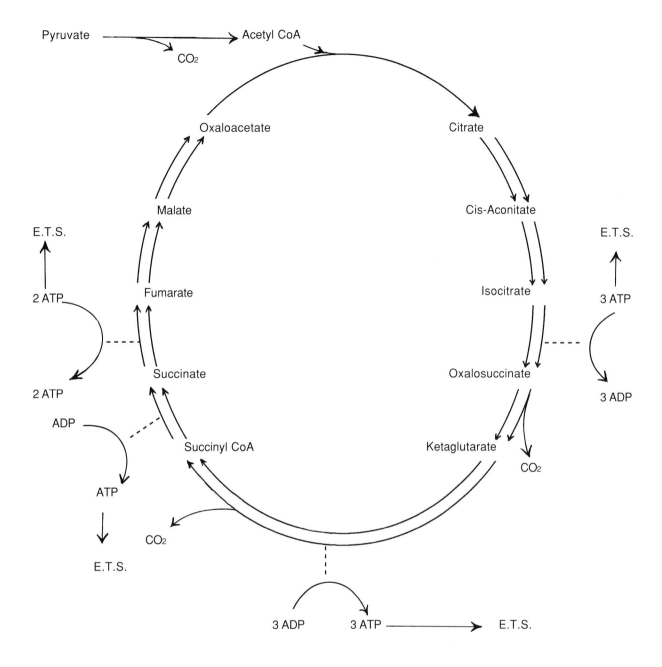

Pyruvate ⟶ Acetyl CoA

$CO_2$

Oxaloacetate

Citrate

Malate

Cis-Aconitate

E.T.S.

E.T.S.

Fumarate

Isocitrate

2 ATP

3 ATP

2 ATP

3 ADP

Succinate

Oxalosuccinate

ADP

Succinyl CoA

Ketaglutarate

ATP

$CO_2$

$CO_2$

E.T.S.

3 ADP    3 ATP ⟶ E.T.S.

E.T.S. = Electron Transport System

**FIGURE 4-11** Krebs cycle. You do not need to memorize this cycle. Only biochemists do. Be familiar with the fact that it is the pathway between the pyruvate generating systems and the final pathway to produce ATP. Glucose > Pyruvate > Krebs cycle > Electron Transport System > ATP.

ment, the differentiated cells of the spiny layer and the granular layer are formed. Finally, the cornified layer is seen in the stratum corneum. It takes about 45 days for a cell to go from the basal layer to the stratum corneum. The stratum corneum is constantly being lost to the environment and replaces itself completely about every 15 days depending on the body location. To

understand turnover rates and proliferation we need to learn the mechanism of the cell cycle.

The cell cycle is a period of time required for the cell to go from the resting stage to the formation of a new cell. There are four periods or stages in the reproduction of a cell.

The **G1 period** (interphase period) is the period in which the cell performs most of its

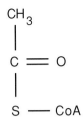

**FIGURE 4-12** Structure of acetyl CoA. This is an extremely important intermediary product essential for many metabolic pathways. The CoA part is the enzyme component which binds to the acetyl group. The complex acetyl CoA enters the Kreb cycle to be further metabolized.

metabolic activities, such as growth of the newly formed cell. The duration of this period may be for a few hours up to many months. Activated by some unknown stimulus the cell enters the next period.

The **S period** (DNA synthesis period) is a period of high synthesis activity in which the chromosomes are replicated.

The **G2 period** (postsynthesis period) is very short, usually lasting only minutes. In this period the cell prepares for division by mitosis.

The **M period** (mitotic period) is the period of actual cellular division with two daughter cells being produced. The cells then enter the G1 period. The cell cycle is diagrammed in **Figure 4-14**. An additional group of cells, called G0, are described as potentially proliferative cells that may be activated into division by a specific stimulus. These cells are not believed to be part of the growing cell pool but are in a "ready phase". As a result not all of the basal cells are proliferating, only a fraction of them, and this is known as the growth fraction (GF). The importance of the GF concept is that it would explain why the epidermis can proliferate at times at a much faster rate, such as in psoriasis. The GF may be as low as 20% in normal skin and move up to 100% in psoriasis.

Cell cycle completion times for various types of tissues:

| | |
|---|---|
| Skin, normal | 13 days |
| Psoriatic | 2 days |
| Mucosal | 4 days |

There are many factors that influence the growth rate of the epidermis. Here we shall mention only a few as we shall touch on this subject later. There is a variation in growth during the day and the night, a so called diurnal variation. There is only a slight increase which occurs about midnight (basis for beauty sleep?).

Hormones affect facial hair and sebaceous gland proliferation. Physiological growth factors, such as chalones, regulate growth by a negative feedback mechanism. This keeps the cell population in homeostasis by counteracting stimulants. Epidermal growth factor (EGF) is a powerful stimulant, as is inflammation from a number of sources. We must keep in mind that when one population of cells is stimulated by a specific factor such as EGF other related cells may be stimulated as well. An example of this is the stomach ulcer sometimes seen in patients with large area burns. As the burns heal much EGF is produced to stimulate epidermal repair. This same EGF also stimulates the cells of the stomach which are also epithelial cells. These rapidly growing stomach cells are less resistant to acid and so they are damaged more easily resulting in ulcer formation.

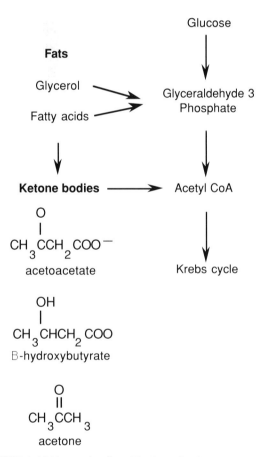

**FIGURE 4-13** Ketone bodies. Blockage in glucose causes fats to be utilized as the major energy source. Ketone bodies accumulate since they can not be further metabolized without additional Krebs cycle components.

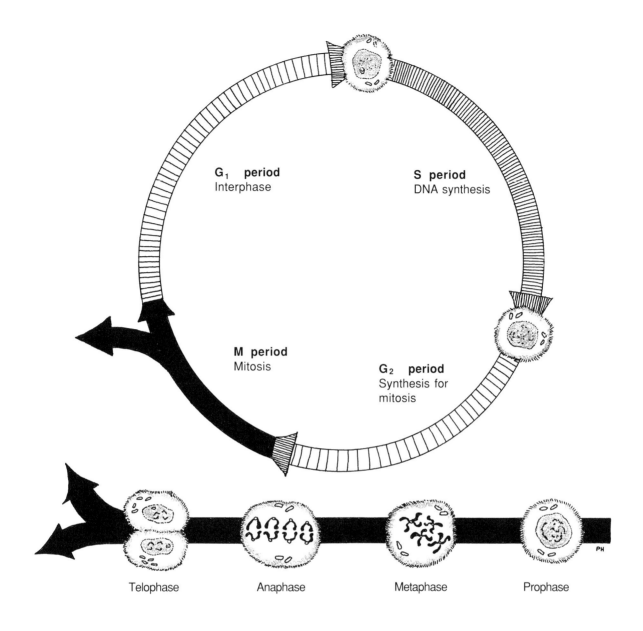

**FIGURE 4-14** The cell cycle. This is a good diagram outlining the various phases of the cell cycle. Mitosis, the M period, is only one part of the cell cycle. The resting stage or G1 Period is an important period where the cell can be acted upon by a number of stimulators.

### The Melanocyte

Here is a truly fascinating subject. A scientist could spend his/her whole life on the study of the melanocyte and not fully understand it. We actually know a great deal about the melanocyte but what we do not know greatly outweighs our present concepts. Melanocytes are responsible for skin color so let's start there.

Human skin exhibits four colors: red, yellow, brown, and blue. Eating foods with the natural yellow color (carotene) accounts for some

of the yellow hue. The red color is produced by the hemoglobin in the blood when it carries oxygen, so called oxygenated hemoglobin or oxyhemoglobin. When the hemoglobin is reduced, that is it gives up oxygen and contains carbon dioxide, as in the veins, it produces a blue color. This blue color accounts for the dark blue color of cyanosis (*cyan* = blue) The brown color is due to the pigment melanin which is the major factor in determining the color of the skin. Let us look at the cell that produces the melanin, and how the melanin colors the skin.

The **melanocyte** produces melanin granules called **melanosomes**. These melanosomes contain the material melanin, a brown pigment. The melanosomes are transferred from the melanocytes to the keratinocytes in the granular layer of the skin. Only when the melanosomes enter the keratinocytes does the skin have color. This is important to know as it is a fundamental principle of skin color. The amount of melanin in the keratinocyte determines the degree of color in the skin or hair. "Be ye blond or brunette, the cause be the same, melanin." In the skin there is about one melanocyte to 36 keratinocytes. This is called an epidermal melanocyte unit. There are a couple of other things you should know about melanin and pigmentation of the skin. We speak of constitutive skin color which is pigmentation generated without exposure to radiation or hormone interaction. Facultative pigmentation is inducible pigmentation that occurs with exposure to ultraviolet radiation, hormones or inflammation. This hyperpigmentation is reversible when the stimulus is removed, as in tanning.

We need also to look at some different types of melanin. Then we can look into the chemistry of how melanin is formed. Here are the known types of melanin that are of interest to us.

**Eumelanin** - a brown to black pigment that is a polymer of high molecular weight. Its chemical composition is unknown. It is almost insoluble in most solvents, and is resistant to most chemical treatments. A very difficult molecule to study!

**Phaeomelanin** - a yellow red pigment that is solublein dilute alkali. The term phaeomelanin literally means gray melanin (*phaios* = gray) so while it is confusing we are stuck with it. Phaeomelanin occurs only in the hair, not in the skin. It is the primary melanin in the red-haired individual.

**Trichochrome** - a red yellow pigment of low molecular weight is also found in hair.

Just one more note before we get into the chemistry of melanin. Once the melanin is in the hair shaft it can not be removed! The color will not change! Maybe fade a little, but no real change. So no one can go gray overnight or from fright. Graying is in some way associated with aging so in some manner melanin must also be linked to the aging mechanism. Think about that.

## Melanin Chemistry. The Dark Pathway.

I have diagrammed the formation of melanin from the amino acid tyrosine (see **Figure 4-15**). You need not memorize all these steps but you must be familiar with the process. Since there will be so many new tanning gimmicks in the future you will be lost without a basic understanding of the process. Here we go.

We start with an amino acid tyrosine and form dopa II. Dopa is shorthand for a complex molecule called 3,4 dihydroxyphenylalanine. Next dopa quinone III is formed by loss of two hydrogens. At this stage the pathway splits to form either eumelanin or phaeomelanin. The presence of sulfur in the form of cysteinyldopa makes the difference. The next steps on the pathway to melanin after the dopa quinone III step are dopachrome to 5, 6 dihydroxylindole to indole-5, 6-quinone and finally to melanin. The controlling step in the synthesis of melanin is the conversion of tyrosine to dopa by the enzyme tyrosinase.

## Melanocyte Physiology and Color Control

Melanin absorbs very strongly throughout the ultraviolet and visible wavelengths of light. This is a protective mechanism. Melanin also contains and absorbs free radicals. This is also a protective mechanism. Melanin production is affected by drugs such as cocaine, phenothiazines and chloroquine (used in malaria prevention). The number of melanocytes varies from region to region in the skin 1000 per cubic millimeter in thigh and 2000 per cubic millimeter in the scrotum (**see Figure 4-16**). The major difference between Negroids and other dark skin races and Caucasians relates to the distribution of the melanosomes. In dark skin races the melanosomes are large and distributed singly whereas in Caucasians they are smaller and packaged in complexes. The melanosomes will vary in size, shape, and degree of melanization, being absent in albinos and being very dense in black skin.

## Tanning and Melanogenesis

There is at present no safe way to tan. The effect of ultraviolet light on the melanocyte is not fully understood. We know that the skin tans in response to light in the range from 280 to 400

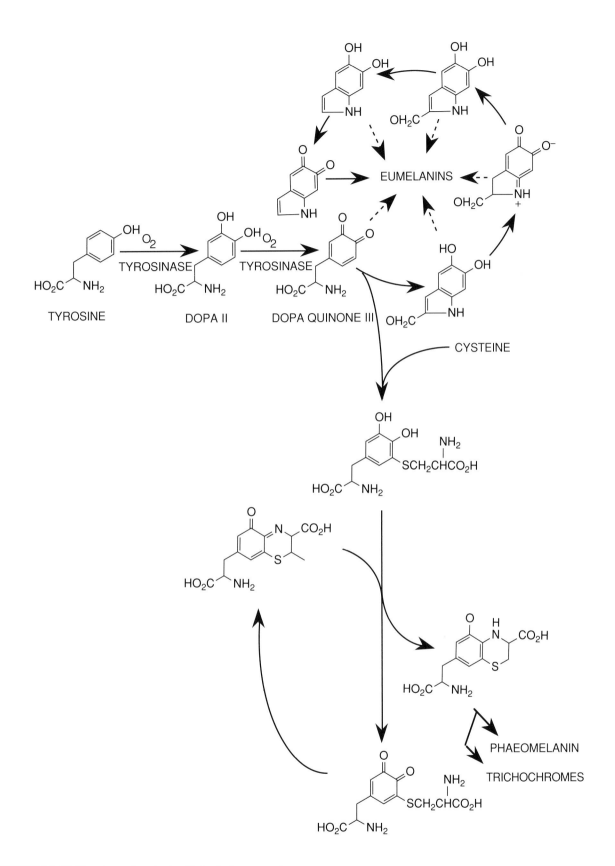

**FIGURE 4-15** Structure of melanin. Melanin is a complex molecule. We do not fully understand its structure. Eumelanins follow the upper pathway while phaeomelanins are combinations of Dopa quinone III and cysteine. This is an imperfect melanin with a tendency to oxidation by ultraviolet light. Trichochromes are phaeomelanins that occur in red hair. They are chemically somewhat different from other melanins. Adapted from Biochemistry and Physiology of the Skin by Lowell A. Goldsmith, Oxford University Press, Inc., 1983.

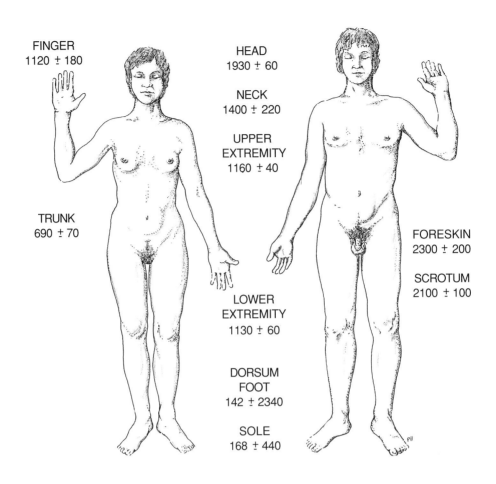

FINGER
1120 ± 180

HEAD
1930 ± 60

NECK
1400 ± 220

UPPER
EXTREMITY
1160 ± 40

TRUNK
690 ± 70

FORESKIN
2300 ± 200

SCROTUM
2100 ± 100

LOWER
EXTREMITY
1130 ± 60

DORSUM
FOOT
142 ± 2340

SOLE
168 ± 440

**FIGURE 4-16** Distribution of melanocytes per square mm of body surface in different body regions.

nm. The shorter wavelengths 280 to 315 nm is known as UVB while the longer wavelength 315 to 400 nm is called UVA. We need not go into more detail at this time as we shall be studying the effects of ultraviolet light when we deal with aging mechanisms. We know that hormones are necessary for tanning. Eunuchs do not tan well. Melanocyte stimulating hormone (MSH) will stimulate pigmentation. MSH is a polypeptide hormone secreted by the anterior pituitary gland. There are two types, alpha-MSH and beta-MSH. These two polypeptides differ in the number of amino acids that they contain. Twenty four hours after injection of MSH the skin will become significantly darker. Another substance called melatonin (5-methoxy-N-acetyl-tryptamine) also causes melanogenesis. It is both confusing and difficult to understand melanogenesis since there are many unknown factors.

What is important to know is that there are multiple ways of influencing pigmentation: increasing the melanocyte number, changing the properties of the melanosomes, or changing their distribution. We shall return to melanocytes when we study disorders of pigmentation.

### The Langerhans Cell, the Macrophages, and the Lymphocytes - An Introduction to Immunology

In the following sections you will be introduced to some new concepts and some concepts with which you may already be familiar. Here, I shall serve as your guide to what are the most important concepts needed for an understanding of the fundamentals of immunology. At first the topic will appear rather complex and the concepts obtuse. Not to worry, for as you read, it will all fit together in a meaningful whole, for like the jigsaw puzzle each piece means little without its proper place in the big picture.

## What is Immunology?

Immunology is the study of the components and functioning of the immune system. The key words are immune system, for this is a system similar to the nervous system or the blood system. The primary function of the immune system is protection. The body must be protected from bacteria, viruses, and from itself. I like Friedmann's analogy of the body as an island surrounded by invading armies (**see references**). In this case the stratum corneum of the skin serves as the first line of defense. If the invaders break through they are met by the sentinels of the skin, the Langerhans cells, which recognize them as invaders and alert the inner defenders - the immune system. Defense and Recognition are the key words. So the function of the immune system is to recognize the enemy and to destroy or neutralize it. (The military speaks of "search and destroy missions" - the same process is happening with the immune system.) A serious problem arises when "friend" is not recognized and is then destroyed. More of this later.

## The Major Components of the Immune System

The four components of the cellular immune system related to the skin are Langerhans cells, macrophages, B lymphocytes, and T lymphocytes. A fifth cell, the mast cell, must also be considered but it does not always function as an immune cell. Now, we must put these together to form the system. We start with the Langerhans cell, but keep in mind this cell is part of a system.

Unlike many cells the **Langerhans cell** (LC) can not be seen easily by ordinary light microscopy. It can be stained with a special histological stain that requires the identification of the ATPase enzyme. This special ATPase is bound to the membrane of the LC and is resistant to formalin. It is a sulfhydryl-dependent ATPase. There are other methods of staining and identifying LC. The LC is a dendritic cell because it is characterized by dendrites, which are cellular projections, see **Figure 4-17**. The LC

occurs mainly in the mid-epidermis and when stained appears as a spider-like cell. Within the cell are mitochondria, lysosomes, microtubules, microfilaments (for cell motility), and a specific organelle called the Birbeck granule (a rod shaped particle with a striated center and a bulged end, much like a tennis racket). See **Figure 4-17**.

Langerhans cells are derived from and continuously repopulated by a mobile pool of precursor cells derived from the bone marrow and thus are of mesenchymal origin. They are motile cells moving in and out of the epidermis within a few hours after stimulation. Here is another key word, stimulation. The LC is stimulated by an antigen, which is any foreign material capable of producing an immune response. The LC activates the other immune cells including the T Lymphocytes to continue the immune system reaction. To repeat this, the LC is stimulated by the antigen and then activates the T-Lymphocytes and other immune cells. These immune cells, the macrophage and the lymphocytes are the next step in the immune system. (You must understand that the last word in immunology has not been written so even as I write this new discoveries are being made.)

The term **macrophage** means "big eater". It refers to a type of cell that shares certain morphological and cytochemical characteristics. It also has common functional properties such as adhering to glass surfaces and immune phagocytosis. They are usually 20 to 40 microns in size. The group of mononuclear macrophages includes monocytes (in the bone marrow and blood stream), free macrophages (in the spleen and lymph nodes), and fixed macrophages (in the connective tissue, lungs, and other tissues). I have always had a certain affinity for macrophages as they were the very first cells that I studied in tissue culture many years ago. Reluctantly, I must leave them now to go onto other cells. Remember that the macrophage has many functions.

**Lymphocytes** (9 to 15 microns in size) are smaller than macrophages, have a large nucleus and little cytoplasm. There are two major types.

The T lymphocyte is capable of recognizing antigen with a high degree of specificity and thus plays a key role in the immune system. It regulates to a large extent the nature and intensity of the immune response. I have listed the

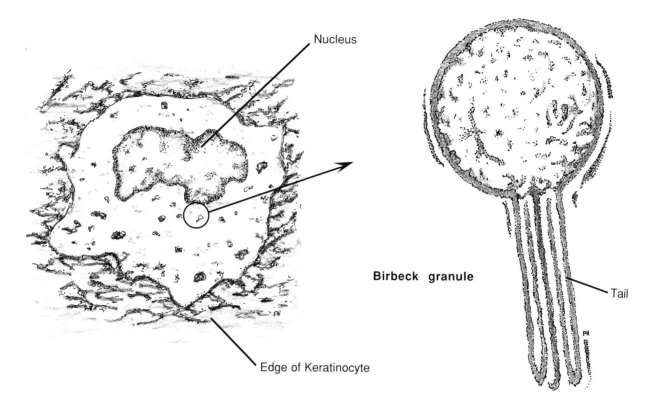

Nucleus

Birbeck granule

Tail

Edge of Keratinocyte

**FIGURE 4-17** Langerhan's cell with Birbeck granule. These are dendritic cells. Note the projections. The Birbeck granule (right) is the visible identity mark of a Langerhans cell. The Birbeck granule on the right is highly magnified.

many functions of the T lymphocyte in (see **Table 4-2**), but the major functions are regulation of B cell antibody production, regulation of T cell growth and differentiation, "killer cell" function, delayed hypersensitivity, cytotoxic reactions, and promotion of nonlymphoid cellular differentiation. You should be aware of the many functions of this cell but you need not commit all these items to memory.

The B lymphocyte is the antibody producing cell. In response to the T lymphocyte it will produce specific antibodies. You may be familiar with the concept of antibodies from your knowledge of gamma globulin. The major antibodies in the blood plasma are IgA, IgM, and IgG. Each of these antibodies has a specific function and arises in response to a specific antigen. When you received immunization as a child you were receiving antigen to promote your immune system to produce antibodies. The complex nature of this system is summarized in **Figure 4-18**.

The **mast cell** is another component of the immune system. They are also derived from the mesenchymal system and appears as two types, mucosal mast cells in the lung and gut, and con-

nective tissue mast cells such as we have in the dermis of the skin. The mast cell responds to a number of stimuli other than immune stimuli. When mast cells are stimulated they release granules that subsequently release their contents to initiate a cascade of reactions. Histamine is one of the major compounds released by the mast cell and accounts for a pronounced inflammatory reaction.

Finally we need to mention the humoral substances associated with the immune system as you will come across these terms frequently:

Lymphokines are regulators of cell-mediated immunity. They are derived from T cells and macrophages. Interleukin I (IL-1) is produced by stimulated macrophages and has many functions. Epidermal thymocyte-activating factor (ETAF) is derived from the keratinocytes, usually damaged cells, and has a similar action to IL-1. Interleukin 2 (IL-2) is a more limited lymphokine. It stimulates growth of activated T cells.

Interferons (IF) are proteins that inhibit viral growth and cell growth. There are three types alpha, beta, and gamma. IF-alpha is anti-viral and can be produced by both T cells and B cells as well as by macrophages. IF-beta is also called fibroblast IF since both fibroblasts and macrophages can produce this IF, which is similar to the IF-alpha. The third type is called IF-gamma, or T-interferon which is distinct from the other two forms. It is produced by lymphocytes in response to antigens or mitogens. The mitogens are substances that cause mitosis and thus cellular proliferation. Currently a large amount of cancer research involves the interferons.

We still have a long way to go to get a handle on the immune system but we have covered much of the basics. We shall go over this again

## T-LYMPHOCYTE FUNCTION

| FUNCTION | PRODUCT |
|---|---|
| T cells | |
| I. Regulation of B- cell antibody production | |
|   A. Helps in its induction | Helper factors and B-cell stimulating factors, (B-cell growth factor, B-cell differentiation factor(s), and T-cell replacing factor(s)) |
|   B. Suppression and its induction | Soluble suppressor factors |
| II. Regulation of T-cell growth and differentiation | Interleukin-2, lymphocyte mitogenic factors, interferons |
| III. Delayed-type hypersensitivity | Lymphokines (migration inhibiton factors, macrophage chemotactic factor, transfer factor) |
| IV. Cytotoxicity | |
|   A. Antigen-specific cytotoxic T cells | |
|   B. Natural killing and antibody- dependent cellular cytotoxicity (activated T cells only) | |
| V. Promotion of nonlymphoid cellular differentiation | Colony-stimulating factors, osteoclast activation factor, factors inducing fibroblast proliferation and collagen synthesis |

**TABLE 4-2** Adapted with permission of McGraw-Hill, Inc. from Dermatology in General Medicine, 3/e, Fitzpatrick et. al., 1987.

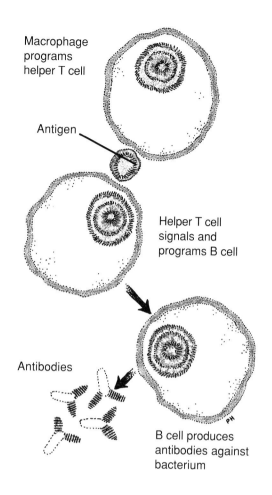

**FIGURE 4-18** Antibody production. Macrophage programs helper T cell. Helper T cell signals and programs B cell. B cell produces antibodies against bacterium.

as we study the processes of diseases in the next chapter, and later when we look at specific treatments. Study the drawings and diagrams as I have tried to simplify these concepts into digestible doses. Particularly look at **Figure 4-19** where I have diagrammed an immunoglobulin. You will come across these terms as you expand your reading so this will serve as an introduction.

### The Fibroblast - A Key to the Future

What a wonder is the fibroblast! It is one of the earliest embryonic cells to differentiate and have an important role in the formation of the skeletal system, the location of muscle cells, the distribution of nerve fibers and the organization

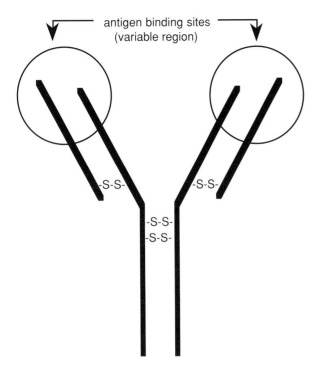

antigen binding sites
(variable region)

-S-S-          -S-S-

-S-S-
-S-S-

**FIGURE 4-19** Immunoglobulin. The shaded areas are the variable areas on the molecule. Note two short "chains" and two long "chains". There are certain diseases of the immune system cells that are characterized by abnormal production of these short and long chains.

gen, which are listed in **Table 4-3**. All collagens are composed of a basic polypeptide chain called the A chain. Three of these A chains unite to form a single collagen molecule called a triple helix, which is composed of repeating triplet amino acids, glycine and two others, most often proline and hydroxyproline. Glycine is always present; every third molecule is glycine. So we have then a three amino acid unit occurring in triplet and twisted into a left handed spiral called a helix, See **Figure 4-20**. At the ends of this helical unit is a nontriple-helical domain called the globular domain. One A chain is in a left helix but when they unite to form a collagen molecule they form a right-handed super helical spiral, this is procollagen. This is the easy part, now for the synthesis.

Collagen is synthesized in the ribosomes of the cell cytoplasm as procollagen but then must be modified by enzymes in the rough endoplasmic reticulum. This is called the post-translational modification stages. It sounds complex, and it is, but it represents one of the major biochemical discoveries of our century. You need to know about collagen synthesis as a skin care specialist. It is so very important in the struc-

of the skin. It is no small wonder that the fibroblast continues to play such an important part in everyday body functions. Yet, with all this importance, fibroblasts do not function as independent cells, they are directed or modulated by specific signals from many cells including T lymphocytes, neutrophils, macrophages, and platelets.

As we learned in skin anatomy the dermis consists of groups of fibrillar proteins which include collagen, elastin, and reticulum meshed in an amorphous ground substance. This amorphous ground substance consists of proteoglycans, glycoproteins, and minor components. These proteins are synthesized by the fibroblast. Let us start with collagen, the major dermal component.

### The Collagen Molecule

Collagen is the most abundant body protein accounting for about one-third of the body weight. Collagen functions to give the body structure and cohesion. So far protein chemists have identified eleven different types of colla-

**CLASSIFICATION OF THE COLLAGENS**

| COMMON NAME | FUNCTION |
|---|---|
| Type I | Structure, skin, bone, organs |
| Type II | Structure, cartilage |
| Type III | Structure, skin, organs |
| Type V | Cytoskeleton |
| Type XI (K or 1α, 2α, 3α) | Chondrocyte cytoskeleton |
| Type IV | Structure, basement membrane |
| Type VI | Myofibril formation |
| Type VII | Anchoring fibril |
| Type VIII | Endothelial cell product function unknown |
| Type IX | Unknown |
| Type X | Structure, hypertrophic cartilage |

**TABLE 4-3** You do not need to remember all the various types. The most common types are I and III. Remember not all collagen is the same. Adapted with permission from Inflammation - Basic Principles & Clinical Correlates, John Gallin, Ira Goldstein and Ralph Snyderman, 1988, pg. 578.

ture of the skin, in aging changes and in maintenance of skin health. There are many steps but we will cover only the essential ones.

The terminal ends of the procollagen molecule are cleaved shortly after translation. Now the hydroxylation process occurs. Hydroxyproline and hydroxylysine are formed by the action of two enzymes, proline hydroxylase and lysine hydroxylase. These enzymes are very finicky and require specific amounts of oxygen, iron molecules, a-ketoglutarate, and ascorbic acid. (Ascorbic acid as you know is vitamin C; it is the lack of this vitamin that caused sailors to develop scurvy at sea.) After the addition of the hydroxyproline and hydroxylysine the next step is glycosylation or the addition of a carbohydrate molecule to the procollagen molecule. Glycosylation begins with the addition of a galactosyl molecule. It is attached first to the collagen polypeptides and then glucose is attached to the galactosyl residue. At the same time the peptide extensions, one at each end of the molecule, receive complex carbohydrate structures consisting mainly of mannose. It is at this stage that the molecule is ready to form the triple helix configuration. The first step is the removal of the nonhelical chains, followed by disulfide bonding which is facilitated by the extension polypeptides that contain sulfur atoms. The enzyme that is responsible for this action is called protein disulfide isomerase. Now the triple helix forms and the molecule is secreted into the intercellular space.

Once in the intercellular space the terminal ends of the molecule are removed by other enzymes and the new collagen molecules will spontaneously assemble and form collagen fibrils. All collagen behaves in this manner but there are specific differences between collagen molecules that account for their functionality. You need not know the chemical differences but you must be aware of the functional differences of the five most common types.

Type I - a structural collagen found in bones, skin, tendons, and other organs. It is the most common type. It is a fibrillar collagen with two identical chains and one different chain.

Type II - a structural collagen found in cartilage and the vitreous humor of the eye. It has three identical chains.

Type III - a "young collagen" occurring mainly in fetal tissues, but accounting for about 10 to 20% of the collagen in the adult dermis. It is made of three identical chains with a high content of hydroxyproline and glycine. It also contains cystine.

Type IV - seen mainly in the basement membranes of the skin. It is different from the other collagens in that it has a molecule with alternating collagenous and noncollagenous domains.

Type V - a ubiquitous collagen found in almost every connective tissue. It represents about 10% of the total collagen but its function is unknown.

Elastin - The Spring of Life

Without elastin life would be very dull. While it makes up only 1-2% of the skin by dry weight it has a very important function in that it provides resiliency to the skin. The dermis in the back of the neck contains 75% elastin which allows us to "rubber neck". (It is a good thing that there is very little elastin in the nose.) Early

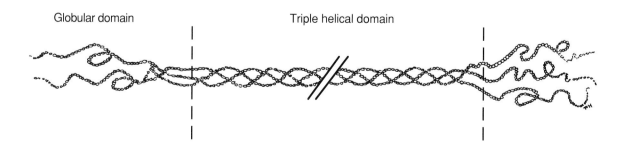

Globular domain          Triple helical domain

**FIGURE 4-20** Procollagen. Collagen product is started in the fibroblast cell and then assembled outside the fibroblast. The two ends of the procollagen are cut off in the final assembly.

research workers had a difficult time with the analysis of elastin since it is so insoluble. Modern technology and persistency have paid off so that now we have a fairly complete picture of elastin.

The basic molecule of elastin is a linear polypeptide of 800 or so amino acids: Chiefly glycine, valine, proline, lysine and alanine with no apparent histidine or methionine. Two key amino acids in elastin are desmosine and isodesmosine. They are involved in the cross linking system that covalently bonds the elastin polypeptide chains into a fibrous network. This unique linkage is formed from four lysine molecules on the peptide chains that come together to form the desmosine molecule. See **Figure 4-21**.

The biosynthesis of elastin is similar to collagen in that only part of the elastin fiber is made within the cellular cytoplasm. After the basic polypeptide is synthesized in the ribosome, post-translational changes occur in the rough endoplasmic reticulum. The molecule next passes to the extracellular space through the Golgi apparatus where the lysyl groups are oxidized in preparation for cross-linkage. One of the key enzymes in this reaction is lysyl oxidase which requires copper and oxygen. In the intercellular space, the elastin molecule is next coupled with a microfibrillar protein which surrounds it. At this stage the whole molecule is brought together by the formation of desmosine and covalent cross-linking.

It is very important for the reader to keep in mind that both collagen and elastin are constantly being produced, destroyed and produced again in response to body needs. It is this feature that allows a great deal of variability in structure and the hope of repair and restructuring of the skin in aging and disease. We shall return to both collagen and elastin when we discuss specific skin disorders.

## THE GROUND SUBSTANCE - BIG WORD - GLYCOSOAMINOGLY-CANS

I believe that a great deal of new knowledge will arrive in the next ten years that will dispel some of the mysteries of the ground substance. We speak of the ground substance as the extracellular material of the dermis. For many

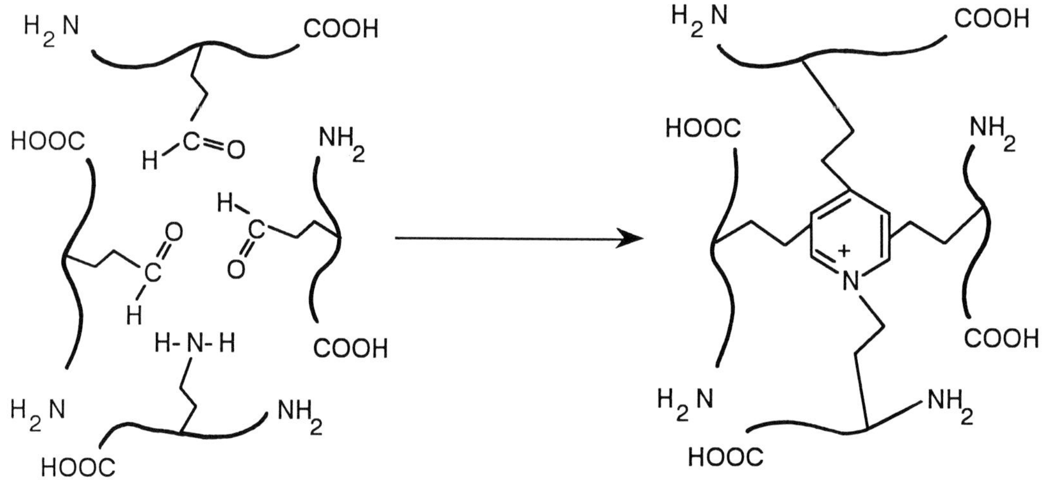

Desmosine

FIGURE 4-21 Desmosine structure. Elastin remains a mystery protein. The concept of a "springy" molecule is terrific but difficult to understand. Desmosine is an amino acid found only in elastin.

years this amorphous material was consider only as "packing" (something to fill up space in the skin). This is not surprising since the brain was at one time thought to be only a sponge used to cool the blood! (In some cases this is not too far off.) We have come a long way to understanding the composition and function of the ground substance.

## The Glycosaminoglycans And Proteoglycans

These compounds are all related by a common structure. The backbone of the group is the glycosaminoglycan moiety. This is a macromolecule consisting of repeating units of disaccharides (two sugar units) which contain either glucosamine or galactosamine alternating with either glucuronic or iduronic acid. The term hexosamine is used to describe any six carbon sugar with an amine group on it. These large molecules are called polysaccharides, being made from as many as several thousand disaccharide units. They can also be small with only a few disaccaride units. So the term glycosaminoglycan is nothing more than a series of amino sugars linked in a long chain. Add to this chain a protein part and you have a proteoglycan. If you dry down the dermis and measure the amount of these glycosaminoglycans you will find only 0.1 to 0.3%. We need to be concerned only with a few of these big molecules. They are as follows:

**Hyaluronic acid** - a superb lubricant for joints. It is a big molecule (some molecules being 5 million molecular weight). Its major components are N-acetylglucosamine and glucuronic acid. Hyaluronic acid is not a proteoglycan since it contains no protein. Hyaluronic acid has a great ability to hold water. It is highly charged being anionic and thus can form gels of various viscosities. Like other macromolecules it is degraded by a specific enzyme, hyaluronidase.

**Dermatan sulfate** (chondroitin sulfate B) - the next most common glycosaminoglycan. It contains proteins along with sulfate groups linked to the sugar molecules. This molecule is formed of alternating residues of glucuronate and N-acetyl-D-galactosamine. The sulfate groups are attached to the galactosamine residues after the protein-chondroitin molecules are synthesized. Little is known about these compounds even today. They are synthesized by many different cells and have diverse functions.

**Heparin** - a proteoglycan that occurs in the mast cells, liver, and lungs. We know heparin mainly as an anitcoagulant in medicine but that is probably not its major physiological function. Being highly anionic in character it has a strong affinity for cations and thus the histamine and serotonin of the mast cells are bound to the heparin molecule. Perhaps heparin acts as a control for the release of these two amines. Incidently heparin comes from the Greek word hepar (liver).

We have now completed our basic review of the physiology and biochemistry of the skin. We still have some areas to discuss, but we will cover them in the chapters dealing with specific disorders and methods of treatment. One of these topics will be thermoregulation and the mechanism of sweating.

Once these bad actors get the run of the place, the scene can get awfully, well, inflammatory. Their terrorist activity can leave a wake of destruction--and even a Wall as tough as this one can't always snap back. We're going to show you how to recognize the major chinks in the armour, tell you what can and can't be repaired, and when to call in the allies.

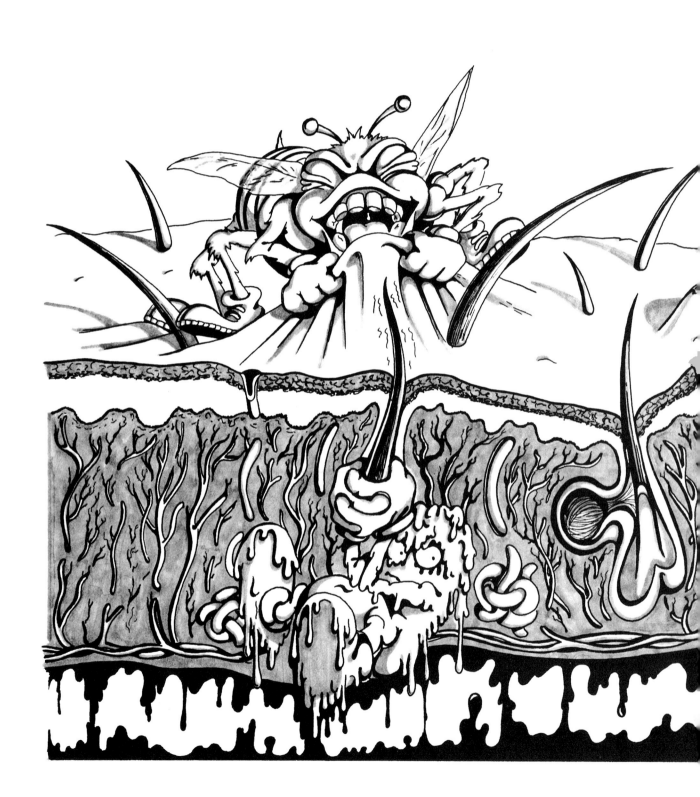

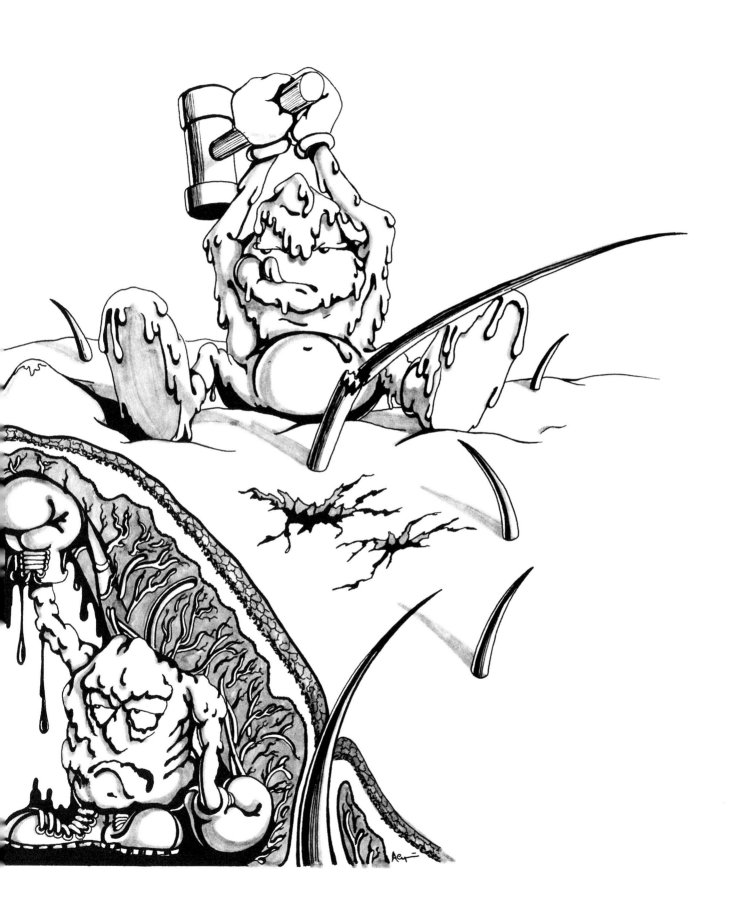

# Introduction to Pathology and the Mechanisms of Disorder

Having studied the skin's normal anatomy, biochemistry, and physiology, the reader is prepared to study disorders of the skin. As the skin responds to the environment (the wear and tear of daily use), assault by infectious agents, and abuse by its owner, changes will occur. Skin care specialists must be prepared to deal with these changes. These changes are the subject matter of pathology (*patho* = disease), the science that deals with the structural and functional changes in tissues and organs that cause or are caused by disease states. Again, we shall concentrate on the concepts of diseases or disorders to arrive at the general principle underlying their mechanisms. For instance, we will start with inflammation as a disease process. You will see that whether it is caused by a bacterial infection, a viral infection, or an auto-immune disease, there are certain common features. At the start I would like to emphasize that we are going to cover those disorders that I feel are the primary concern of the non-physician skin care specialist.

While we shall cover some malignant disorders, they are included only for the purpose of identifying them so that they may be referred to a physician for treatment. After we complete this chapter we will be ready to put this new knowledge together to develop a systematic approach to diagnosing abnormal skin conditions.

There are several systems of classifying disorders of the skin. They may be broadly divided into disorders of the epidermis or the dermis. They may also be divided into immunological, inflammatory, proliferative, or neoplastic. They may be further divided into physical, biochemical, biologic, genetic, metabolic, nutritional, developmental, degenerative, or psychological disorders. For our purpose we shall use a more limited classification, disorders of importance to the skin care specialist.

## INFLAMMATION - THE CORNERSTONE OF DISEASE STATES

The student of skin pathology must first learn that while the skin is composed of epidermis, dermis, and subcutaneous tissue components, these components generally react together rather than separately when challenged by a disease. So it is with inflammation. The best definition of inflammation that I have read comes from the book <u>Inflammation, Basic Principles and</u>

Clinical Correlates, edited by Gallin, Goldstein and Snyderman. "**Inflammation** is a localized protective response by injury or destruction of tissues, which serves to destroy, dilute, or wall-off both the injurious agent and the injured tissue." The classical signs of acute inflammation are redness (**rubor**), swelling (**turgor**), heat (**calor**), and pain (**dolor**). The red, hot, swollen, painful boil is an example. When we examine the tissues in the inflamed area with a microscope, we find dilated arterioles, capillaries, and venules associated with increased permeability (leakiness) and increased blood flow. There is **exudate** or a pouring out of fluid and white blood cells. The white blood cells or leukocytes are key players in the inflammatory response.

The **leukocytes** are made up of five types of cells: **neutrophils**, **basophils**, **eosinophils**, **lymphocytes**, and **monocytes** (macrophages). Together with the exudate of plasma proteins, these cells form yellow **pus**. The first defense of the body involves the leukocytes. Most infections, however, recruit both humoral (**B cell**) and cellular (**T cell**) components of the immune system regardless of the cause of the inflammation. We shall look into this in detail. In this discussion you will meet some new terms. As you continue reading these terms will become "friendlies".

(As an aside, my wife, Joanne, classifies all the noises she hears while driving the car as "friendly" or "unfriendly". While not too scientific, somehow she has managed not to have a mechanical disaster.)

Three stages of cutaneous inflammation can be identified whether the inflammatory process is acute or chronic. **Acute** and **chronic** are terms that refer to time. We may substitute short for acute and long for chronic. There is no absolute time span defined for either of these terms, so additional terms are used: **subacute** (between acute and chronic) and **subchronic** (between subacute and chronic). For example, something that comes on quickly such as a pimple has an acute onset. If it lasts for a week or more it is subacute. If it lasts for a month it is subchronic. If it lasts for months it is described as chronic. Arthritis pain is an example of chronic pain, however, the person may have acute flare-ups that last for a few days. These terms refer both to the time of onset of the inflammation and how long it lasts. Now, back to the stages of inflam-

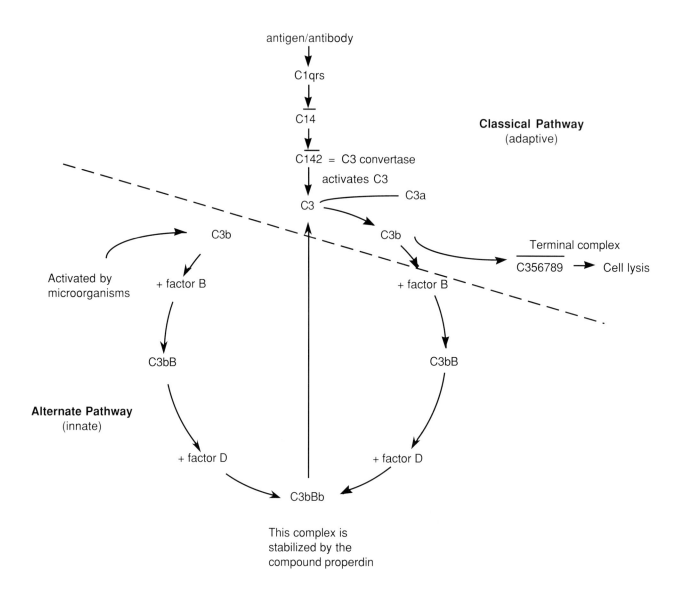

antigen/antibody

C1qrs

C14

C142 = C3 convertase

activates C3

C3

C3a

**Classical Pathway**
(adaptive)

C3b

C3b

Terminal complex

C356789 → Cell lysis

Activated by
microorganisms

+ factor B

+ factor B

C3bB

C3bB

**Alternate Pathway**
(innate)

+ factor D

+ factor D

C3bBb

This complex is
stabilized by the
compound properdin

**FIGURE 5-1** Alternate and classical complement pathways. The complement system is a group of circulating proteins that provide defense against microorganisms and other antigens. The system is activated by a complex series of protein and enzyme reactions. Both systems end up making C3b which forms the complex that lyses cells.

mation.

The first stage of injury to the skin is a transitory decrease followed by increase in the size of the blood vessels (**vasodilation**). This phenomenon accounts for the redness of the skin. As the vessels dilate the blood flow increases for a few seconds to a few hours and then slowly decreases. During this stage the leukocytes have moved from the blood to the inner lining of the blood vessel (**endothelium**). Once there they become adherent (or stick). The second stage also includes the escape of fluid from the blood vessels, and the passage of the leukocytes into

the tissues from the vessels. This occurs when the endothelial cells of the small veins (**venules**) contract leaving gaps between the cells, allowing both plasma and leukocytes to pass. Only the venules do this. Arterioles and capillaries do not exhibit the endothelial contraction. The three leukocytes (neutrophils, basophils, and eosinophils) migrate to the scene of the disorder and are the first to start the body's defense.

During the third stage the cells are doing their thing, eating (**phagocytosis**) and destroying the invaders, and the plasma becomes filled with potent humor factors that also enter into the inflammatory process. Let's look at these agents.

## THE COMPLEMENT SYSTEM

Many years ago as a medical student I thought that this was a very complicated system. Today it is even more complicated as there are many more pieces. Like all puzzles, however, you can put it together with patience and diligence. The complement system consists of a series of proteins that become active in steps, one following after the other, called sequential steps. A number of new substances are generated which influence the response to inflammation. Just to let that sink in, a series of proteins undergo change in the presence of the inflammatory process and result in additional active substances being produced. Inflammation initiates this process, otherwise the complement system is inactive. There are two pathways that activation of the complement system can follow, the classical pathway and the alternate pathway.

The **classical complement pathway** is activated by antibody-antigen complexes and by target cells that are sensitized with immunoglobulins such as IgG and IgM. There are three units: C1 (**the recognition unit**), C4, C2, C3 (**the activation unit**), and C5 thru C9 (**the membrane attack unit**). The membrane attack unit is the one which will rupture red blood cells that have been sensitized.

The **alternate complement pathway** can be activated by polysaccharides which include endotoxins and zymosan which are the components of bacterial cell walls. Other cells may activate the alternate system such as leukocytes or red blood cells. There are three factors in the alternate pathway to learn: **Factor B**, **Factor D**, and **properdin**. The effect of the alternate pathway is the same as the classical pathway, that is, an effect on C3 to form C3b. In **Figure 5-1** I have diagrammed the two systems and their various components.

The key concept to learn is that the complement system is a complex of proteins which mediates important biological reactions which include cytotoxicity of antibody-sensitized cells, viruses, and bacteria. In addition, the complement system mediates the humoral portion of inflammation and stimulates phagocytes and lymphoid cells. So it plays a key role in the body's defense.

Remember that there are three steps to the complement system function: initiation, activation, and recognition and attack. In the classical pathway you need antibodies such as IgG and IgM to initiate the system. To initiate the alternate system you can have antibodies such as IgG and IgM and bacterial endotoxins, bacteria, fungi and both lymphocytes and red blood cells. We move now to the other systems and factors in inflammation.

**Hageman Factor** is the activating protein in a second system of soluble proteins that are involved in the inflammatory process. Hageman Factor is activated when it binds to a particle or a negatively charged surface such as glass, cell membranes, or endotoxins. When activated, Hageman Factor leads to the formation of **bradykinin** (a potent vasodilator) that both increases cell permeability and degranulates mast cells. It also produces **plasmin**, a substance that degrades fibrin into small peptides. This causes the neutrophils to migrate (**chemotaxis**).

## THE PROSTAGLANDINS AND THE ARACHIDONIC ACID CASCADE

Here again there are new terms to learn, but like new friends they may prove exciting. One of the most interesting aspects of the prostaglandins is that they are one of only four families of natural compounds that exhibit profound biological activity. (The other three are steroid hormones, polypeptides, and biologic amines.)

**Prostaglandins** were named after the prostate gland (*prostatus* = one who stands before), a gland located in front of the bladder in males. The prostaglandins were first found in the fluid from the prostate gland. Remember, when we speak of prostaglandins we are speaking about a family of biological products.

The origin of the prostaglandins is in the lipid of the cell membrane, particularly with a polyunsaturated fatty acid called **arachidonic acid** (Gr. *arachis* = peanut). This is a fatty acid with twenty (20) carbon atoms and four double bonds. Its shape is shown in **Figure 5-2**. In the presence of oxygen, under certain circumstances, arachidonic acid will start a cascade of reactions that will form many products, including the prostaglandins. This reaction is often referred to as the arachidonic acid cascade. I have listed all of the steps, however, for our purpose we need to learn only the following steps.

Step one is the action of **Phospholipase A$_2$** on the cell membrane to free arachidonic acid.

Step two is the action of **cyclooxygenase** on arachidonic acid to form **endoperoxides**. These are the precursors of prostaglandins.

Step three is the formation of the following prostaglandins which are designated by the initials PG followed by a letter and number:

**PGF$_2$** causes vasoconstriction and muscle contraction, as in labor and menstrual pain.

**PGD$_2$**, **PGE$_2$**, and **PGI$_2$** dilate most vascular beds and increase pain.

The prostaglandins also mediate or modify the release of other cellular substances which are involved in inflammation. They are related to both the immediate and the delayed immunological reactions. **Cortisone** and other anti-inflammatory drugs can in turn block the action of the prostaglandins. The term **NSAID** (non-steroidal anti-inflammatory drug) refers to drugs such as **aspirin** and **ibuprofen**.

Now look at **Figure 5-3** to see another pathway that is quite active in inflammation. When arachidonic acid is formed it may be acted upon either by the enzyme that forms the prostaglandins or it can be acted upon by another enzyme called **lipoxygenase** to form a new pathway. This is known as the lipoxygenase pathway which results in potent agents of inflammation including the following products called **leukotrienes**. The important leukotrienes are:

**LTB$_4$** appears to promote leukocyte recruitment (accumulation) to the injured site.

**LTC$_4$**, **LTD$_4$**, and **LTE$_4$** have edema promoting activities and increase vascular permeability. They are also known as **SRS-A** leukotrienes (slow reacting substance for anaphylaxis).

Anaphylaxis (Gr. *an* = excessive + *phylaxis* = protection) is an unusual or exaggerated response of the body to a foreign substance. This

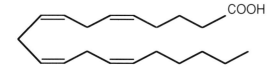

**FIGURE 5-2** Arachidonic acid structure. This is the basic structure. Notice the four double bonds in the molecule which allow versatile chemical changes.

reaction is so severe that it can cause death in a matter of minutes from respiratory failure.

Now you have been introduced to many new terms which like the trees in a forest can obscure the whole, or big picture (a commonly used military term which most of us never understood). Let's put this all together in a diagram that will allow you to see it all at once and help you to put the these pieces together. Without a fairly clear understanding of the inflammatory process you will have even more difficulty in understanding other pathological reactions of the skin. Look at the diagram in **Figure 5-4** and follow the steps. These terms will occur again and again as we study the pathology of the skin.

## DISORDERS OF THE SKIN ASSOCIATED WITH INFLAMMATION

We shall now look at specific disorders of the skin which are related to the mechanisms of inflammation. The most common are seborrheic dermatitis, eczema, bacterial and viral infections, fungal infections, contact dermatitis, and acne.

### Seborrheic Dermatitis

The cause of this common skin disorder is unknown. It is more common than psoriasis. It affects between 2 and 5% of the population with males being slightly more afflicted than females. It can occur at any age but it is seen most frequently in the first three months of life and again at ages 40 through 70 years. It is believed that the active large sebaceous glands of the newborn may be a major factor in the early affliction.

APPEARANCE - The skin appears oily, pink, edematous, with yellow to brown crusts on the face, around the ears, on the upper trunk, and in the hair. It is frequently confused with eczema and psoriasis.

PATHOLOGICAL FINDINGS - **Staphylococcus aureus** and **Corynebacterium acne**, and yeasts, including **Candida albicans** and **Pityrosporum orbiculare** have been found to be associated with this disorder. Many other causes have been proposed by investigators including emotional stress, physical stress, zinc deficiency, and certain diseases of the nervous system. It is well known that cold weather and

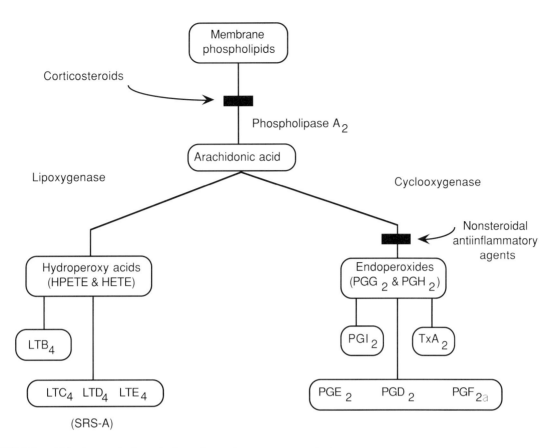

**FIGURE 5-3** Arachidonic metabolism. In the cell membrane the phospholipase A2 (an enzyme) acts to produce arachidonic acid. The two pathways that arachidonic acid may follow are complex processes related to the inflammatory process. The black boxes indicate where the reaction can be blocked by antiinflammatory agents.

low humidity in over heated motel rooms tends to exacerbate the condition.

### Eczema

The word eczema is from the Greek word *ekzein* meaning to boil out. I think that this is an apt description of a disease which is quite confusing to all who come in contact with it. It is a true inflammatory disorder, responding to both internal and external factors. This disorder is more accurately called **eczematous dermatitis** to distinquish it from other types of dermatitis. It is a very common condition, occuring in about one-third (33%) of the patients visiting the office of a dermatologist.

APPEARANCE - Eczematous dermatitis, in the acute form, is characterized by areas of erythema, edema, and tiny clusters of vesicles (blisters) which may ooze serum and form crusts. The chronic form is associated with minimal erythema, however, there is **lichenification** (a thickening of the epidermis with deep markings). The chronic form can be confused with psoria-

sis.

PATHOLOGICAL FINDINGS - The causes of eczematous dermatitis are many. We need to look at a few to get an idea of the variable forms of this disorder. **Allergic contact eczematous dermatitis** is caused by chemicals from plants, fabrics, metals, cosmetics, and medications. **Photoallergic contact eczematous dermatitis** is caused by a combination of ultraviolet light and a causative chemical. **Polymorphous light-induced eruption eczematous type** is caused only by exposure to ultraviolet light without the presence of a chemical. Another more common type is **infectious eczematous dermatitis** which is seen with open draining wounds. This type clears when the wound, the primary cause, is treated. There are many other types, too numerous to mention, of importance to the dermatologist.

### Bacterial Infections

From the start, I must state that the skin specialist must be able to distinquish a minor bacterial infection of the skin from a serious infection. In many cases this may be a question of the area involved, the stage of infection, and the causative organism. In any case, **if you have the slightest doubt as to the nature of a skin infection**, **refer the client to a physician**. This must be your unfailing rule. In this section I shall provide a brief review of the essential bacteriology of the skin. Most readers will recall their basic courses in bacteriology and be able to remember many of the definitions and terms. If you have not had a basic course in bacteriology, you will need to review a more basic text before going on to this section. First, a few general remarks about skin and bacteria.

The skin is normally very resistant to a wide variety of bacteria. If the skin is intact, infection is difficult to produce. The bacteria are unable to penetrate the skin. The skin pH (5.5) does not appear to be an important factor since the bacteria can grow at pH values well below 5.5 . I believe that high pH values above 8.5 or 9.0 may have an effect on the normal resistance or produce breaks in the lipid barrier. I believe, as do many other skin physiologists, that the most important element is the state of moisture on and in the skin. Most infections occur in the moist areas of the groin, between the toes, under the breasts, around the mouth, and in the nasal folds. A dry intact skin is difficult to infect.

**Stage 1.  Vascular Phase**

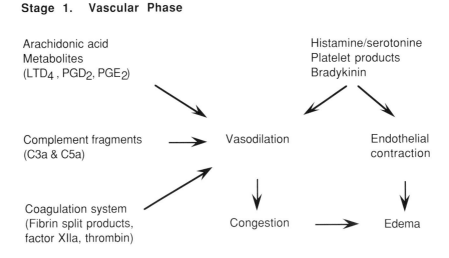

Arachidonic acid
Metabolites
(LTD$_4$ , PGD$_2$, PGE$_2$)

Histamine/serotonine
Platelet products
Bradykinin

Complement fragments
(C3a & C5a)

Vasodilation

Endothelial
contraction

Coagulation system
(Fibrin split products,
factor XIIa, thrombin)

Congestion

Edema

**Stage 2.  Cellular Phase**

a. Leukocyte migration
b. Inflammatory infiltrate

Cellular chemotaxis

- Prostaglandins
- Leukotrienes
- Fibrin
- Collagen
- Transfer factor
- Neutrophil chemotatic factor
- Platelet activating factor

c. Resolution
d. Organization

**FIGURE 5-4** Stage I and II of the inflammatory process. View inflammation as a two stage process. The Stage I is the initial contact of the offending agent with the body defenses. The net result is a vascular response resulting in redness and heat on the skin. Stage II is the cellular stage which is characterized by movement and action of white cells and macrophages. This stage results in healing of the inflammatory process after the offending agent is removed or neutralized.

## Common Bacteria of the Skin

Now let us look at some of the most common bacteria that we shall encounter on the skin. You will recall from basic biology that you classified bacteria as **Gram positive** and **Gram negative** based on their staining characteristic with **Gram's Stain** (Hans Christian Gram was a Danish physician who lived between 1853 and 1938. He was interested in bacteriology and developed the staining technique that bears his name.) The details of the Gram stain are readily available. Bacteria will turn either red or blue with this stain.

We further divide the bacteria into two groups, **cocci** or **bacilli**. The cocci are round bacteria that occur in clusters such as Staphylococcus (S.) (Gr *Staphyle* = a bunch of grapes), as chains or pearl strings such as Streptococcus (Gr *Streptos* = twisted). Bacilli are rod shaped bacteria. We shall limit our discussion to Gram positive and Gram negative bacteria on the normal skin. Normal skin contains **Propionibacterium acnes**, **Aerobic diptheroids** (**the Corynebacterium group**), **Staphylococcus epidermis**, and **Micrococcus** (anaerobic staphylococci). Gram negative bacilli generally make up a small part of the resident flora of the skin, except in certain areas. In moist areas one may find **Escherichia coli** (**E. coli**), **Proteus**, **Enterobacter**, and **Pseudomonas**.

## Pathogenicity of Bacteria

Bacterial infection of the skin is determined largely by the ability of the bacteria to invade the skin and the relative toxicity of the bacteria. The capacity of a bacteria to resist or avoid the body's defenses (phagocytosis and immunological response) conveys a virulent aspect to it. Certain toxins released by the bacteria contribute to its ability to produce local lesions. **Bacillus anthracis and Corynebacterium diptheriae** are two bacteria with this ability. The mechanism of invasiveness of many organisms remains a mystery. Ultimately the interaction of the bacteria and the host is the basis of pathogenicity. You are familiar with **toxic shock syndrome** which is produced by a bacterial **exotoxin** of Staphylococcus aureus. **Exotoxins** are produced by bacteria and are not a part of their structure.

Gram negative bacteria present a different problem. They contain complex **endotoxins** that are a part of the bacterial cell wall. These endotoxins are a complex of both phospholipids and polysaccharides which produce the toxic effect. It appears that the lipid portion is the toxic component which results in many of the manifestations of shock, hemorrhage, and fever. Generally the toxins raise havoc with the tissues, causing destruction by cell death. See **Table 5-1** for the classification of toxins.

**Group A Streptococci** are uncommon on the skin. Typical Group A strep infections are characterized by edema, rapid spread through the tissue planes, and a thin exudate. The clinical course is rapid. The spread of Group A Streptococci is usually from one person to another person. The major source of infection is usually the upper respiratory tract. Thus, many individuals are carriers of this organism. **Staphylococcus aureus** is found widely distributed in the skin and nasal passages. Many individuals are carriers of this organism, too. The virulence of this organism, however, is related to both intrinsic and extrinsic factors. For example, the staphylococci contain toxins and coagulase (enzymes) that account for their high toxicity, but the state of the skin and the overall state of health of the person has a large influence on the nature of the infection. Preexisting wounds, diabetes, treatment with cortisone, a depressed immune system, and a debilitated body all add to the total effect of the staphylococcus infection.

**Impetigo** is a superficial infection of the epidermis characterized by both vesicles and pustules forming just beneath the stratum corneum. The causative agents are usually the Group A Streptococci or Staphylococcus aureus. This is an easy lesion to treat, provided you can keep your clients fingers away from the lesions. I will describe treatments later on.

**Folliculitis** is an infectious condition of the hair follicle. Superficial folliculitis appears as small, round pustules at the hair openings. The causative agent is principally S. aureus, however, sometimes gram-negative organisms may be involved. Deep folliculitis is usually caused by S. aureus and is characterized by redness, swelling, and pus formation.

**Furuncles** are common boils. They appear as deep seated infections around hairs. Since they are deep in the skin, they are confined and

## CHARACTERISTICS OF EXOTOXINS AND ENDOTOXINS

| PROPERTY | ENDOTOXIN (Heat Stable) | EXOTOXIN (Not Heat Stable) |
|---|---|---|
| Origin | From bacterial cell wall | By-product of metabolism of bacteria |
| Chemical composition | Liposaccharides | Protein materials |
| Degree of toxicity | High levels required | Toxic in minute levels |
| Immune response | Weakly immunogenic | Highly immunogenic |
| Typical action of toxins | Fever, weakness, shock | Paralysis - either spastic or flaccid, variation in protein metabolism, cell membrane injury |

As an example, toxic shock syndrome from tampons was produced by a bacterial endotoxin.

**TABLE 5-1** Exotoxins are synthesized by the bacteria while endotoxins are actual parts in the wall of the bacteria.

can produce pain by pressure. They do not occur in areas where there is no hair. The causative agent is S. aureus.

**Carbuncles** are large, deep seated infections which spread from furuncles through the fibrous tissue septae. They are very painful and not easy to treat. S. aureus is the most frequent causative agent.

**Cellulitis** is an acute deep infection of the skin characterized by a redness of the skin with indistinct borders. The causative agent is S. aureus. The infection follows, most often, a puncture wound or ulcer in the skin. This must be distinguished from **erysipelas** (Gr *erythros* = red + *pellas* = skin) which is caused most frequently by Streptococcus pyogenes and has a red swollen appearance with sharp margins. It is a more superficial infection than cellulitis.

**Erythrasma** is a common infection occuring in the intertriginous areas and is characterized by well defined, irregular, brownish-red spots. It is more common in men and occurs more often in warm climates. The causative agent is S. aureus.

Gram Negative Infections

(Infections with Bacilli as causative agents)
**Pseudomonas aeruginosa, "the blue pus organism"**, is a frequent inhabitant of the skin. It is seen in the ear canal, in the spaces between the toes, and in the nails. This organism gains entry into the skin through a breakdown of the tissues. Serious infections can result. In some cases the organism can enter the skin even though it is intact. This is usually under moist conditions such as in hot tubs and swimming pools. In nursing homes, where debilitated patients are confined to bed for long periods of time, serious infections can occur. Once in the skin the organism can invade the blood stream and produce **septicemia**. Septicemia means putrefied blood, the common name is "**blood poisoning**". Any bacteria can produce an invasion of the blood stream once it enters the skin, so this danger is always present.

**Hemophilus influenza** is a small pleomorphic bacillus which causes cellulitis in the upper part of the body, most frequently the face. Mainly it is a causative agent in young children but it can also be found in adults. It is seen as a single circumscribed area with indistinct margins. Usually this infection is preceded by an upper respiratory infection.

Other gram negative organisms that cause cellulitis include **E. coli, Proteus, Klebsiella, Enterobacter, Serratia marcescens**, and **Bacteroides**. These organisms are frequently cultured from the bowel and are not considered as being normal pathogens. These infections are most frequently seen in individuals with **diabetes melitus (sugar diabetes)**, bowel inflammatio, perineal inflammation and trauma, and in elderly patients. Like cellulitis, these infections of the skin present with redness, swelling, and pain. Gram negative bacilli, however, may also produce gas. These are particularly nasty infections.

There is one other gram negative infection of interest. Produced by a coccus in the genus **Neisseria**, this is the organism that most commonly causes **meningococcemia**, an extremely serious disease. This results in thrombosis and necrosis of dermal vessels. Petechiae may appear on extremeties, trunk, head, palms and soles, and mucous membranes. Another infection caused by Neisseria is **gonorrhea**, a venereal or sexually transmitted disease. The lesions occur mainly within the sexual organs. Chronic infections such as those associated with septicemia may also produce lesions on the skin. These are usually few in number and are often seen in and around the joints of the knees and elbows. They may be pustules, papules, or vesicles.

Modes of Transmission

With the advent of AIDS there has been a renewed interest in viral infections and the contagious aspects of viral caused disorders. Of prime importance to the skin care specialist is the prevention of the spread of disease. Because it is extremely important that the skin care specialist does not become infected by the client, here is a good place to concern ourselves with the possible routes of infection and try to understand the modes of transmission of infectious agents and prevention.

You must first come into contact with the infectious agent in order to become infected. This very simple statement is at the heart of both the spread and prevention of infection. The possible routes of infection are: 1. person to person, 2. contact with infected animals, 3. contact with **fomites**, 4. contact with **vectors**, 5. ingesting contaminated food or water, and 6. inhalation of airborne agents. Let's look at these closely.

**Person to person contact** has many avenues such as sexual contact, hand contact with contaminated materials or nasal secretion, open wounds, pimples, and other sores that drain. Kissing is notorious for spreading **infectious mononucleosis** and **herpetic infections** of the lips (**fever blisters**).

**Animal contact** when the animal is infected can result in conditions such as **ringworm**, **rabies**, **tularemia**, and **anthrax**. Bats carry rabies, as do cats and dogs. Mice and rats carry many diseases.

**Fomites** are cups, glasses, instruments, and other inanimate objects. These objects can include combs, floors of showers, and, yes, even toilet seats. Infectious mononucleosis can be transmitted by contaminated cups and glasses. Ringworm is easily transmitted from fomites, particularly ringworm of the scalp. Combs and the backs of upholstered chairs can hold and innoculate the skin with the spores of the disease.

**Vectors** are animals that transmit diseases to man or other animals. This is a loose interpretation of the word vector. In the strict sense it refers to **arthropods** (insects) as real vectors. The mosquito is required for the propagation of **malaria** since the sexual development of the malarial parasite occurs in the mosquito before it is transmitted to man. **Rocky Mountain Spotted Fever** requires a tick called **Dermacentor andersonii** to harbor the germ that causes this disorder. This germ is not a virus or bacteria, but a Rickettsia which has the characteristics of both. **Mechanical vectors** are agents that carry disease from one animal to the other without the need for maturation in the carrier. For instance, the disease called **toxoplasmosis** is caused by a parasite which is common in cats. Flies carry the parasite from kitty litter to food which is subsequently eaten by humans. Contaminated food and water transmit many diseases including poliomyelitis, cholera, hepatitis, and typhoid fever. Trichinosis, tape worms, and salmonella infections are all transmitted by food and drink. Many of these are related to the fecal-oral route, where the feces of the infected person contaminates the food of others. The Great Cholera Epidemic of England and the notorious Typhoid Mary are two examples of this mechanism of disease propagation.

Airborne infection results from coughing or sneezing with the resultant dissemination of millions of microbes. Large droplets fall to the floor. In some cases tiny droplets dry and remain airborne and infective for long periods. The most famous case of this was Legionnaires' disease in Philadelphia that was spread by an air conditioning unit.

The methods for preventing the spread of disease are well known. Wash your hands, wear masks, and wear gloves. Be careful of open wounds, sterilize your equipment between clients. All of these are known, but they must be practiced to be effective. Now, on to the viral diseases.

## Viral Diseases of the Skin and Viral Infections

Viral infections have always been with us. It is only recently that successful methods for growing viruses have been found and can now be used to study viral biology and viral diseases. Everyone is familiar with **measles** and the development of the measles vaccine, a triumph of modern viral biology. A virus is not a bacterial organism. It is incapable of reproduction outside of a living cell. They are **obligate parasites** of living cellular organisms.

### How Viruses differ from Other Organisms

The virus consists of a single type of nucleic acid, either DNA or RNA (you will recall that all other organisms have both). Some viruses have no cell wall but rather a protein called the **capsid**. Together the nucleic acid and the capsid are called the **nucleocapsid**. The information needed to invade the cell and reproduce the virus is contained in the nucleocapsid. Most animal viruses have a type of membrane called the **envelope**. The combination of the nucleocapsid and the envelope is called a **virion**, however, some virions do not have the envelope. Viruses are classified by their host. The **Phage** group of viruses attack bacteria. They are complex viruses that may contain a genome of 50 to 200 proteins for a double stranded DNA type. Phage is a short term for Bacteriophage since these viruses destroy bacteria.

Plant viruses are almost all single-stranded RNA types with three exceptions. They are transmitted from plant to plant by insects, worms, fungi, and man-made machines.

Animal viruses are both RNA and DNA types and they may be either single-stranded or double-stranded. Most are enveloped and have single-stranded RNA or double-stranded DNA. Viruses replicate in the cell after invasion of the cell membrane. They utilize the protein machinery of the cell to replicate the virion and assemble the virus structure. The virus can also make the cell produce other proteins which are not a part of the virus structure. The importance of this type of synthesis is that these proteins may signal the host cell to produce abnormal protein which can cause the cell to enlarge or divide abnormally.

The basic steps in the infection of a cell and the replication of the virus include the following sequence: 1. attachment of the virus to the cell, 2. penetration of the cell membrane, 3. uncoating of the virus, 4. protein biosynthesis of viral components, 5. viron assembly, and finally, 6. release of the new viruses. It is of interest that cells have to have specific receptors for viral attachment, otherwise the virus cannot infect the cell. In addition, only certain cells can replicate a given type of virus. For example, the virus that causes warts (**the human papillomavirus**) can only infect certain differentiating epidermal cells. As in the bacterial infections, it appears that the host is the determining factor in the severity of the infection. The severity relates to the individual's immunological competence and general state of health.

### Common Viral Diseases of the Skin

While there are many skin diseases which are primary viral diseases, we must limit our interest to those that are of importance to the skin care specialist. Many viral disorders are systemic in origin with skin manifestations. We shall limit our study to the **herpes group, papovirus** and **retroviruses**.

**Herpes virus** is the common fever blister virus. This is a double-stranded DNA type virus that is manifested by many diseases: **fever blisters**, **shingles**, **genital herpes**, **chickenpox**, **mononucleosis**, and **cancer**.

**Herpes simplex type 1** may occur anywhere on the body. It is frequently seen in childhood about the face, particularly around the mouth. Infection occurs from direct contact or exposure to mucocutaneous contact with another infected person. There is no case of infection from a fomite. The infection is ushered in with fever, sore throat, painful vesicles, and ulcerated areas around the mouth and lips. The condition lasts from 7 to 10 days. Painful or persistant cases should be referred to a physician, but most cases are self-limiting.

**Herpes simplex type 2** is the virus that causes genital herpes. This occurs following sexual exposure in 95% of all cases within 3 to 14 days after sexual relations with a partner that has an active genital lesion. The first sign is the appearance of a group of small vesicles which rupture in 2 to 4 days forming an ulceration. In females there is pain, itching, dysuria (painful urination), and vaginal discharge for 6 to 7 days, peaking at 8 to 10 days. The disease continues for 18 to 21 days with new lesions forming during this period. The recurrency of genital herpes is a major problem. It is estimated that there are 30 million people in the United States infected with herpes simplex type 2. About 50% of the males who are infected have a recurrent infection within 4 months while about 50% of females will have a recurrent infection in about 8 months. The average number of recurrent infections is 3 to 4 per year. 15% of the infected population will have 8 or more per year. Recurrent infections are more painful in the female.

**Herpes zoster** is the virus type which causes shingles. It is the same virus that causes **chickenpox**. It is a localized disease, limited in distribution to one dermatome which is innervated by one spinal or caudal sensory ganglion. It infects the nerve, and the pathway of that nerve is the single site of involvement. It affects both sexes equally. It affects people predominantly over 50 years of age. The young may be affected, but they comprise only about 10% of the reported cases. In individuals with immunosuppressed disorders such as AIDs, the incidence is 20 to 100 times more frequent.

**Varicella** or chickenpox occurs mainly in the young. Chickenpox has nothing to do with chickens. The word seems to have come from the old English word *gican* which means to itch. I believe that nearly everyone is familiar with chickenpox. Most physicians never see a case of chickenpox as medical students. They may have experienced one in their own family or they must rely on the expertise of the mother or that paragon diagnostician of childhood diseases, the

grandmother. Chickenpox is highly contagious, with 87% of siblings contacting the disease in a household. The disease has an incubation period of 14 to 15 days and the initial contact is infective from 2 days before the rash appears until the lesions crust over. One sees macules, papules, pustules, and crusts all occuring on the patient's skin. This disease is important to know as it does occur in adults, even though it is rare. As a skin care specialist you must be careful if you have a child with chickenpox as this disease can be spread by indirect contact.

**The Papovavirus Group (The wart group)** is a double-stranded DNA virus. Warts have been known since antiquity. There are many types but all are caused by the same virus family. Eighteen types have been identified so far, but we shall limit our study to only two types, **common warts** and **flat warts**. Common warts are caused by type 1, 2, and 3 HPV (human papillomavirus). They may be palmar or plantar, mosaic, oral, or anogenital. Warts are most frequent in the young, occurring between the ages of 10 and 39 years in 79% of the cases. Warts are contagious, but with the exception of the sexually transmitted ones we do not know how they are spread. Breaks in the skin and macerations are two possible routes of infection.

Common warts are known as **verruca vulgaris**. They appear as rough, raised, scaly papules or nodules that occur in groups or singularly. Any area of the skin may be infected, but they are most often seen on the hands.

Flat warts are called **verruca plana** and are seen as tiny 2 - 4 mm, very slightly raised papules on the face and hands of children. **Plantar warts** are seen on the soles of the feet or as **palmar warts** on the hands. They are thick hyperkeratotic warts that produce pain on pressure. **Mosaic warts** are a type of plantar or palmar wart that by coalescence have formed large plaques.

**The Retrovirus Group - AIDS Group** are single-stranded RNA viruses. This group of viruses is responsible for much human misery. They are known to cause cancer, hepatitis (non A and non B), and of course, AIDS. We shall look only at AIDS as this is the most likely disease which you will come into contact with as a skin care specialist. We shall spend more time with this virus because of the importance of prevention of transmission of the disease agent. Retroviruses are so named because they have **reverse transcription**. This is a process where viral RNA enters the cell and synthesizes a double-stranded DNA molecule which then enters the nucleus and eventually becomes a part of the host's genome. The retrovirus contains an envelope that fuses with the cell after it is taken in by a process called **pinocytosis**. A reverse transcriptase then makes the DNA molecule and the infection progresses. These viruses can cause cancer if they carry a gene called an **onc** or an **oncogenic gene** which induces the transformation of cells into tumors. Since normal cells have a limited number of divisions and are contact inhibited, they are well controlled. The onc genes, however, produce a protein kinase which causes the cell to phosphorylate certain plasma membrane proteins and prevents this control. The cells may continue to divide and more importantly move about the body (**metastasis**) where they have no business being. Not only are they non-functional but they are also harmful. These transformed cells are cancerous and when they spread throughout the body they are said to be metastasized.

AIDS is short for **acquired immunodeficiency syndrome**. First recognized in 1979 it is now quite prevalent with hundreds of thousands of cases in the United States. The major risk groups for this disease includes homosexuals, intravenous drug users, hemophiliacs, people requiring blood transfusions, and people of Haitian origin. The skin manifestations of AIDS are a result of the **T-cell** immunodeficiency and are related to infections by opportunistic organisms. These are organisms that under normal conditions would not be infective, such as the yeast **Candida albicans**.

### Fungal Diseases of the Skin

Fungi cause many infections of the skin. Fungi are eukaryocytes that obtain their nutrients from the decomposition of dead organic matter. They are neither plants nor animals, but have their own kingdom called Fungi. The fungi have characteristic filaments called **hyphae**. These are elongated cells or a series of cells with common cytoplasm. The hyphae give rise to spores which are the reproductive structures. The hyphae contain chitin or cellulose which are large polysaccharide molecules. When a mass of hyphae come together they form a **mycelium** which is the heart of the fungus colony, the **thallus**. Some fungi do not produce hyphae. One of these is the yeast fungus. Fungi are usually haploid cells but during sexual reproduction in the cycle they may be diploid. In this process two cells fuse to form a diploid cell called a **zygote**. The zygote divides and forms haploid cells that start new colonies. Most reproduction by fungi is by simple cellular division with new cells forming new colonies. One other characteristic of fungi is that they may be **dimorphic** (having two forms). They may be filamentous in one stage and bud-like in another stage.

**Tinea nigra** is an asymtomatic and superficial fungus of the stratum corneum which occurs in the palms of the hands as brownish-black macules that spread centrifugally. This condition responds to simple **antifungals** and **keratolytic agents**.

**Tinea versicolor** is a superficial fungal infection which is characterized by scaly hypopigmented areas and hyperpigmented irregular macules. They are common on the trunk and extremities. A significant number of people have this condition. It is especially easy to observe during the tanning season. The fungus responsible is **Pityrosporum orbiculare**, a dimorphic fungus. The fungus is recurrent but responds to simple treatments such as 2.5% selenium sulfide solution (Selsun Blue).

The **dermatophytes** are a group of 39 species that are implicated in superficial fungal infections of the skin. There are three major grous: **Microsporum**, **Trichophyton (T.)**, and **Epidermophyton**. All of the dermatophytes appear to follow a similar pathogenesis. First, the skin is innoculated with the fungus. This is followed by a period of incubation in which the fungus is growing in the stratum corneum. This is followed by the spread of the organism. The growth rate of the fungus must exceed or equal the turnover rate of the stratum corneum, otherwise it will be shed. This is why the lesions of dermatophytoses have a circular appearance. There are a few organisms in the center of the lesion and the major inflammatory action is at the perimeter of the lesion. **Tinea capitis** is a fungal infection of the scalp and the hair. Most infected individuals are children between the ages of 4 and 14 years. Males are more affected than females, and there is a higher incidence in persons living in overcrowded conditions. Tinea capitis can be spread by combs, brushes, pillow cases, and by upholstered chairs. Fortunately, this is a self-limiting disease and will rarely extend beyond puberty. The pathogenesis of this infection is fairly well understood. During anagen the infection begins in the stratum corneum, and following a period of incubation spreads into and around the hair shaft. The hyphae descend to the level of the keratogenous zone, stop at the fully keratinized zone, and never enter the nucleated zone. Tinea capitis may be caused by many different organisms including Microsporum and Trichophyton. The clinical signs are familiar to anyone who has worked with hair. Woods Lamp is effective as a diagnostic aid since most species of Microsporum will produce a bright greenish fluorescence when illuminated by this light. If doubt remains the hairs may be examined using a 5 to 10% solution of **Potassium Hydroxide** (KOH) and a microscope. Scrape the scalp with #15 scalpel blade and put the scrapings onto a microscope slide. Add a drop or two of the KOH and cover the mass. The hyphae will become visible in and around the hair.

**Ecothrix** infections are characterized by arthospores outside the hair shaft, while **endothrix** infections show arthrospores inside the hair shaft in a mosaic pattern.

**Tinea favosa** is a chronic infection of the scalp and glabrous skin and/or nails. It is characterized by yellow crusts within the hair follicle. They may eventually produce scars. This infection is mostly limited to families and is rarely epidemic since close, prolonged contact is needed to produce infection. There may be two or three causative organisms, most common are **T. schoenleinii** and **T. violaceum**. A common finding in this disease is a scutula (*scutum* = shield). This is a disc-like concentration of hyphae and keratin with a yellow-red color and a single hair at the center.

**Tinea barbae** or "barber itch" is limited to the coarse hairs of the face of males. The most common causative agents are **T. mentagrophytes** and **T. verrucosum**. Other organisms may be found. There are three forms of the disease; 1. inflammatory (**kerion type**), 2. superficial (**sycosiform type**), and 3. spreading (**circinate type**). This infection must be distin-

quished from a bacterial folliculitis as it responds well to antifungal agents such as **griseofulvin**.

**Tinea corporis**, or **tinea circinata** (the common **ringworm** group) occurs on all areas of glabrous skin. It is spread by direct contact from man to man or from animal to man. The causative agents are most commonly **T. mentagrophytes**, **T. rubrum**, or **Microsporum canis**.

**Tinea imbricata,** caused by T. concentricum, occurs in the Far East, South Pacific, and South and Central America. This is a chronic infection which may last for life and may be related to a genetic susceptibility.

**Tinea cruris** or "jock itch" is almost exclusively found in males, though I have seen it in obese women. It occurs in the groin and can extend to the scrotum and perianal areas. The infection is spread by direct contact or by fomites such as towels. The causative agent is usually **Epidermophyton floccosum** but almost any other dermatophyte could be involved, particularly **T. rubrum**. Drying the area helps to reduce the infection, however, at times griseofulvin is required.

**Tinea pedis** or **athletes foot** is world wide. It was apparently unknown until man began to wear shoes and is still unknown in shoeless people. The causative agents are **T. mentogrophytes**, **T. rubrum**, and **E. floccosum**. The clinical picture is well known. The intertrigenous areas between the fourth and fifth toes and between the third and fourth toes are most frequently involved. Fissures, maceration, and scaling are the classic findings. There are variants of this disease and the diagnosis should be accomplished by the KOH test. Infection is most common during the summer months and is spread by swimming pools, locker rooms, wash rooms, and walkways. The infection requires warm moist areas to propagate. Treatment is well known and there are several effective preparations available over the counter. Sometimes the period of treatment must be extended for 90 days.

**Tinea ungulum and onychomycosis** - The difference between these two is that the first is a nail plate infection caused specifically by a dermatophyte, while onchyomycosis represents any infection of the nail caused by any fungus. Fungal infections of the nails are limited to adults

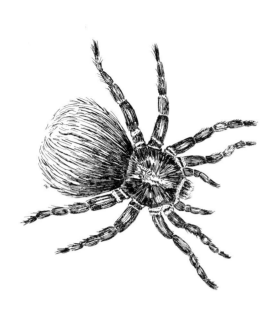

in almost all cases and infect men more than women. Candida or yeast infection of the nails called paronychia do affect women more commonly due to wet working conditions. Women are becoming more susceptible to toenail infections which may be related to the types of restrictive footwear which is characteristic of modern dress. The causative agents are many but the most common are **T. rubrum**, **T. mentogrophytes**, and **E. floccosum**. The clinical picture and the treatment is complex. These patients require referral and follow up, for while the cure is not hopeless there is a need for strong supportive therapy.

Finally, let us discuss the yeast infections or **candidiasis**. This is a most common disease and affects many areas of the body. The mouth, vagina, and rectum are the major sites. The causative agent is **Candida albicans** which means "glowing white or white". Candidiasis may also be caused by **Monilia albicans.** There are more than 80 species in the genus Candida, but only a few have been found to be pathological in man. The two most common (occuring in 80% of infections) are **C. albicans** and C. tropicalis. The colonization of C. albicans requires warmth and moisture. It therefore usually resides in the mouth, gastrointestinal tract, and vagina. In fact it is very difficult to initiate a skin infection with C. albicans without occluding the surface of the skin. There are predisposing factors which help to initiate the infection: 1. mechanical factors,

such as burns, trauma, obesity with occlusion, 2. nutritional factors such as avitaminosis, iron deficiency, and malnutrition, 3. physiological condition, aging, pregnancy, and menses, 4. systemic disease such as diabetes and uremia, 6. iatrogenic factors such as catheters, x-rays, and medications, and 7. oral contraceptives. The clinical manifestations of candidiasis are many. In the mucous membranes we find the disease in the mouth and in the vagina or penis (**balanitis**). Skin manifestations can include: 1. intertrigo fingers, toes and under the breasts, 2. folliculitis, almost anywhere, 3. paronychia and onychomycosis, 4. external otitis, 5. skin abcesses and 6. cellulitis. Look for the disease in skin folds and moist areas such as the diaper area, the armpits, gluteal folds, abdominal folds, and folds in the groin. Look for it on the fingers and behind the ear. The treatment requires removal of the predisposing factors and local or systemic medications. **Gentian violet** 2.5% has been used for many years, but now we have **nystatin**, **clotrimazole**, and **amphotericin**. Most superficial infections are easily treated but systemic infections require referral.

### Insect Related Diseases - The Arthropod Group

Man is host to a large number of parasitic infections. One of the horrors of studying medicine is to be aware of some of these diseases, particularly the tropical parasitic diseases. Unless you work or live in the tropics there is little need to learn this aspect of parasitology, but you will need to know some of the more common parasites. For our purpose we have limited this section to the arthropod group of insects, since they are rather common problems in both the United States and Europe. (See **Figure 5-5.**)

Arthropods are a group of invertebrates that are characterized by a chitinous exoskeleton, a bilateral symmetry, jointed appendages (*arthros* = joint and *podos* = foot), and true segmentation. There are nine classes that are of importance to us.

The **Arachnida** contain four pairs of legs and breathe through lung sacs of special tubes. The more important are the ticks and mites (**Acari**), the spiders (**Aranae**), and the scorpions (**Scorpiones**). The only important class for us is the Acari. There are three suborders of mites:

1. **Trombidiiformes** include the **chiggers, grain mites**, and **follicle mites**. The follicle mite, called Demodex, is usually found in the sebaceous glands and hair follicles. There are no known disorders caused by this mite with the possible exception of allergies.

2. **Food mites** are of several types: grain mite (**Acarus**), **cheese mite** (**Glycyphagus**) and the **grocery mites** (**Tyrophagus** and **Tyroglyphus**). These mites cause itching and a rash with papules and vesicles. Grain mites known as **Pyemotes ventricosus** are a cause of an epidemic characterized by systemic symptoms of fever, diarrhea, anorexia, and malaise. The skin may show red macules.

3. **Fowl mites** occur with people who keep birds or who work around pigeons; even office workers can contract them through air conditioning systems. They also produce a rash. The most common fowl mites in the USA are **Dermanyssus gallinae** and **D. avium**.

The lowly **chigger** or harvest mite (**Trombicula splendens**) is associated with summer outdoor activity. The familiar red itchy legs and itchy belt line are signs of infestation. This is the common "**red bug**" of the Southern USA.

The bites may result in a papular urticaria or vesiculation. Scratching may lead to a secondary infection by the normal skin flora.

The **scabies** mite is known as **Sarcoptes scabiei**. It is the best documented of the mites, having a history far back into antiquity. This mite is frequently missed as a cause of skin rashes. The typical lesion is the burrow with associated papules and vesicles. These burrows are S-shaped or straight with small vesicles at the site of the female mite, a small gray speck at the bottom of the vesicle. The condition is easily treated. Scabies are common in crowded areas and can be transmitted with clothing exchange and through bodily contact.

**Ticks** are classified as hard ticks (the **Ixodidae Group**) and soft ticks (the **Argasidae Group**). Ticks are active in the spring and summer, and are inactive in the winter. What separates a tick from all the other mites is the barbed **hypostome** used for feeding. The ticks that cause **Rocky Mountain spotted fever** and **Colorado tick fever**, **tularemia**, and **Lyme Disease** are all hard ticks. Tick bites show intense pruritis and an erythematous ring. Ticks should be removed. The time honored method is to use petroleum jelly or gasoline over the tick. This in-

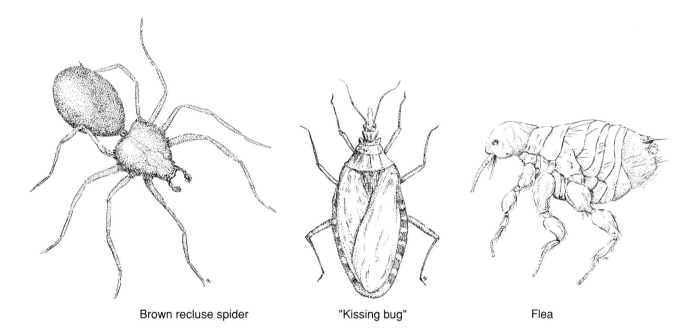

Brown recluse spider          "Kissing bug"          Flea

**FIGURE 5-5** Common arthropods. The most common "critters" you are likely to see trespassing on your skin are ticks and chiggers (picked up by walking through wooded areas, or from pets); fleas (mainly from pets); mites (from rugs, clothing, pets); head and body lice (clothing, bedding, combs and brushes, towels); pubic lice (mostly through sexual contact). The brown recluse spider and the "kissing bug" may inflict a painful bite. (Figure 5-5 continued on next page.)

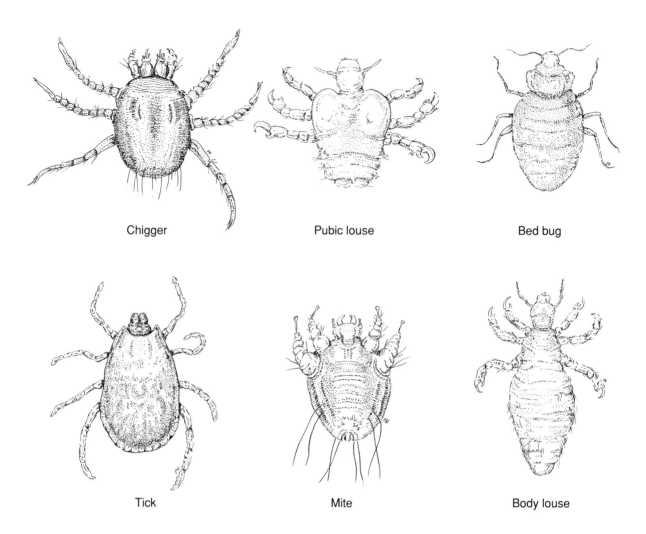

Chigger          Pubic louse          Bed bug

Tick          Mite          Body louse

**FIGURE 5-5** (cont.)

terferes with the breathing apparatus of the tick, the spiracles. The tick will then remove its hypostome (its anchoring device) from the skin by itself. If the hypostome remains in the skin after tick removal, it should be removed surgically.

**INSECTA** - The Insecta comprise several orders, of which Anoplura is the worst, for they suck blood. These parasites infect the head, body, and pubis of mankind. Two villians are responsible, **Pediculosus humanus** and **Phthirus pubis**.

Pediculosus humanus has two forms, **var. capitus** (the **head louse**) and **var. corporis** (the **body louse**). It is well known that age, sex, or social status cannot prevent infection. Five to 30% of the people in certain populations can be infected. Anyone working with hair is familiar with this condition. Body lice are rare in the higher economic strata. The findings of red macules with multiple exorciations and hives should suggest this disease.

The **crab louse** or Phthirus pubis is usually transmitted by sexual contact but may also be transmitted by clothing or hairs. You can find these lice all over the body even to the edge of the scalp. The eyelashes and eyebrows do not escape infestation. They appear as yellowish-brown small spots which move when pulled out of the skin. The nits are fastened to the hair shaft in a manner similar to hair lice. Treatment is easy and effective. Kwell lotion or shampoo is available by prescription. It is wise to consult with a physician to verify the diagnosis and obtain the prescription.

**Hemiptera** - There are two families of Hemiptera that feed on the human. The most common is the **bedbug (Cimex lectularius)** which feeds at night by bloodsucking the victim. The bites are not painful but they do form red papules that itch. These bugs live in old houses, furniture and bird's nests.

The "**kissing bug**" (**Reduviidae**, found

mostly in the Southwestern USA) can transmit serious diseases such as **Trypanosomiasis**. The bites are very painful. Red papules may also be seen. 80% of cases present with a red, inflamed eye. Edema and tumor-like lesions may later appear on the chest, back, and legs. This disease is often fatal.

### Allergic Contact Dermatitis

You will recall that I mentioned allergic contact dermatitis when we were discussing eczematous dermatitis. Allergic contact dermatitis is part of a larger group of eczemas. The distinction is this. Eczematous dermatitis is produced by irritants. Allergic dermatitis is produced by an inflammatory reaction initiated by the immune system in response to a specific substance. Let's take an example; **poison ivy dermatitis** is a true allergic contact dermatitis. The maddening thing about poision ivy is that you can come in contact with it for many years without inflammation and then all of a sudden you blister after contact. Why? Because you are now sensitized to the allergen poison ivy. Any time that you come in contact with it again, your immune system, now primed for action against the allergen, will respond with a poison ivy rash. It is important for you to know the difference between an irritant and an allergen.

Here are the steps required to produce a contact allergic reaction. Step 1 - the inception phase. When you touch the poison ivy leaf, the chemicals from the leaf begin combining with the proteins of your skin at the point of contact. This stimulates the Langerhans cells. An antigen-cell complex is formed and reacts with the T-lymphocytes. Now the T-lymphocytes are activated and they differentiate into new cells with a specific weapon against the poison ivy chemical. These new T-lymphocytes are called supressor lymphocytes and you have become sensitized. Step 2 - the elicitation phase. Now that you have supressor cells in your blood stream, they circulate around, like policemen, looking to make sure that there is no trouble. On comes the poison ivy chemical, again binding with the Langerhans cells, but this time the supressor cells spring into action. Two to four days after contact you begin to itch, get erythema and blister at the point of contact.

At this point you should recall all the things we discussed in the immune response phase of inflammation. The diagram shown in Figure 5-4 shows the steps. Remember anything which will bind with proteins will produce an allergic response.

Here are a few clinical signs which can help you in this diagnosis. Contact dermatitis is not "catching". If more than one family member presents with a similar condition you are most likely dealing with an infectious disorder. Children under four to five years of age and pre-teens usually do not get contact dermatitis although they are not excluded. The most common allergic contact dermatoses in children are exposure to plants, metals, and shoes. The pattern and location of the dermatitis along with a history of exposure are helpful in arriving at the diagnosis. Confirmation requires a positive patch test to the offending agent.

### Acne

Acne is the scourge of mankind and the travesty of youth.

Acne is the most common skin disease facing mankind. It afflicts 89% of seventeen year olds to some degree. Nodular cystic acne is exceptionally bad and is much more common in white males than in black males of the same age (15 to 21 years). Acne tends to persist, and flare up from time to time in 8% of men and 6% of women in their 30's. We will spend some time studying the pathogenesis of acne as it is understood today.

The definition of **acne vulgaris** is that it is a self-limiting disease primarily of adolesents that involves the sebaceous glands. There are usually a variety of lesions consisting of comedones, papules, pustules, nodules, cysts, and sequelae, such as pitted or hypertrophic scars. Here I have quoted from Dr. John S. Strauss, as he is an eminent authority in this field.

The word acne is from the Greek word *akne* meaning a point, or *achne* meaning chaff (seed covering-very itchy when contacted).

Four etiological factors have been associated with the pathogenesis of acne:

**Altered keratinization** - The first sign of acne is usually a blackhead (comedo). For a long time it was believed that the comedo was a plug of dry sebaceous oil filling the duct of the sebaceous gland. We now know that this is not

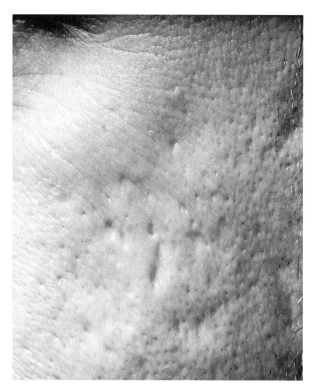

**FIGURE 5-6** Healed comedone scar formation. These are linear depressed scars and some punctate or "ice pick" scars seen in this photograph.

true. The comedones are a combination of keratinized material and lipid material. There is a change in the keratinization pattern seen in the comedo. Initially there is a large amount of lamellar-granular material followed by an increase in keratohyaline granules and dense keratin material. Why and how this occurs is unknown. We do know that the proliferative rate is increased in the keratinocytes of the sebaceous follicles. This increased rate plus the tenaciousness of the lipid keratin complex makes a dandy plug for the sebaceous duct.

**Lipid abnormalities** - We know also from the work of Dr. Strauss that acne patients excrete more sebaceous lipids onto the surface of the skin than people without acne. There is, however, a large variation in the amount of sebum produced within an acne group. Without the sebaceous gland activity there is no acne. One of the culprits identified in the sebum lipids is the free fatty acid content. You will recall that free fatty acids are the product of hydrolysis of triglycerides. When free fatty acids are injected into the skin, they produce marked inflammation. The amount of linoleic acid found in the sebum of acne patients is lower than that found in the sebum of acne free individuals.

**Bacterial actions** - These are the culprits which cause the ugly pustules. The most commonly found organism is **Propionibacterium acnes**. A second bacterium, P. granulosum, is found frequently in the hair follicles associated with acne lesions. A yeast, Pityrosporum ovale, has also been found in acne lesions. The action of the bacteria is to produce the inflammatory response by the lipolytic activity within the ducts. The end result of this process is to set off leukocyte migration and the complement system. Redness and pus follows this reaction.

**Hormones** - In both males and females the androgens become dominant and acne results. Males with acne show an increased level of serum testosterone. Females with acne show an increased level of urinary androgen metabolites. Some newer findings show that increased levels of testosterone metabolites are found in both men and women with acne. When men or women with acne are given androgens, cortisone, or anabolic agents the acne will be aggrevated. All of these agents work through the hormone chain reaction of the pituitary-adrenal axis. The pituitary is the master gland of the body. It sends out messages to the target glands including the adrenals, ovaries, testicles, thyroid, and breasts. An important consequence of this system is the effect of psychological stress on the body. Since the pituitary is located in the brain, it is subject to a great deal of cortical control from the higher brain. Do not underestimate the role of mental stress on the etiology of acne.

The picture of a comedo is not a pretty sight. The comedo starts in the middle of the follicle as an expanding mass of keratin and lipid materials. As it grows in size the follicle walls become thin and the follicle itself dilates. Eventually most of the sebaceous cells are replaced by undifferentiated epithelial cells. The keratin is permeated with lipids and bacteria. A cross section of a comedo shows concentric layers of laminated material centered around a hair or hairs. The open comedo differs from the closed comedo in that the orifice is open and the material is more compact. Open comedones do not appear to become inflamed unless traumatized. The closed comedo forms an inflammatory process by the action of lipids rupturing into the dermis. This step is followed by the entire comedo mass breaking into the dermis and producing a full inflammatory response. The result is either a nodule, a pustule or a combination of both of these lesions. The healing process results in the scar formation (see **Figure 5-6**).

Above is the description of acne vulgaris, which is the most common type of acne. There are other types, based on either the appearance of the lesions or on the etiology. Some skin specialists do not distinquish between these various types preferring to lump them all together as acne of different severities. Here are some types that you may see or read about.

**Drug Induced Acne** - This is most common with steroid therapy, appearing as a folliculitis about two weeks after steroids are initiated. Comedones and scarring may occur.

**Halogen induced acne** - Induced by iodides and bromides. Not usually caused by topical exposure but more likely by ingestion.

**Tropical acne** - Usually a flare up of acne vulgaris appearing on the chest and buttocks. This is a highly resistant type and often requires removal of the patient from the tropics.

**Acne conglobata** - A severe form of acne. It is related to acne vulgaris in that the etiology appears similar, however, it occurs later in life. The lesions are multiple and occur on the back, buttocks, and chest. There are also lesions on the face, neck, upper arms, and abdomen. Abscess formation is common and draining sinus tracks are often present.

**Rosacea** - A chronic disease usually in middle aged men which is manifested by an erythema and telangiectasia. The presence of hyperplasia of the skin of the nose, known as rhinophyma may be present. We shall discuss this disorder later.

## Aging

The greying of America and Europe is a fact of our times. The shift in population age is upward. For the skin care specialist, this is not only a challenge, but an opportunity. The importance of understanding aging as a biological process can not be overstated. This is why we should consider some of the theories of aging and what happens to an individual. There are two main theories of aging:

**Genetic** - The terminal or final step of tissue differentiation which is genetically coded.

**Environmental** - Aging is understood as an accident resulting from many errors that have occured during the lifespan of the individual (eg. DNA replication, translation, etc.).

Many scientists now believe that aging is a composite of these actions. There is some genetic coding, however, the organs do not all age at the same time. Many studies have shown this. On the cellular level aging is seen by molecular biologists as 1. a change in the genetic program, 2. a coding error of point retention in DNA, 3. an impaired control of transcription and post-translation, 4. a reduced transport of m-RNA, and/or 5. protein synthesis errors. Other findings at the cellular level are a decrease in the number of cells in organs, and a decrease in the number of mitochondria per cell. The cell becomes larger in size as do the mitochondria. I believe that the mitochondria play an important part in cellular aging.

The effect of the environment is critical. Poor nutrition in childhood is devastating to the body and may cause rapid aging. Stress, smoking, and sunlight add to the destruction of the skin and other body organs.

Skin care specialists need to understand the mechanisms of aging in general and of the aging of skin in particular. The best book that I have seen covering this topic is Aging and the Skin , Bahlen, A. K. and Kligman, A. M. (Eds.), Raven Press, New York, 1988. Much of the following is a summary from that text. I would recommend that the student purchase this book.

Our skin has both a chronological age and a physiological age. We will be judged to be old or young by the condition of our skin. The hair is also used in age evaluation, however, rather it is grey or colored, it has less weight to the judgement if the skin is in good condition. We appraise skin by color, reflectivity, texture, and plumpness. Young skin is viewed as pink, shiny, smooth, unblemished, and resilient. Old skin is viewed as grey, dull, mottled, wrinkled, blemished, and lax. What are the events in skin that lead to this devastation? As a physician I have seen the early depression reaction in a woman's eyes as she studies the first lines on her face. Over the next years there comes despair and finally resignation. Contrasted to these women are the women in their 80's and 90's that still have their hair dressed and wear makeup. The psychological effects of aging are profound and extensive.

Now let us look at some of the physiological and anatomical changes seen in aging skin.

**The epidermis** - Many students of aging skin consider a thin epidermis to be the hallmark of aging skin. This appears to be true. The rete pegs flatten and the normal undulations of the basement membrane dampen into a smooth line. Fewer basal cells are found and less keratin is produced.

There is no apparent disorder of keratinization; however, in histological sections one sees changes in cell size, shape, and staining characteristics. Disorder is the key word. Thus, aging skin follows universal decadence by becoming disordered.

**The appendages** - Sweat gland function is diminished in older skin. We know that heat regulation is more difficult for the aged and they suffer more easily from heat stroke. Both the size of the sweat glands and number of sweat glands appear to decrease with age. Histological findings show changes in the secretory coils, such as shrinkage and involution. Dry skin in the elderly may relate in some way to the decrease in sweating.

The apocrine glands show diminished secretory function, however, there is less damage and disorganization than is seen in the sweat glands.

The sebaceous gland secretion is controlled by hormones so that we find a sex difference in the rate of secretion in an aging population. Sebaceous gland secretions increase with puberty reaching a maximum in adolescence, maintaining this level throughout adult life, and diminishing after age 50 in women and age 70 in men. While there is a decrease in the output of sebum, these glands will respond to androgen injections at any age. The sebaceous glands enlarge in the elderly, particularly on the face and forehead. Thus, we see the large pore problem in women. The effect of the decreased sebum on the condition of the skin in the aged is unknown. I am of the school that it has no real effect.

Hair growth remains a mystery. Why hair grows well in some areas and not in others is unknown. We know that the hair follicle in both men and women will respond to androgen at any age. The amount of hair, the texture of hair, and the thickness of hair, are all difficult to relate to an aging group because of the enormous variations among individuals.

**The dermis** - The dermis plays a major role in the appearance of aging skin. We learned in the biochemistry and physiology of the skin that the collagen and elastin provide the basic support structure of the skin. It is the elastin that supplies the snap and the collagen that supplies the strength. Knowledge about the dermal changes in the aging skin remains inconclusive. We know that the dermis is thinner, the collagen more disorganized, with less collagen per unit area even though the bundles are thicker. Since men have a thicker dermis than women, there is less facial sagging in males.

Elastin is greatly increased in sun exposed skin. In other areas there is a loss of elastin in the papilary and lower dermis. Upon microscopic examination there are some partially formed elastin fibers, mostly tubular, without the necessary matrix to make them functional. The upper reticular dermis shows a number of thickened elastin bundles which are not elastic. Mention is made of the role of the ground substance which is diminished in aging skin, but this is a marginal finding.

The water content of the dermis is not decreased in aged skin.

The cellular content of the dermis is decreased, in particular the mast cells, making the onset of inflammation more difficult. There is regional loss of fat deposits. The loss of fat on the back of the feet, the back of the hand, and the pretibial area account for the thin appearance of these areas. Other areas increase in fat deposits such as the wrist, abdomen, and suprailiac.

The microcirculation is decreased in aging individuals. There are serious problems with thermal regulation. One important observation by Dr. Kligman is the reduced clearance rate of aged skin. With this reduced blood flow, the ability to clear drugs from the skin is reduced. We should rethink the need for frequent applications of products to the skin of the aged.

Aging skin does not appear to be more or less permeable than young skin. The real barrier to skin penetration resides in the lipid composition in each area of the skin. Wound healing is not significantly reduced in the aged person although time is a factor. Both wound healing and skin permeability relate to the microcirculation of the skin. The immune response is reduced in the aged. There is a reduced number of Langerhans cells, and a decrease in T-cell dependent responses. There is a decrease in mast cells, and in the inflammatory response.

The skin care specialist needs to constantly be updated in these various areas. More shall be discussed when we study treatments.

When I see the Wall crumbling, you know, I look around this place and figure it can't just happen for no reason. One day the structure looks wobbly, and you gotta figure out if you're headed for a collapse. We know how slick our enemies are, but like fingerprints on a cookie jar, they're gonna leave some clues. You gotta get up close to figure out whodunit, and how tough they are.

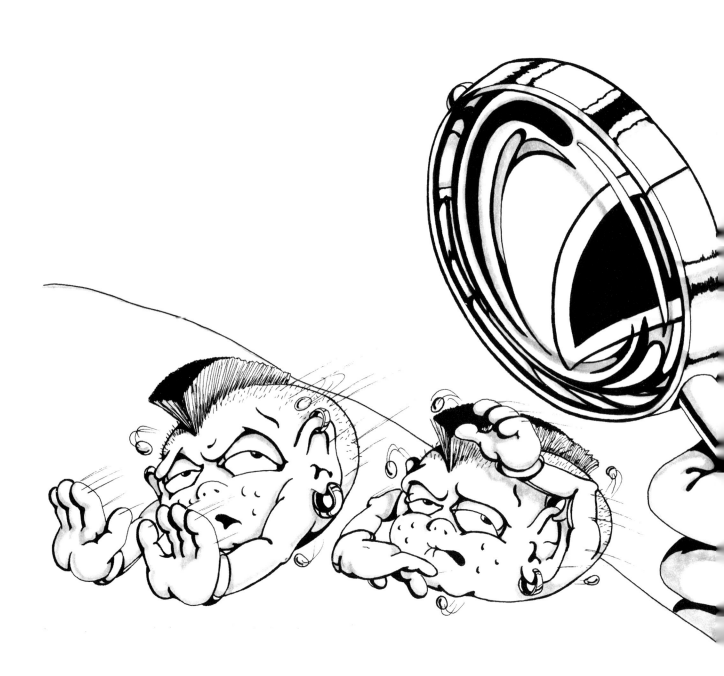

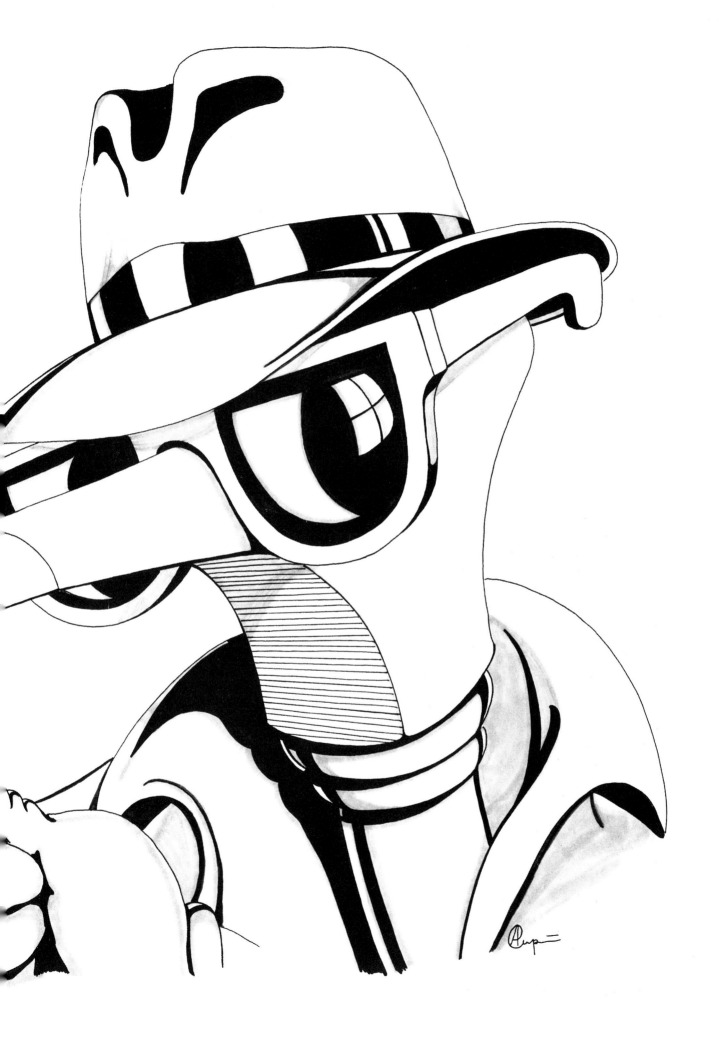

# Diagnosis of Skin Disorders

At one period (a very long period) diagnosis was the real thing and almost the only thing in medicine. Few therapeutic agents of proven value existed and there was little understanding of the cause of most diseases. Reading the old medical textbooks makes one feel the frustration of the physicians of the past, yet one develops respect for their observational skills and their therapeutic heroics.

Today there are vast arrays of both diagnostic and therapeutic options available to the physician. Sadly, many of these choices do not extend to the non-medical skin care specialist, or even to the dermatologist. In this chapter it is my aim to introduce the reader to the fundamentals of diagnosis as it applies to the non-medical skin care specialist. It is inevitable that we borrow techniques from medicine, for we study the same territory. Bear in mind that being able to diagnose a disorder does not necessarily qualify you to treat that disorder. **One of the greatest and most harmful actions is the wrong diagnosis or failure to diagnose a serious treatable disorder**. Fortunately, many non-serious skin disorders are self-limiting and the body graciously helps us to remedy our errors of diagnosis and thwarts our treatments by curing itself. Remember that a fever is a sign of a potentially serious illness. A fever and a general rash always indicate a serious illness that requires the immediate attention of a physician. Any skin condition manifested by hemorrhagic changes (either **purpura** or **petechia**) must be referred to a physician.

The skin care specialist has four basic instruments for diagnosis: the eyes, the ears, the nose, and the hands. These four tools are tied into the brain, where the information they gather is assessed and interpreted. Any additional device that has been devised by man is only an extension of these basic instruments. The finest microscope, the best x-ray system, or the finest laboratory all yield information that must eventually pass through one of the basic four instruments. The key steps are: 1. observe the person, 2. listen to the person, and 3. examine the person visually and tactily. There are a large number of nerve fibers per unit area in the fingertips. They are extremely sensitive. The fingers, eyes, and ears are able to distinguish minute quantities, qualities, or changes therein. As time passes and your experience grows, you will develop your own individual diagnostic methods and habits. Habits may be good or bad. Strive for excellence in the beginning stages of the learning process.

Now let us examine some basic lesions and definitions. Many of these are old friends, but a little review is never wasted.

## COMMON LESIONS

**Lesion** comes from the Latin word *laedere* (*laesio* meaning to hurt). A lesion is defined as any pathological or traumatic discontinuity of tissue or a loss of function. A scar is a lesion, a pimple is a lesion, a cut is a lesion, a black eye is a lesion, and a paralyzed hand is a lesion. The common lesions of the skin are grouped into three types (flat, elevated, or depressed) based on their relationship to the surface of the skin.

### Flat Lesions

A **macule** (Latin for spot) is a flat circumscribed area of change in skin color. It is not raised or depressed. There is no change in the surface texture of the skin. Due to the color change the macule is visible. The cause may be the results of a pigment change, blood, or blood products. Examples are **freckles**, **petechiae** (small, pinpoint, purple or red spots due to blood), and **ecchymoses** (large areas of blood leakage into the skin resulting from bruises).

**Telangiectasia** are bright, red, branching lines seen through the skin and are the result of dilated capillaries. Remember that *telangiectasia* is Greek for "dilated blood vessel". Sometimes they blanch with pressure.

**Infarcts** are macules that result from an area of cutaneous necrosis due to the occlusion of a blood vessel. They are irregular, gray, variegated, or dusty-red. Occasionally they may be slightly depressed.

### Elevated or Raised Lesions (The Largest Group)

**Papules** are small, solid, raised lesions less than one (1) centimeter in diameter. A classic sign is a papule that can be felt with the finger tips. They come in many shapes and colors. Red papules are seen in **psoriasis**. In **miliaria rubra** (**prickly heat**) they may be pointed. A **pimple**

is a papule before it is a pustule.

**Plaque** is an elevated, plateau-like lesion that has a flat surface. It may cover a wide or a small area. In patients with **psoriasis**, you will see plaque as a red, raised, scaly lesion. **Lichenification** or scarring due to scratching of **eczema** is a type of plaque that may look like tree bark.

**Nodules** are larger than papules, usually over one (1) centimeter and result from collection of cells or metabolic materials. Nodules are classified as to depth and anatomical components. They may be epidermal, epidermal-dermal, dermal, dermal-subdermal, or subcutaneous. **Warts** are epidermal nodules and **lipomas** are subcutaneous nodules of fatty tissue.

**Wheals** are slightly rounded, plaque-elevations due to edema. The common **hive** is a wheal. They are usually red or deep pink. The borders are not sharp and, in fact, may move about. The epidermis is not involved in a wheal. Stroking the skin with a fingernail produces a wheal known as **dermatographism**. **Angioderma** is a wheal that occurs in loose skin such as the lips, eyes, hands, and feet. It may be massive and disfiguring. When you see this condition make sure the person is breathing well, for **laryngeal edema** sometimes occurs with angioderma on the skin and may severely compromise breathing. Most cases of angioderma subside with mild treatment, but nevertheless take every case seriously.

**Vesicles** and **bullae** are essentially the same lesion, differing only in size. A vesicle is a circumscribed, fluid-filled, elevated lesion that looks like a bubble. Vesicles are smaller than 0.5 centimeter, when larger they are called **bullae**. The walls are thin and mostly translucent revealing the fluid inside, which may be serum, blood, or extracellular fluid. Viral diseases cause both vesicles and bullae. Vesicles and bullae form from a separation of the skin between certain planes; for example, **impetigo** vesicles and bullae cleave below the stratum corneum. **Blisters** are bullae formed from heat, friction, or chemical reactions.

**Pustules** are elevated circumscribed lesions that contain **pus**, a purulent exudate. Pus contains leukocytes and may or may not contain bacteria. Pus may be of various colors - yellow, white, green, or red being the most frequent. Pustules are seen in many diseases associated with infection of both viral and bacterial origin, but some are sterile, as in **pustular psoriasis**. We spoke of huge pustules like **furuncles** and **carbuncles** and now we add **abscess** which is a deep localized collection of purulent material. The location of an abscess is usually a red, swollen, tender, area on the skin. When an abscess drains on the skin from a deep structure, the tract connecting the two is called a **sinus**.

**Cysts** are sacs that contain fluid or semisolid material. The most common cysts are **epidermal cysts** which are often called **wens** by the public. **Sebaceous cysts** form in the hair follicles and grow quite large at times. They contain keratin and sebaceous material and at times become infected, particularly when squeezed by dirty fingers.

**Scales** are wild stratum corneum cells that are thickened and flaked. They are silvery, rarely being colored. When scales shed spontaneously the process is called **desquammation**.

**Crust** is dried surface blood, serum, or pus. It may be thin, thick, friable, or very adherent. Crust may also be any color. **Ecthyma** is a condition in which the entire epidermis is crusted over.

### Depressed Lesions

**Excoriations** are superficial excavations of the epidermis. They are due to scratching or abrasion and may be finger-nail shaped or quite linear.

**Erosions** are moist lesions that are circumscribed and depressed into the epidermis. If you remove a bullae covering, the base is called erosion.

**Ulcers** are moist lesions that penetrate beyond the epidermis and at least into the papillary dermis. Two advanced forms of ulcers are **stasis ulcers** and decubitis ulcers.

**Scars** are the result of the healing of an ulcer or a dermal wound. Scars may be in the epidermis, as **stretch marks** (striae), or in the dermis. They may result from any disorder that involves the dermis (**acne** scars are an example).

**Atrophy** is a condition in which a cell, tissue, or organ decreases in size. In the skin we can define **epidermal atrophy** as seen in the elderly and in sun-damaged skin. The epidermis is almost transparent and has few, if any, markings. **Dermal atrophy** occurs when there is a loss of connective tissue from the papillary and reticular dermis. Two common causes are inflammation and trauma, though many others exist.

## MOLES AND NEVI

A **nevus** is a circumscribed growth of skin appearing at birth, or shortly thereafter. A nevus may be composed of almost any type of tissue such as keratinocytes, sebaceous gland components, dermal components, or melanocytes. They are benign growths of almost any color. The red ones are called **hemangiomas** and the melanin pigmented ones are called **moles**. The histological name for a mole is a **pigmented cellular nevus**. They may be junctional and occur only in the intraepidermal area, or compound involving both the epidermis and the dermis. Hemangiomas may be very large and flat as in the **port wine stain**, or large, soft, and elevated as in the **strawberry hemangioma**.

**Senile hemangiomas** are small, raised lesions. They can be red or purple, and are seen mostly on the trunk in older persons. They are also called "cherry spots".

A **spider angioma** consists of a central punctum (point) with radiating "legs" or branches, resembling a spider. They are common in pregnancy.

**Lentigines** are small, flat, pigmented lesions, usually a uniform brown or black color. They may occur anywhere on the body. They are not related to sun exposure in early life.

**Freckles** are well circumscribed brown macules that are related to sun exposure. In fact, freckles can not occur without prior exposure to the sun. They are harmless.

The above descriptions are morphological short cuts used to describe a skin condition. To this group let's now add the following terms.

**Configuration or arrangement** is the position of the lesion in relation to others of its kind. They may be linear (in line), annular (ring-shaped), confluent (touching or coalescent), etc.

**Distribution** refers to where the lesions are and what pattern they take. Are they distributed on the head and hands, or only on the abdomen? Are they generalized (all over the body), or are they localized?

With these new terms you can begin to characterize a skin disorder by describing it. Let us take an example from a textbook of dermatological diseases. This description is from <u>Dermatology in General Medicine</u>. "The primary lesion is either an erythematous papule, an urticarial-like plaque, or most commonly, a vesicle; however, large bullae may infrequently be seen. Vesicles, especially if they occur on the hands, may be hemorrhagic. The continual appearance and disappearance may result in hyperpigmentation and hypopigmentation. Occasionally, patients will present with only crusted lesions and a thorough search will reveal the primary lesion. The herpetiform (herpes-like) grouping of lesions is often present in areas, but patients have many individual non-grouped lesions." This is the description of the clinical findings of Dermatitis herpetiformis.

## ANATOMICAL SITES OF COMMON DISORDERS

Common skin disorders and their associated lesions do not always appear uniformly distributed over the body. In the diagrams in **Figure 6-1** I have shown the most common skin disorders, their associated lesions, and their most probable sites. In the diagnosis of skin diseases the four important descriptive terms are **type**, **shape**, **arrangement**, and **distribution**. We shall repeat these from time to time as they are the tetrad of skin diagnosis. We are continuing to push into the area of dermatology, but there is no other way.

I have grouped the diagnosis by region of the body as follows:

**The head and face** - acne, rosacea, seborrheic dermatitis, melasma, solar keratosis, xanthelasma, perleche, spider angioma, cancer, psoriasis.

**Chest, abdomen and back** - psoriasis, senile keratosis, senile angioma, cafe-au-lait, acne, tinea versicolor, seborrheic dermatitis.

**Groin and perineal area** - pruritis ani, psoriasis, fungal infections, intertrigo, venereal warts.

**Hands and feet** - fungal infections, warts, eczematous dermatitis, solar keratosis.

**Arms and legs, elbows and knees** - psoriasis, antecubital and popliteal atopic dermatitis; dermatofibroma (usually upper legs).

**Head and Face**

1. Acne - chin, nose, cheek, forehead
2. Rosacea - nose and cheeks
3. Seborrheic dermatitis - scalp, corner of nose
4. Melasma - forehead, cheek
5. Solar keratosis - no specific site
6. Xanthelasma - eyelid
7. Perleche - corners of mouth
8. Spider angioma - no specific site
9. Cancer - nose, top of ears, neck
10. Psoriasis - hairline and scalp

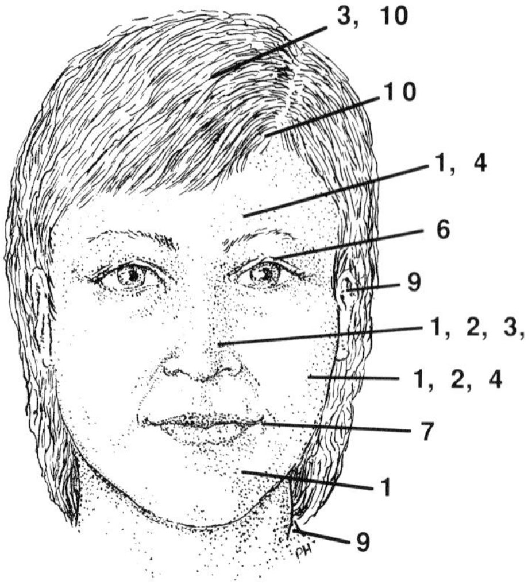

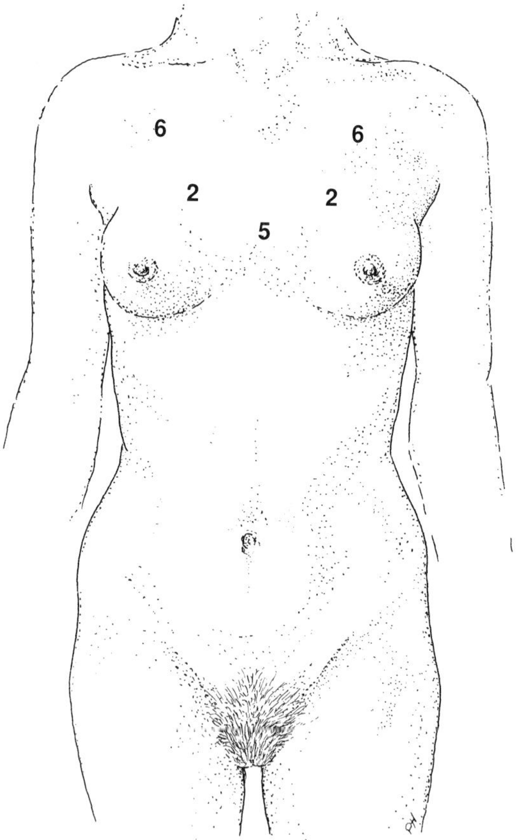

**Chest, abdomen and back**

1. Psoriasis - trunk, no specific site
2. Solar keratosis - upper chest and back
3. Senile hemangioma - trunk, no specific site
4. Cafe au lait - trunk, no specific site
5. Acne - upper back and chest
6. Tinea versicolor - upper chest and back
7. Seborrheic dermatitis - between shoulder blades

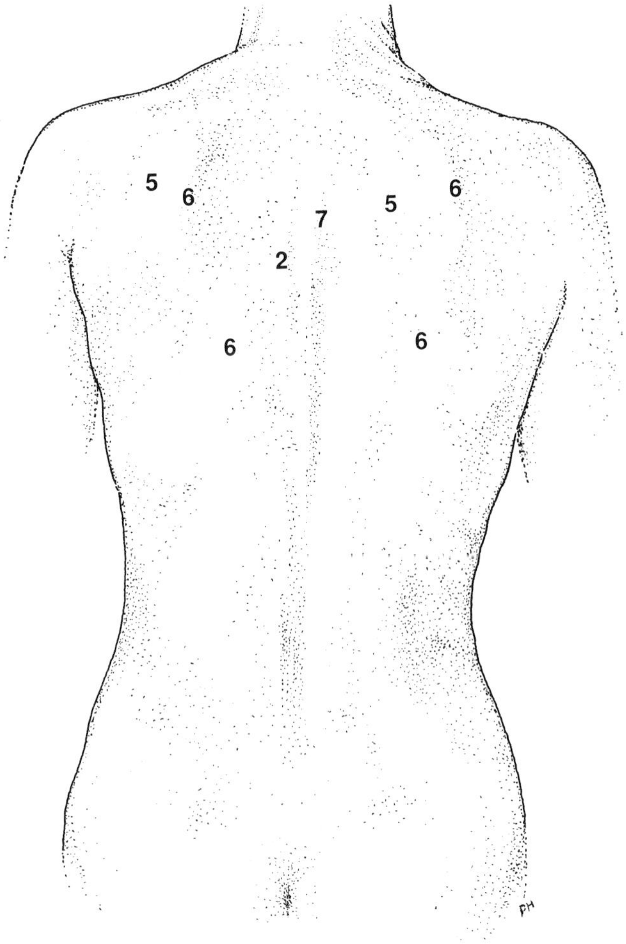

**FIGURE 6-1** Diagnosis of diseases in body regions. The numbered diagrams indicate the regions of the face and body where a disease is **most likely** to occur. This does not mean, of course, a disease will not occur elsewhere, but you can use this as a guide to aid you in diagnosis.

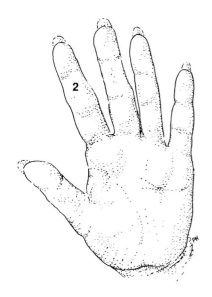

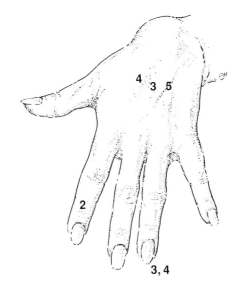

**Hands and feet**

1. Fungal infections - between toes
2. Warts - heel, ball of foot, fingers
3. Eczematous dermatitis - fingers, around nails, dorsum and hand around around nails
4. Psoriasis - dorsum, around nail of hand
5. Solar keratosis - dorsum of hand

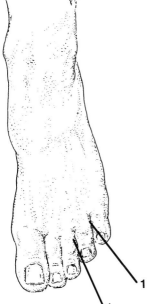

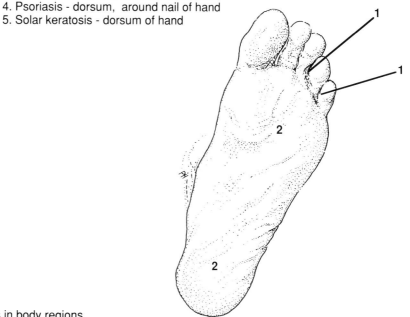

**FIGURE 6-1** (cont.) Diagnosis of diseases in body regions.

One must bear in mind that while the lesions cited above are commonly present on the sites listed they could occur elsewhere. It is important when examining the face to look behind the ears and in the nasolabial folds, at eye margins and at the hairline.

Often the back is neglected as are the buttocks. It is important to turn the client over and to look at the back with a good light. Finally,

make sure as you examine that you make notes of your findings.

## A METHOD OF SKIN EXAMINATION AND DIAGNOSIS

### History Taking

"Listen to the patient, he is telling you the

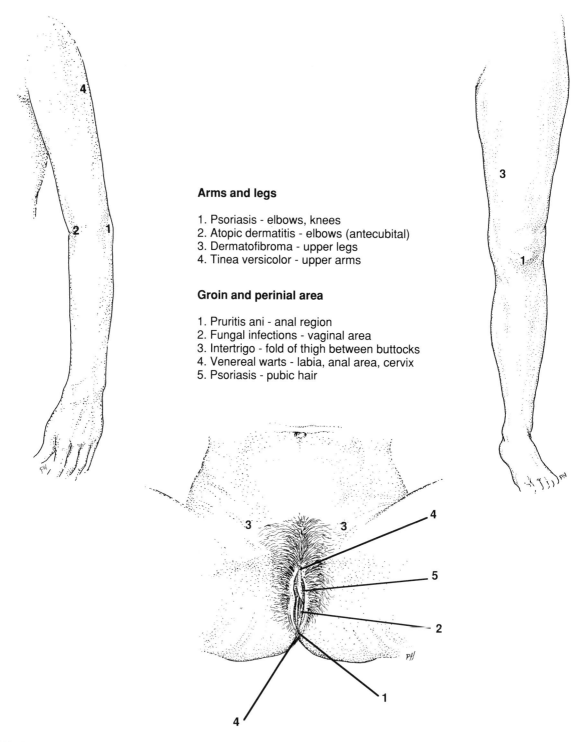

**Arms and legs**

1. Psoriasis - elbows, knees
2. Atopic dermatitis - elbows (antecubital)
3. Dermatofibroma - upper legs
4. Tinea versicolor - upper arms

**Groin and perinial area**

1. Pruritis ani - anal region
2. Fungal infections - vaginal area
3. Intertrigo - fold of thigh between buttocks
4. Venereal warts - labia, anal area, cervix
5. Psoriasis - pubic hair

**FIGURE 6-1** (cont.) Diagnosis of diseases in body regions.

diagnosis." Every medical student has heard this sentence more than once in preclinical years. Learning to take an adequate history is one of the most difficult of all disciplines in medical practice. Many physicians either take too brief or too extensive a history. The tendency of most of us is to arrive at a diagnosis quickly and then ask questions that will support our diagnosis.

At times this can be a foolish and dangerous practice; at other times, as in acute medical or surgical emergencies it is necessary. You learn how to take a history by working with experienced history takers, by reading medical reports and by practicing. For the skin care specialist, the principles are the same as for the budding physican. I have outlined below the essential areas you will need to cover, along with a few notes. Keep in mind that this is only a guide. At the end of the history you must be able to summarize the person's condition in a single paragraph or you have missed the point, and most likely the diagnosis.

### The Lesion

When and where did the lesion appear?
Is there itching?
Has it changed?
How has it changed?
Did anything provoke the lesion?
Was there any previous treatment?

### General History of Illness or Condition

There are many questions that may be asked, but they all relate to the onset, duration, and circumstance of the present condition. For instance, if a client appears in your clinic with a chief complaint of acne, you want to know a great deal about his general state of health as well as the history of his acne. The history of the present illness need not be long. Do a system review in order to relate any systemic condition to the onset of illness, which could influence your treatment program.

### System Review

Eyes, ears, nose, and throat - ask about tearing, redness, pus in the eyes, visual changes, hearing loss, nasal conditions, sore throat, etc.
   **Respiratory** - ask about difficulty in breathing, chest pain, cough, sputum.
   **Cardiovascular** - ask about chest pain, swelling of the feet, high blood pressure.
   **Gastrointestinal** - ask about diet, bowel habits, stools, vomiting, nausea.
   **Endocrine** - ask about history of thyroid disease and diabetes or menstrual problems.
   **Neuromuscular -** ask about painful joints, muscle pain, and tingling or loss of sensation.
   **Genitourinary** - ask about dysuria, frequency of urination, and hematuria (blood in the urine).
   **Psychological** - ask about nervousness, anxiety, depression, fears.

### Past Medical History

At this stage you should begin a survey of past medical history. You will want to know about previous illnesses, operations, allergies, medications, smoking habits, and drinking habits.

### Family History

Married, single, widowed, divorced, children, family diseases, causes of death of deceased members of the family.

### Social History

Occupation, hobbies, travel.

All of this effort may seem like a lot of time and trouble to diagnose acne vulgaris, but experience has taught me that sometimes only one piece of information is needed to arrive at the correct diagnosis. With a detailed medical history you are trying to uncover that important piece of information.

Starting with your knowledge of anatomy and adding skin pathology, you now must acquire a systematic approach to skin evaluation or **diagnosis**. The word diagnosis is from two Greek words: *dia* meaning through and *gnosis* meaning knowledge. You can not diagnose without knowledge of anatomy, pathology, and the clinical picture. As mentioned above, you also need the history of the present illness, past medical history, occupational and social history, and a system review. All of these elements put together allow you to arrive at a conclusion or impression of the person's condition.

### The Examination

Have your client undress, then properly drape them, as partially undressed examinations are difficult and incomplete. Preserve the dignity and modesty of the individual. Your behavior must be professional and your conduct of the examination completely objective. No jokes or sly remarks. Do not talk to yourself or say words that will alarm the person. Be considerate and conscientious.

Provide adequate light. Daylight is best. Avoid fluorescent lighting unless it is color corrected for daylight tones.

Start with the hands. Look at the fingernails, the palms, and the back of the hands. Note color changes and the types and distribution of lesions. Look for sweating palms. (Make allowances for the nervous person.) Many skin care specialists as well as general physicians start with holding and examining the person's hand as it helps to establish a non-threatening contact with the examiner.

Make mental or written notes. With experience you will perform a complete examination without taking written notes except for recording occasional measurements.

Examine the head. Feel the head with your fingers, run them gently down and over the scalp and note any lumps or bumps. Tender areas need to be examined more carefully by spreading the hair. Carefully examine the eyes for pus, blood, swellings, and tearing. Feel the ears as you look for swellings, redness, and lesions, especially on the tops of the ears. Be sure to check the ear canal. Next is the nose. Look for swellings, telangiectasia, large pores, or comedones. Examine the lips and the mouth. Look for ulcerative lesions, vesicles, cracks, or fissures. Have the client open the mouth and look for lesions inside the mouth. Check the corners of the lips for fissures. Stand back and look at the skin in terms of laxity and color. Have the person turn on his/her side and observe the changes in the facial skin. See if it flows or if it is turgid. Run your hand down the sides of the neck and feel for lumps. Do the same for the back of the neck. The front of the neck rarely has any significant dermal lesions but look for any abnormal swelling or redness. Many skin tags appear on the neck. Look at the state of the platysma muscle as this is a cardinal sign of the degree of aging.

The chest and the back should now be examined. I prefer a supine position for the initial examination of the anterior chest. If you are examining a female, observe the nipples for fissures or cracks. Check for acne or abscesses on the breast or hairy areas. You will not need to feel the breasts. What is under the skin will require a physician to diagnose and treat. Look for intertrigo beneath the breasts, especially in obese women or women with pendulant breasts. Examine the chest again in the sitting position and then examine the back. At this point have the person stand so that you may examine the buttocks. Look for lax skin in this area. It is a sign of advanced aging.

Finally, examine the arms, the legs, and the feet. Do not neglect the soles of the feet, particularly the spaces between the toes. Fungal infections and plantar warts are two common disorders in this area. If the person you are examining is diabetic, take particular notice of the condition of the feet.

**Simple Diagnostic Tools**

The **diascope** is used to distinguish between red lesions caused by dilated blood vessels, leaking blood, or pigment. A diascope can be prepared using a microscopic slide and a 3X magnifying lens. If you press the slide against a red lesion and the color disappears, this indicates that the blood vessels have collapsed and you are dealing with an inflammatory lesion, or a noninflammatory vascular lesion (such as telangiectasia). If it does not disappear, the blood has leaked into the tissue. Lesions with color due to pigment will not change with the pressure of the slide. If you press the slide against a papule and it does not disappear, you know that the papule is most likely a dense accumulation of cells. It takes experience, but you will find this tool useful.

The Wood's Light emits ultraviolet light at wavelengths of 320 to 400 nm. Fungi infections such as Microsporum or P. orbiculare can be detected with this light. Certain disorders of pigmentation may be separated and identified with this light. Pigmented cells in the epidermis become more intense under Wood's light. Dermal cells that contain pigment do not change. Vitiligo, or loss of pigmentation is seen as white skin under Wood's light.

We are now ready to look at the most common skin conditions seen in otherwise normal people. Since the skin care specialist will deal mostly with well people, we need to study these conditions. The dermatologist, however, deals with sick skin and sick people.

**DISORDERS OF THE SEBACEOUS GLANDS**

**Acne vulgaris** is so common that some physicians consider it a physiological response to hormones at puberty. The onset is usually at puberty for boys, though in girls it may precede puberty by as much as two years. Let me describe the clinical picture. Acne starts with comedones, then progresses to papules and pustules. In an acute flare-up all three lesions may be present. The face, back, chest, and shoulders are the most commonly affected sites. The comedones may be present as open blackheads which are flat. The black color is believed to be due to melanin in the keratinocytes. The closed comedones, or whiteheads, have a slight papular appearance and are the major source of inflammatory lesions. These inflammations may be quite large. They extend down to the dermis producing scar tissue on healing. The typical acne scar is a punched-out pit.

**Acne rosacea** has vascularity as well as acne lesions. The age of onset is between 30 and 50 years of age. It is more common in women, but more severe in men. The darker pigmented races rarely have acne rosacea. The vascular component (blotchy and diffuse erythema) appears first in the central part of the face that comes and goes but eventually stays. Telangiectasia appears and is followed by acne lesions. Comedones are not usually found and cysts and scars are rare. This helps to distinguish it from acne vulgaris. Long standing rosacea can result in an irregular, lobulated, bulbous enlargement of the nose known as **rhinophyma**. It is believed by some that vasodilating agents such as alcohol exacerbate this condition, thus the term "**whiskey drinker's nose**". There appears to be an abnormal flushing type reaction associated with rosacea causing the face to become dusky red, a condition called **erythrosis**.

**Seborrheic dermatitis** is seen in the scalp, face, chest, and back. There is a scaly, erythematous eruption present without papules or pustules. It occurs in infants as "**cradle cap**" in severe cases. It next appears after puberty and can continue for a lifetime. The cardinal sign is a greasy, scaly erythema of the face. The most common cause of the red butterfly lesion on the face is seborrheic dermatitis.

## HYPERPROLIFERATIVE DISORDERS

We spoke of hyperproliferative disorders in our discussion of skin pathology. They are characterized by an increased rate of cell growth, or

the opposite, a decreased shedding of cells from the stratum corneum.

One of the most common skin disorders seen by the dermatologist is **psoriasis**. This skin disorder occurs in 1 to 2 percent of the population, in the United States alone. This means that nearly one in fifty (1 out of 50) can have this disorder. It is known that psoriasis is a genetically determined disease with an onset in childhood or early adulthood, though the pattern of inheritance is unknown. The course of psoriasis is unpredictable in that it may remain localized to a few areas or spread rapidly to become generalized. The lesions in psoriasis are elevated, erythematous, scaly, sharply demarcated plaques. The knees, elbows, scalp, and trunk seem to have a predilection to psoriasis. Oddly, **pruritis** is not a major problem. It occurs in only one-fifth of the people having this disorder. This is interesting in that the word psoriasis comes from the Greek *psora*, which means itch . While the scales appear to be unusually thick, they are made up of loosely stacked cells which flake off fairly easily. Nail involvement is not uncommon. The periunguinal area may show marked involvement. Remember that this is a chronic disease for which there is a treatment but no cure.

**Keratosis pilaris** is characterized by a fine papular involvement of the hair follicle openings. It is scattered irregularly over the upper arms and thighs. The skin feels rough to the touch. The condition is noninflammatory. It occurs more commonly in dry climates and can last for many years.

**Solar or senile keratosis** is characterized by warty lesions that are premalignant. As the name implies, these lesions occur on sun exposed skin of the face and hands in aged individuals.

**Ichthyosis (fish skin)** is really the name for a group of diseases, all characterized by an accumulation of stratum corneum scales. These are genetic disorders that have no known cause and can affect one in three hundred (1 in 300), as **ichthyosis vulgari**. The disease starts as small, white scales on the extensor surfaces of the extremities and spreads to the trunk, forehead, cheeks, and scalp. The creases of the arms are usually spared but the palms are frequently markedly involved. One often finds keratosis pilaris along with the ichthyosis. Both conditions become worse in cold, dry weather and improve in the summer. Ichthyosis in the newborn is most commonly seen as the **collodion baby**. The child is encased in a transparent parchment-like membrane which breaks up and peels off in about two weeks. This is relatively rare and is mentioned for those of you who will become associated with hospitals.

**Epidermolysis hyperkeratosis** occurs shortly after birth. It is frequently localized but can become general in distribution. The lesions are dark in color and often give off an unpleasant odor. The palms and soles are frequently involved.

**Dermatofibrosis** is characterized by slowly growing, benign skin nodules (dermatofibromas) consisting of cellular fibrous tissue surrounding collapsed capillaries.

**Darier's disease** is characterized by small, firm papules scattered over the flexor surfaces of the extremities, the trunk, and the face. There is no specific pattern and the condition is without symptoms. Lesions are usually pink to flesh colored. They coalesce into plaques and assume a tan to brown color with a greasy appearance. A distinguishing feature of this disease is that the nails and mouth might become involved.
**Reiter's syndrome** is not uncommon. This syndrome is characterized by urethritis, conjunctivitis, arthritis, and ulcerative skin manifestations. These manifestations are hyperkeratotic plaques of the scalp or extremities. Scattered pustules and scaling lesions of the palms and soles may be present. While the cause is unknown, many cases appear to be acquired sexually.

## ECZEMATOUS DERMATITIS CLASSIFIED DISORDERS

**Atopic dermatitis** is an allergic disorder. There is usually a history of allergies in the family of the client with atopic dermatitis. This disease is characterized by an early erythema and edema that may progress to vesiculation and oozing followed by crusts and scaling. This is frequently followed by lichenification, often with hyper- or hypopigmentation. The pruritis that accompanies this disorder often leads to excoriations from scratching. Look for the following features in the atopic individual:

1. An increased number of markings on the palms with cross-hatched lines.
2. A line under the margin of the lids of both eyes (**Dennie's line**).
3. The skin is dry and blanches easily when scratched with a nail (**white dermatographism**).
4. There is some indication that sweat and sebum production are reduced.
5. The itch threshold is low and many things can produce itching, such as heat, cold, low humidity, exercise, friction, foods, allergens, soaps, or tension.

Clinical findings are quite variable from mild, slightly involved to severe, generalized involvement. The condition is seen most commonly in male children and female adults. In infants the lesions appear first on the face and the scalp at about three months and then spread to the extremities. In older children or adults the disease starts on the flexor surface of the neck, the antecubital fossa, and the popliteal space. One of the cardinal features of the disorder is the waxing and waning of involvement. You must look for complications from contact dermatitis and infection. There is a hypersensitivity to topical agents. Atopic individuals are usually tense, aggressive, and resentful. This is a life long disease without cure and it is not easy to adjust to.

**Nummular eczema (coin-shaped eczema)** is characterized by typical round patches located on the buttocks, legs, extensor surface of the arms, and the dorsum of the hands. It is chronic and attended with intense itching. The cause is unknown.

**Phompholox (dyshidrotic eczema)** is relatively common. It is helpful to remember that the term phompholox is from the Greek word for bubble. The clinical picture is one of vesicular eruption of the palms and soles with intense itching. The condition is recurrent, noninflammatory, and is not associated with the sweat ducts. The cause is unknown.

**Hand eczema** is nothing more than eczema of the hands. It looks so awful, however, that it is given special attention. The dorsum of the hand is usually involved first, followed by the fingers, and then the palms. The condition is usually most severe, showing cracks, fissures, edema, erythema, vesiculation, weeping, crusting, and scratch markings. There are many causes of hand eczema. The most common are low relative humidity, irritants, and frequent hand washing. Look for this disorder in housewives, cooks, bartenders, nurses, nurses' aids, and occasionally doctors.

**Neurodermatitis (lichen simplex chronicus)** is a disorder resulting from frequent scratching or rubbing of the skin. It begins with pruritis followed by scratching. The scratching is characteristic. Look at the areas which can easily be reached by the hands. The most common sites are the nape of the neck in women, and the outside lower leg in men. The lesion appears as a circumscribed area of lichenified plaques with or without scales or hypopigmentation. This disorder is cured by removing the irritation process. These individuals are often resentful and angry and are not easy to treat.

## DISORDERS OF THE SWEAT GLANDS (MILIARIA)

When sweat cannot flow to the surface of the skin, the sweat is retained in the sweat duct and a condition known as miliaria results. This word comes from the Latin *milium* which means millet, a type of grain.

Various manifestations are produced based on the level of the obstruction. The types most commonly seen are **miliaria crystallina** which occurs with obstruction of the duct in the stratum corneum. A group of small vesicles appear on the skin. There is no inflammation and no treatment is required.

**Miliaria rubra** is commonly called **prickly heat**. This occurs with a deeper obstruction, at the level of the epidermis. This lesion may appear as an erythematous papule or vesicle. Examination of the lesion with a 3x power lens will reveal no hair follicles at the site of the lesion. The erythema comes from vasodilation in the upper dermis. These lesions sting and burn. They become worse with sweating.

When pustules are present the name changes to **miliaria pustulosa**. The disease is the same except for leukocyte infiltration into the papules and papulovesicles.

**Miliaria profunda** occurs when the duct is obstructed deep in the dermis. There is no inflammation and there are no symptoms. This disease is marked by the absence of sweating. It is of concern because of the necessity to regulate heat.

Miliaria occurs when the weather is hot and humid, if the skin is occluded, injured, infected, or sunburned. Damage to the sweat ducts is the usual cause. Treatment is usually concerned with removing the causative environment.

## DISORDERS OF PIGMENTATION

As we studied the biochemistry of melanin, we noted that this important biochemical is not well understood. Many substances can promote or retard the appearance of melanin. We shall look at a few disorders now, but we will reserve our discussion of the serious condition, melanoma, for later in our discussion of neoplastic diseases.

**Melasma (chloasma** and also **mask of pregnancy)** is a hyperpigmentation of the cheeks and forehead characterized by patchy, tan or brown, macular lesions. This condition is seen in women who are pregnant or taking birth control pills. It is more prominent in the darker skinned individual. Exposure to the sun will increase the melanization. There are no symptoms. The hyperpigmentation may be permanent or it may disappear and reappear with subsequent pregnancies or contraceptive usage.

**Cafe au lait** macules are well-circumscribed pale brown macules. They can be from 2 to 20 cm. Generally they appear at birth or soon after, and tend to disappear with age. Cafe au lait macules are themselves common and benign; occasionally, however, they may be indicative of systemic disease.

**Vitiligo** is hypopigmentation of the skin in localized areas. This is a genetic disease of no known cause. The skin shows no melanocytes in the involved area. Vitiligo is seen most often in patients with hyperthyroid disease, pernicious anemia, diabetes, and diseases of the adrenal glands. The treatment is cosmetic. This is a serious social disease. It has profound effects on both men and women. You can do considerable service to these clients by applying corrective make-up skills and providing personal support.

**Tinea versicolor**, a fungus infection by P. orbiculare, can cause hyper- or hypopigmentation of the skin. It is characterized by finely desquammating, pale, tan colored patches on the trunk and upper arms. These patches do not tan. In dark skinned individuals there may be a lessening of pigmentation in the affected area. The fungus fluoresces under Wood's lamp. Scrapings may be easily identified under a microscope. Treatment usually consists of cleaning the infected area and applying selenium sulfide. This disorder is quite common. Discoloration can last up to a year after the fungus has been removed. Recurrence is also common.

## OTHER BENIGN DISORDERS THAT YOU WILL SEE

**Lichen planus** is an itchy inflammation of the skin that occurs on the flexor surface of the wrists, the ankles, the knees, the mouth, and the glans penis. The lesions on the skin appear as flat, purplish papules or plaques having gray lines on the surface. Their shape can be rather odd, in that they are polygons which may be discrete or confluent. In the mucous membranes the lesions are quite tiny and are often covered with lacey, white lines. Curiously, this disorder is seen around the mouth in transplant patients. It is also seen in patients with liver disease (eg. biliary cirrhosis and hepatitis). Often drugs will produce lichen planus type eruptions (eg. anti-diabetics, heavy metals, phenothiazine, diuretics, beta blockers). Some have suggested that this disease may be an immune response disorder secondary to antigens on the skin.

**Pityriasis rosea** is an acute, self-limiting, annulo-squamous eruption occurring on the trunk and the proximal extremities. The history is the key to recognizing this disease. It occurs usually before the age of 35. Generally, a large (1 to 5 centimeters) erythematous disc (**herald patch**) appears on the chest. This is followed by the appearance of many satellite lesions after 7 to 10 days. These lesions are pink and scaly. The scales start in the center of the lesions. The disease lasts about 6 to 8 weeks. It can spread anywhere on the skin. In my experience the worst cases are seen in nurses, doctor's wives, and strip tease artists. The individual is usually alarmed. The disorder must be distinguished from other more serious disorders such as psoriasis, drug eruptions, and secondary syphillis. It is apparently not contagious, and its cause is unknown.

## SERIOUS OR LIFE THREATENING CONDITIONS

Every skin care specialist must be familiar with the signs and symptoms of life threatening skin conditions. Recognition of these disorders is an essential part of your training.

**Signs** are any objective evidence of disease. This could be any objective finding by an examiner such as a fever, rash, sound in the chest.

**Symptoms** are any functional evidence of disease usually as perceived by the patient, such as pain. **Primary symptoms** are associated with the disease process while **secondary symptoms** are caused by the disease process.

**Syndrome** is a collection of signs and symptoms which indicate a particular disease.

Often you will see "sign" used for "symptom" in the medical literature.

We will examine a few of the more serious conditions so that you will be alerted to their existence and the need for referral.

## SKIN MANIFESTATIONS OF SYSTEMIC DISEASES

Dry skin (**xerosis**) is generally a benign disease of the elderly, but it may also be an early sign of hypothyroidism, sarcoidosis lymphoma, or essential fatty acid deficiency.

**Pruritis** (**itching**) can be associated with many systemic diseases (eg. drugs, biliary obstruction, kidney failure, pregnancy, blood disorders, malabsorption syndrome, or psychiatric problems).

**Hives** (**urticaria**) can be associated with a few serious disorders, but in general it is allergic in nature either to foods or drugs. If it persists for over 6 weeks, chances are it is psychogenic in nature.

**Alopecia** (**hair loss**) is a frequent sequela of pregnancy or the use of cytotoxic drugs such as in cancer chemotherapy. Many other conditions such as thyroid diseases and connective tissue diseases can also contribute to alopecia.

**Purpura** (**skin hemorrhage**) is often associated with primary blood disorders frequently induced by drugs. Any purpuritic finding deserves referral to a physician.

**Painful red nodules** (**erythema nodosum**) are seen in disorders of the intestinal tract, such as ulcerative colitis. A condition known as Crohn's disease is associated with ulcers in the mouth, erythema, and edema in the anus, and nodules on the skin.

**Xanthomas** are yellow nodules or plaques composed of lipoproteins deposited in skin, subcutaneous tissue and tendons. It is almost always indicative of vascular disease (high cholesterol). Xanthelasma is xanthomas on the eyelid.

**Connective tissue diseases** are seen most frequently in women. These disorders are believed to be autoimmune in origin and are characterized by skin manifestations. The major involvement is elastin and collagen. The skin is often hard and shiny. The major disorders are:

**Systemic lupus erythematosis** (SLE) usually presents as a discoidal lesion on the skin. The butterfly lesion on the face is often an early sign but only in a third of the clients. There may be both macules and papules present along with purpuric areas that may resemble a drug eruption.Ulcers of the fingertips and telangiectasia under the nails is not infrequent. Four times more women than men have this disease.

**Dermatomyositis** is characterized by inflammation of the muscles and a dermatitis of a variable nature (usually pruritic or eczematous inflammation of the skin). A finding that is fairly consistent and often diagnostic of the disease is edema of the eyes attended with a purple to red discoloration of the upper lids. A scaly, macular erythema of the knuckles may be present. The disorder appears similar to SLE except for the painful muscles. The syndrome without the skin manifestations is called **polymyositis**. In children the disease may be self limiting.

**Scleroderma** is characterized by shiny, tight, leathery, hard skin frequently seen on the hands and the face. It can progress to involve all connective tissues including those of the internal organs. This is called **systemic progressive sclerosis** and, fortunately, is relatively rare. **Morphea** (**Addison's keloid**) is a form of localized scleroderma, which while uncommon, is seen more frequently than systemic progressive sclerosis. Women are afflicted three times more often than men. Onset is within the second to fifth decades. The lesion appears as a circumscribed, hard plaque with an ivory center and a surrounding violaceous halo. There may be a lack of both hair and sweating in the plaque area. The presence of the violaceous border indicates an active lesion.

## MALIGNANT NEOPLASIAS - CANCERS OF THE SKIN

The term **neoplasia** means "new growth".

It applies to both **benign** and **malignant** tumors. **Cancer**, however, only applies to malignant neoplasias. Cancers that spread are difficult to treat and frequently lead to the death of the client. The spread of a tumor is called **metastasis**, which means it has gone beyond the original site. This may be by direct spread or by cells breaking off of the original tumor and floating in the blood or lymph to new sites where they continue to grow. The cancerous cell has escaped the normal growth regulatory mechanism of the body and has circumvented the immune system of the body. As a result it is free to grow throughout the body, wrecking havoc on the essential organs as it spreads. When a tumor is localized to one area it may be surgically removed or treated with radiation, thereby affecting a cure. Metastatic cancer, however, requires far more drastic treatment.

### Squamous Cell Carcinoma

**Squamous cell carcinoma** arises from the **prickle layer** (**stratum spinosum**) of the skin. It has the ability to grow rapidly and to spread. The incidence is 12 per 100,000 for men and 6.7 per 100,000 for women. There are many causes, but sunlight, chemicals, chronic sores, and scars are among the more common. The lesion is variable, but look for a hard nodule with indistinct borders. There may be some scaling or ulceration. As the lesion develops, it becomes more firm and affixed to the dermis. Rolled edges of normal epidermis with a central area of ulceration and vegetative growth may be seen, but scaly, abnormal keratinization is more common. These lesions must be referred to a physician. Look for these lesions on sun-damaged areas of the hands, neck, face, and legs. Scars and chronic ulcers can also give rise to these lesions.

### Basal Cell Carcinoma

**Basal carcinomas** arise in the basal layer of the epidermis. They are probably the most frequent of all cancerous tumors and certainly the most common skin cancer. These tumors grow slowly and rarely metastasize. They do, however, invade deeper tissue and bone. They are most common in fair skinned individuals who work in the sun, and in the elderly. The tumor is described as a **noduloulcerative** lesion that starts as a slowly enlarging papule. The papule grows and the borders become "pearly" appearing like ground glass. The center begins to erode. This is the so called "rodent ulcer" appearance. Telangiectasia is present and the skin markings are erased by the tight, smoothing action of the tumor. The tumor's appearance is fairly characteristic, but the wide variety of lesions and their destructive nature requires a histological examination for diagnosis. Look for these lesions on skin that has been sun exposed. THE RULE IS REFERRAL TO A PHYSICIAN IF THERE IS THE SLIGHTEST SUSPICION OF A SKIN CANCER.

### Malignant Melanoma

**Melanoma** arises from melanocytes. Malignant melanoma is a cancerous lesion that has a relatively high potential for invasion and metastasization. The tumor occurs frequently on sun exposed areas, but it can occur anywhere on the body, including the eyes. While it is rare before puberty, it can occur anytime in life. In the USA, the incidence of malignant melanoma is rising. In whites, both males and females are affected equally. In blacks ,the incidence is 6 to 7 times less frequent. The incidence in orientals falls somewhere between the other two. The distribution also differs among the races. In whites, the lesions may be spread over the body. In blacks and orientals, the lesions are mainly found on the palms, soles, the nail beds, and the mucous membranes. In whites, there is also a sexual difference in the distribution. Males have more lesions on the back, while females have more lesions on the lower legs. There is a definite relationship of incidence of melanoma to sun exposure. The classic findings are:
1. Variegation of color. Look for brown and tan but also blue, red, white mixture half tones of pink, purple, and gray.
2. Irregularity of the border. Look for notches and decrease of skin mark. See if a satellite lesion is present.
3. Irregular surface. Look for uneven elevations, loss of markings, irregular topography.

Some of the precancerous lesions associated with malignant melanoma are:

**Lentigo maligna** is a flat, pigmented lesion occurring almost exclusively on the sun exposed skin in the elderly person with actinic damage. It begins as a tan, freckle-like lesion of irregular shape on the head, neck, or upper extremities. They usually appear late in life (fifth to sixth decade). The pattern and pigmentation are irregular. Only about 5 percent develop into melanoma.

**Congenital melanocytic nevi** occur at birth. They may be quite large, covering a large area such as the arms, buttocks, or trunk. They may be raised and may contain papillomatous projections and hair. The color may vary from brown to black. The presence of a congenital nevus of this type increases the risk of melanoma.

**Dysplastic melanocytic nevi** have irregular borders, variegated color (usually shades of brown, red, and flesh tones), and a flat to slightly raised surface. They are relatively rare, having an incidence of only 1 to 8 percent in white postpuberty individuals. Compare this to the incidence of nevocellular nevi in the same group (75 to 80 percent). THESE LESIONS SHOULD BE REFERRED TO A PHYSICIAN.

### AGING SKIN

This subject has recently aroused a great deal of interest, since the reported reversal of wrinkled skin by retinoic acid. This is considered a significant breakthrough in the treatment of aging skin, even though it may not be the final answer. The diagnosis of aging skin is not difficult in the later stages, but in the early stages it is easy to overlook the subtle changes that are taking place. There is a large difference between **chronological age** and **physiological age** in most individuals. It is important to know the physiological age of the client in order to provide proper care. I have arrived at the following scheme based on my own clinical experience (see **Figure 6-2**). In this scheme I group aging signs by periods of years.

### Stage One (10 to 20 years)

HISTORY - Puberty occurs earlier in females than in males. Early onset of menses can indicate a tendency for a faster aging rate. A history of severe prolonged illness will leave signs of debilitation and wear. A congenital

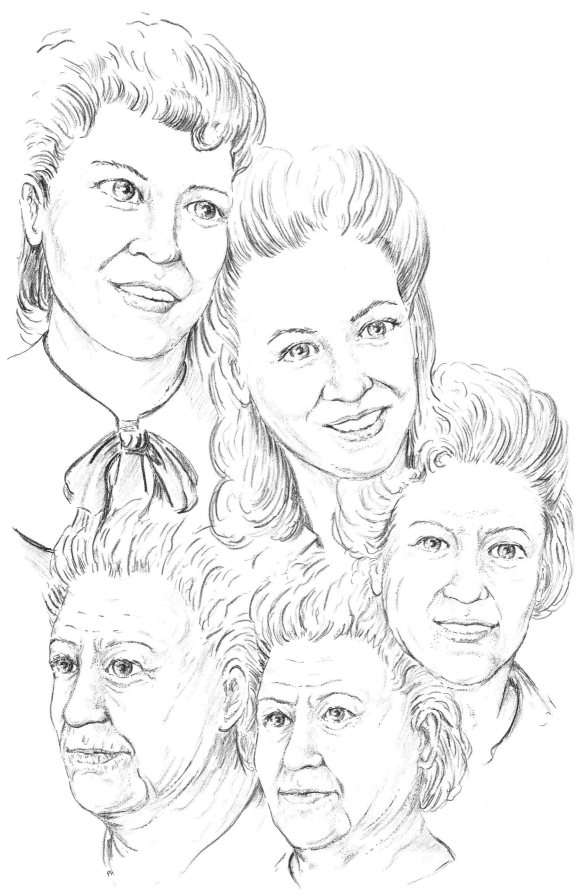

**FIGURE 6-2** The Stages of aging. Aging occurs in some individuals in a subtle manner. Look for the lines around the eyes, mouth, and neck for early signs. If you see vertical lines around the mouth in a person under thirty this is an indication of dermal destruction.

metabolic disease such as juvenile diabetes will produce subtle changes in the skin. Orphans, runaways, abandoned chidren, and physically or sexually abused children will all exhibit signs of stress related damage in their skin. Smoking, drinking, and illegal drugs will have severe adverse effects on the skin. The sunbather, the skier, and the beach bum will all show early signs of skin damage.

PHYSICAL FINDINGS - The face will show both changes in color and tone as well as in visible lesions. Look first at the mouth. Ask the person to purse their lips. Examine the mouth area with a 3 power lens. Look for small linear wrinkles running perpendicular to the orbicularis oris. Also look at the nasal labial folds and under the columella for similar wrinkles. Next examine the eyes, particularly the outer canthus and lower lid. Fair skin and blue eyes are an indication of a potential for faster aging. Look for freckles and telangectasia on the face. Examine the neck and the platysma muscle for the appearance of "drooping chin" and linear markings. Look for any congenital pigmented lesions. Look at the hair. Gray hair at this age is very rare and would not portent well for the individual as graying is a consistent sign of aging. Thin hair is also associated with aging, but it is not a reliable sign. Finally, look at the general deportment of the posture and the psychological attitude of the client, remembering that some people think old. Examination with a UV lamp will show hidden damage as a deeper pigmentation scattered over the face and fine wrinkles around the mouth, nose, and under the eyes. Average findings in this age are a few pigmented lesions, a few lines at the outer canthus in the 18 to 20 year olds and in avid sunbathers. There will also be fine mouth-area wrinkles in this age group. The skin should be smooth and firm with good snap and no drooping.

**Stage Two - Ages 21 to 35 Years**

At this period of life many changes have already taken place. Heredity and environmental effects are more apparent. It is significant that the period of 30 to 35 years of age was the upper limit of life for mankind for many hundred thousands of years. It is at this period that changes in the connective tissue are manifested by visible skin changes. Let us look at the po-

tential findings in the twenties age group. The changes are subtle and related mainly to the face,the neck, the and hands. You will not see these changes in a person who does not smoke or whose alcohol consumption is low. Fine lines in the skin and decreased "spring back" in pinched skin can be noted. Color changes may be noticed as mottled areas of pigmentation on the face. The "**smokers line**" may be visible as a pronounced increase in the nasolabial crease.At thirty-five look for laxity of the skin under the chin with small wrinkles about the mouth and eyes. Tiny crow's feet are present. All these signs will be exaggerated in smokers, drinkers, and sunbathers. The hands will show some early thinning in sunbathers and women with heavy exposure to detergents and water. Males with outdoor occupations will show increased pigmentation on the hands. Some gray hair may be present.

**Stage Three - Ages 36 to 50**

From the age of thirty-six to fifty are the worrisome years for both men and women , but more so for women. The major change is the laxity of the skin. At forty, the nasolabial fold is deeper, the forehead shows wrinkles that are moderate, the mouth creases are more evident, the neck skin shows more sagging, the platysma muscle begins to lose tone, and the subcutaneous fat decreases. In men, eyes show fat protrusion and crow's feet with wrinkles under the eyes. At forty-five things continue to get more loose and lax. The chin sags, the cheeks sag, the lower lids get more baggy, thc crow's fcct become worse, the mouth lines are accentuated. Lipstick "runs" are a big problem. The hands begin to thin and show more bone and less soft flesh. In males the baggy eyes are more advanced, the crow's feet increased, and the cheeks continue to sag.

**Stage Four - Ages 50 to 65**

I call this period the fixation period, because it is a time of physical and mental change that can result in a permanent "old age attitude" and appearance. Look for the bony changes in women and the early dowager's hump that begins to appear due to a lack of the female hormone, estrogen. Now the cheek bones become

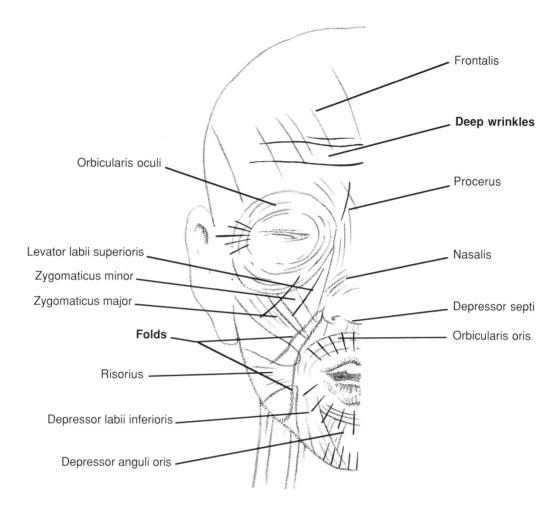

Frontalis

**Deep wrinkles**

Orbicularis oculi

Procerus

Nasalis

Levator labii superioris

Zygomaticus minor

Zygomaticus major

Depressor septi

Orbicularis oris

**Folds**

Risorius

Depressor labii inferioris

Depressor anguli oris

**FIGURE 6-3** Facial wrinkles. Front. Notice the directions of the wrinkles. They occur over the muscles in a perpendicular line to the long axis of the muscle; smiles and frowns will make the lines deeper and larger.

more noticeable as the skin sags and the fatty tissue atrophies. The neck assumes a hatched pattern, with deep vertical folds and horizontal lines. The sternocleidomastoid muscle becomes more prominent giving rise to the "cords" in the neck. In males the same changes are present, but usually to a lesser degree. At age sixty there is a still greater "retraction" of the skin as the bony skull becomes more visible. The jowls become prominent and the nose appears longer. Many folds appear in the neck. The eyes show a heavy-lidded effect with extra loose skin folding over the lids. At sixty-five, the resorption of bone makes the head appear smaller and the nose to appear even longer. The skin is in complete disarray as the folds increase due to a greater laxity of the skin. At this time the "turkey neck" appears. In males this is also present, again to a lesser degree. The hair is gray in many individu-

als and coarse facial hair appears on women. Sebaceous glands on the nose and forehead become more prominent, resulting in more noticeable pores. Comedones may be seen anywhere on the face, but particularly about the outer canthus of the eye.

### The Fifth Stage - Ages 66 and Older (The Period of Resignation and/or Adjustment)

The years after age 65 are only now becoming the subject of more serious study. Thirty years ago, the amount of research on aging skin was quite limited, but it has grown steadily since then. By age seventy the skin shows creases in all directions vertical, horizontal, and oblique. Deep wrinkles and creases are mainly in the direction which is transverse to the long axis of

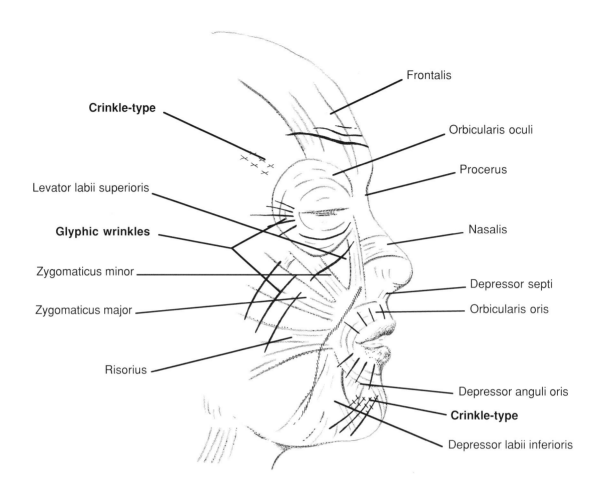

Crinkle-type

Levator labii superioris

Glyphic wrinkles

Zygomaticus minor

Zygomaticus major

Risorius

Frontalis

Orbicularis oculi

Procerus

Nasalis

Depressor septi

Orbicularis oris

Depressor anguli oris

Crinkle-type

Depressor labii inferioris

**FIGURE 6-3** (cont.) Facial wrinkles. Side. Crinkle-type wrinkle- fine wrinkles formed from folded skin. Usually seen in persons 75 years and older and in sun damaged individuals with post-inflammatory changes in the skin called elastosis. Glyphic wrinkle - has a crisscross pattern and is frequently seen on the cheeks and neck. Deep wrinkle - forms a major line or deep groove that is long and straight. This is the most troublesome wrinkle because it is so visible and so difficult to eliminate.

the facial muscles. The appearance of crow's feet at the outer canthus of the eye is an example of an oblique crease, however, the rule of transverseness to a long muscle holds, as the orbicularis oculi is a circular muscle (see **Figure 6-3**). Vertical wrinkles are seen between the the eyelids and the eyebrows, with a deep vertical crease appearing in front of the ear. A major crease is seen at the angle of the mouth and the nasolabial fold, extending at times down to the chin. Knowing the anatomy of the facial muscles will help you to appreciate these changes.

The lips show further thinning, almost receding into the interior of the mouth, and many small, fine vertical lines appear on the lips. Lipstick now "feathers", causing embarrassment and dismay. The hair is usually gray to white, and thin. The skull is smaller with prominent

ears and nose. Coarse facial hair appears more often.

Fortunately, not all individuals age uniformly. Great variation is observed. Many of the signs listed above are absent in individuals who have attained the age of ninety. It is, therefore, important to determine both the chronological and the physiological age of an individual.

The above physical features must be viewed with other conditions that one frequently observes in an aging population. The most common conditions are:

1. Benign and malignant tumors
2. Dermatophytoses
3. Seborrheic dermatitis
4. Disorders of the sebaceous glands
5. Seborrheic keratosis
6. Contact dermatitis

7. Atopic eczema
8. Vitiligo

These conditions should be considered as part of the total picture in the evaluation of the client. All too often we tend to see each condition as a separate entity divorced from the total person. When care is given in this manner it is fragmented and less effective. One of the major forces that has evolved in non-medical professional skin care is the **holistic approach** to the client. This is a strong point and should not be played down.

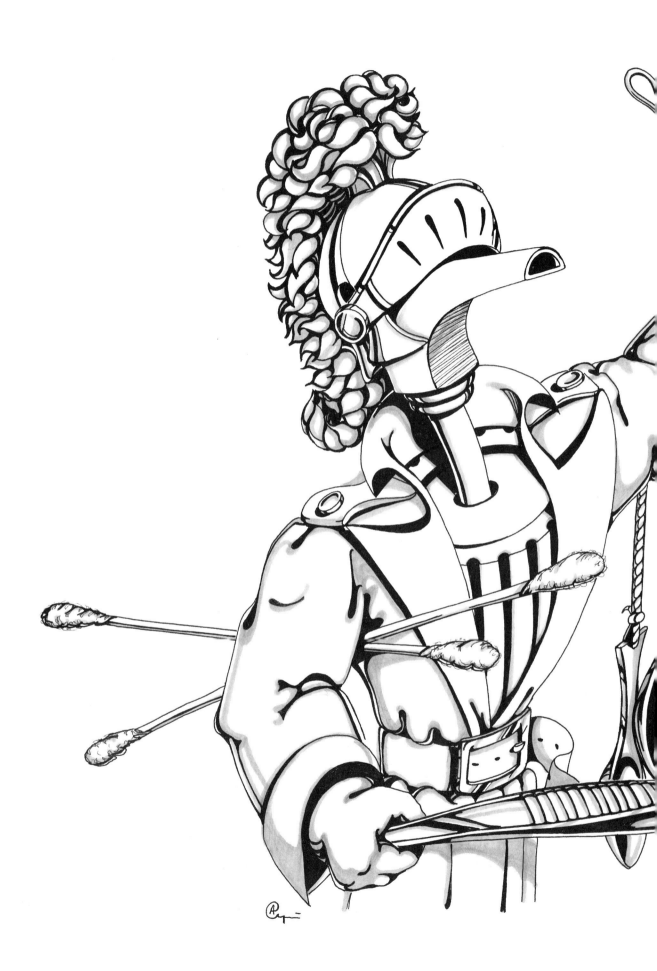

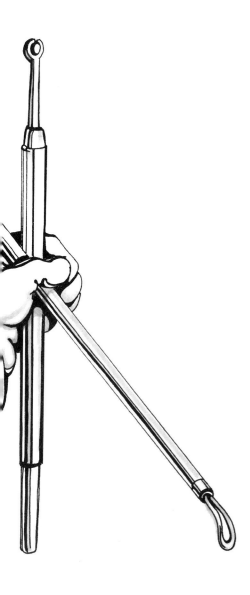

Like I told you before, Gramps and Dad did their bit to preserve the Wall with patching and painting, because that's all they could do. We know what this place is made of now, and my job is to dive in a little deeper and try to restructure the mess inside, before the cracks start happening. Smooth as I am, though, I know even I may need the assistance of another pair of hands.

# Physical Modalities

This chapter will review basic principles of physics and introduce the student to new concepts. The purpose of this chapter is to provide information permitting the skin care specialist to understand the underlying principles behind instruments and what can be expected from the use of physical modalities. There are some tough concepts in this chapter, many new terms, and some mathematics. Advanced mathematics is not needed to understand this chapter and anyone with high school algebra should have no problem.

We shall cover four basic modalities: heat, pressure, electricity, and electromagnetic energy. Some methods use a combination of two or more of these modalities. For instance, massage with wrapping uses heat and pressure.

Specific application of these treatment modalities is reserved for the chapters on treatment of specific conditions.

## HEAT

The use of heat in the treatment of diseases is as old as antiquity. Hot springs and hot mud have been used from the earliest days of man.

Homer wrote in 1000 B.C. of the medicinal use of hot baths but it wasn't until 1840 that the first serious medical article appeared. Since then many articles have been written which establish the use of heat as a therapeutic modality. This science is called **thermotherapy**.

### Basic Physics of Heat

On first impression **heat** and **temperature** are often considered the same things, that is, they are identical quantities. Unfortunately, this is not the case, each is a separate measurement. The unit used to measure heat is the **calorie**. The calorie is the amount of heat required to raise one gram of water one degree Centigrade. Temperature is defined as the total translational kinetic energy of individual molecules. Heat measures the total quantity of energy in a given mass of material while temperature measures the quantity per molecule. Here is an example. To heat a cup of water for tea to 100 degrees Celsius takes a lot less heat than it would to heat a bath tub full of water to the same temperature. They are both at the same temperature but the tub of water contains a lot more heat than the cup of tea. Heating a little house is less expensive than heating a big house, as everyone knows. The study of heat transfer and work is the science of **thermodynamics**. In living tissue it is difficult to apply strict thermodynamic laws. In living systems there are many irreversible reactions that occur at certain rates. For example, you burn up food and the food changes to other products giving off energy as heat. This is an irreversible reaction as the original food is gone forever. The rate of these reactions is extremely interesting to scientists who study energy relations in biological systems. I have included this topic in our discussion on heat since it is a very basic concept. When you study a biological reaction system as a function of temperature you have a very nice method of quantifying the reaction system.

**Some Thermal Properties of Tissues**

Two additional terms necessary to understand the relationship between heat and living skin are **specific heat** and **thermal conductivity**. Specific heat is the amount of heat in calories necessary to raise the temperature of one

gram of material one degree Celsius (from 15 to 16 degrees C.) Thermal conductivity is the transfer of energy by the interaction of molecules. Thermal conductivity is measured in millicalories/centimeter/second/degree C. When you measure the conductivity of a material you are measuring the behavior of the material which comprises the conducting layer. You can relate the thermal conductivity of the skin to blood flow in the skin. For example, the blood flow in skin is 1 microliter/square centimeter/second which produces a thermal conductivity of 3.5 millicalories/centimeter/second/degree C. The amount of water and fat in a tissue greatly affects the thermal conductivity and the specific heat of that tissue. The thermal conductivity of skin is changed by moisture and fat content. Now let us look at skin temperature and see how all this fits together.

**SKIN TEMPERATURE**

The temperature of the skin under normal conditions is usually 3 to 5 degrees lower than the interior body, or **core temperature**. The skin temperature varies by region due to the amount of blood circulation and thickness of the skin. The forehead skin may show a temperature of 33 degrees C while the big toe will show only 30 degrees C, provided the room temperature is 22.8 degrees C and the rectal temperature is 37.25 degrees C (rectal temperature is the core temperature). The body loses about 60% of its heat by **radiation** (infrared radiation). These infrared waves average about 9 microns long and can be seen by infrared detectors. Some snakes detect warm blooded animals in this manner.

Skin temperature is regulated by blood flow since the body heat is brought to the skin surface by the blood and then transferred to the environment. As the environmental heat increases the blood flow increases. This is the basic principle of using heat for therapy. Blood flow alone can compensate for the increase in skin temperature by the **heat radiation mechanism** in an environmental temperature up to 31 degrees C, but beyond that temperature the mechanism of **evaporative heat loss** must come into play.

Evaporative heat loss is based on the use of body heat to change liquid water into water vapor. It requires 580 calories to evaporate one gram of water at body temperature. The rate of loss of heat by evaporation is less in still air than in a mild breeze, but a 2 mile/hour breeze will double the heat loss from the skin. (Oh, for a cooling breeze!). This is fine for us but for animals the wind disturbs their fur and causes greater heat loss. This is why animals tend to huddle in windy cold weather. Humans have 100 to 600 sweat glands per centimeter on the body depending on body part. These glands can produce 2-3 milligrams of sweat per square centimeter every minute which means that the body can lose more than 10 to 15 millicalories of heat per square centimeter every second. In terms of water loss that is about a gram of water from every square centimeter of skin each minute.

Humidity has a great effect on the amount of heat loss due to evaporation because of the relationship between the water saturation ability of air and the temperature. When the air is nearly saturated with water little fluid can be evaporated into it. As you well know hot humid days are very uncomfortable even in a breeze. Remember that humidity is always relative, it is expressed as a percentage of water saturation of the air.

## MAJOR FACTORS DETERMINING PHYSIOLOGICAL REACTIONS TO HEAT

The major factors that determine the number and intensity of physiological reactions to heat are:
1. The tissue temperature - therapeutic range 40 to 45 degrees C.
2. Time of temperature elevation - therapeutic range 3 to 30 minutes.
3. Rate of temperature rise.
4. The size of the area being treated.

## USES OF HEAT AS A THERAPEUTIC MODALITY

We mentioned that as the skin's temperature increases, so does the blood flow in the skin. The metabolic activity of tissue increases as well.

**Do not apply heat to:**
1. Poorly vascularized tissue, that is, tissue with poor blood flow.
2. Bleeding surfaces, as bleeding tendencies are increased with heat application.
3. The gonads, testicals or ovaries.
4. Individuals with sensory loss, except with extreme care, as they are unable to determine excessive heat.

### Types of Heat Transfer

Heat can be transferred to tissue by the following methods:
1. **Conduction**, the direct contact of a warm and a cold body.
2. **Convection**, passing a hot air current over the skin.
3. **Radiation**, using a heat lamp or the sun or by conversion of one energy source to heat, as in ultrasound waves converted to heat in the tissues. Remember that heat is generated when the tissues resist the flow of energy. When the tissues are heated beyond the therapeutic limit they are destroyed.

### Metabolic Reactions

You know that increasing the temperature of a reaction will increase the rate of the reaction. In tissues, increasing the temperature by 10 degrees C will increase the metabolic rate two or three fold. Now here is an important factor: as the tissues heat up the energy expenditure is increased, so that over 45 degrees C the energy requirements to repair the tissue damaged by this heat is in excess of what the body can produce to make the repair. Thus, the tissue is destroyed. Oxygen uptake is increased if the tissue is heated within the therapeutic range which allows more nutrients to be available to promote tissue healing.

### Vascular Effects

While skin blood flow will increase with skin temperature this reaction is somewhat more complex. The skin is unique in that it has specialized blood vessels (vessels with arteriovenous anastomoses). These vessels play an important role in heat loss. The arterioles can shunt blood directly to the venules and thus to the venous plexuses which bypass the capillary bed. This blood flow mechanism is under the control of the nervous system and is triggered partly by the warmed blood in the brain. You will find this system of arteriovenous anastomoses, or A-V shunts, in the palms and fingertips of the hands, in the soles and toes of the feet, and in the ears, lips, and nose of the face. Heat applied to the skin stimulates cutaneous thermoreceptors that trigger a reflex arc in the spinal cord which causes vasodilation. Remember, when one area of the skin is heated this vasodilatory reflex is not limited to the area heated. It is well known that heating the back can cause an increase in blood flow to the feet.

### Neuromuscular and Connective Tissue Effects

Raising the dermal tissue by a temperature of 1.2 to 4.23 degrees C with infrared radiation increases the sensory nerve conduction velocity. The pain threshold in certain peripheral nerves is elevated by surface heat. Muscles are rarely heated by surface methods. The effects of heat on the underlying muscles is not well known but muscle endurance and strength appear to be decreased. Heating connective tissue increases the elastic qualities. This occurs at temperatures between 40 and 45 degrees C.

### The Biophysics of Heat Application to the Skin

The intensity of the heat applied, the duration of application, the thermal conductivity, the specific heat, and the density of the tissue are all factors in the final skin temperature produced. The tissues, at a depth of 0.5 centimeter (cm) are usually affected most by superficial heat. Tissues at 1 cm or more will require greater heating time, about 30 minutes, while at 3 cms there is hardly a 1 degree C increase in temperature. Fatty tissue is a poor conductor of heat. Fat and tissue below the fat layer are usually not heated by superficial heat. This is important to know since the joints of the hands and feet contain little fatty tissue and can be easily raised 9 degrees C with only twenty minutes of heat at 47 degrees C.

### Heating Agents

**Hot packs** transfer heat by conductance. They can be as hot as 71 degrees C, then wrapped in towels prior to application with 6 to 8 layers. **Never put the hot pack directly on the skin! The patients should never lie on the hot packs even with towel wrapping**. Check and observe the patient's skin after five minutes of heating for mottled erythema or blotchy areas as this indicates uneven heating.

Paraffin wax with mineral oil will remain liquid at 47.8 degrees C, but melts at 54.5 degrees C. Individual tolerance to paraffin varies between these two temperatures. **Do not apply paraffin over open wounds or infected areas.**

Infrared radiant heat is administered with lamps, usually made of tungsten or carbon filaments, which are heated when an electrical current is passed across them.

We speak of both **near infrared** which is in the wavelenth range of 700 to 1500 nanometers, and **far infrared** which is in the range of 1500 to 12,500 nanometers. You can distinquish the difference between the two types of lamps. Near infrared is luminous or visible. Far infrared is non-luminous and thus invisible. (Your eyes can see only to about 800 nanometers in the infrared light).

The depth of penetration for far infrared energy is about 2 millimeters while near infrared may penetrate 5 to 10 millimeters. Heating with an infrared lamp is by radiation so there is no need for a conducting material to be placed between the lamp and the skin. Placing the lamp directly over the skin will yield greater energy to the surface because perpendicular light is reflected less from the skin than light which strikes the skin at an angle. The amount of energy delivered to the skin is related to the distance of the lamp to the skin, which typically is 45 to 60 cm.

Again you must bear in mind that as you bring the lamp closer to the skin you will increase the intensity of the heat considerably. The **inverse square law** operates with light. This law states that the intensity of light at a surface varies inversely as the square of the distance. For example, if you reduce the distance of the lamp from the skin by one-half you will increase the intensity of the energy by four times. The choice of near or far infrared is more a matter of equipment availability since the physiological effects of both energy levels are similiar.

We shall learn how to use the various forms of heat in the chapters on treatment.

## PRESSURE - WHAT IT IS AND HOW IT IS USED IN SKIN CARE

Pressure is important in skin care since it is a factor that relates to the flow of blood and lymphatic fluid in the skin. Pressure is used therapeutically in the form of massage, bandages and stockings. Combined, the arterial, venous, and lymphatic systems are called the vascular system (all terms that will be used frequently in this discussion).

**Pressure** is defined as force per unit area. We use the term "pressure" whenever we speak of fluids. Pressure in the teapot, pressure in the cooker, blood pressure, and oil pressure are examples. We are speaking of a certain force that is delivered over a defined area. These units are pounds per square inch (psi) or newtons per square meter. The metric system uses newtons per square meter. A newton is a unit of force which will produce an acceleration of one meter per second per second when applied to a mass of one kilogram. Now to make this a little more confusing there is still another system that is used and that is the centimeter gram system (cgs). In the cgs, the dyne is the unit of force and is equal to a force that will produce an acceleration of

one gram of material one centimeter per second per second. This is written as dyne = gm-cm/sec. A force is always exerted by something and upon something. Physicists need to express force in mathematical terms in order to measure things. Force is not the same thing as weight, but it is weight (or more accurately mass) that is moving. If an object is not moving it has weight but no force. Now we can relate a newton to a dyne by saying that one newton is equal to 100,000 dynes. The newton is a bigger force. Keep in mind that pressure is force distributed over an area, so we must always speak of dynes per square centimeter or newtons per square meter.

### Fluid Dynamics - How the Blood Flows

We spoke about the blood flow to the skin in the arteries and capillaries and also about the lymphatic system and how it relates to the blood. It is time to put these bits of information together and to understand how these systems affect the skin. Paramount to understanding the effects of blood flow on the skin is an understanding of the capillaries. It is at the level of the capillary that fluid exchange between the tissues and the blood vessels occur. Look now at the diagram in **Figure 7-1** and note the structure of the capillaries. First you will see the small arteriole from which arises a more narrow metarteriole. Notice that the metarteriole has small muscle fibers scattered near the proximal end and that the metarteriole passes through the network of capillaries to the venous side where it joins with a venule. These muscle fibers control the flow of blood into the capillaries. Notice also that the capillaries are not on the direct route from arteriole to venule but arise from the metarteriole, and that a precapillary sphincter muscle controls the flow of blood to the capillary.

Now we can look at the lymph or tissue fluid that baths the cells. Certain elements of the blood are able to move out of the capillary vessels through the walls and once they move out they are called interstial fluid and lymph fluid. The difference is that interstitial fluid bathes the tissue but when it flows in the lymphatic vessels it is called lymph. The lymphatic vessels are somewhat like capillaries in that they have single cell walls, but unlike capillaries they are blind-ended. See **Figure 7-2**.

Minute openings in the lymphatic capillaries allow fluid to pass into the capillary but not out. In the case of edema, or tissue swelling, this system serves to direct proteins back into the vascular system from the interstitial spaces. The lymphatic capillaries are anchored to the surrounding tissue which serves to open the capillaries further and when the tissues swell, it permits more fluid to flow into them.

Remember, the lymphatic system is a separate system from the blood vessels, although the lymph fluid empties into the venous system in the area of the neck. So while they are separate they are interconnected. See **Figure 7-3** for a view of the location of the principle components of the lymphatic system.

### Blood Flow

From basic anatomy and physiology you know that blood flow is the amount of blood that passes through a blood vessel in a given period of time. We call this the volume of blood per unit time, or for example, milliliters per second. In a minute the blood flow would be 60 times that or 300 ml per minute. There are only two principal factors that determine blood flow, blood pressure and resistance. Resistance is due to the force of friction of the blood on the blood vessel walls. Let's look at both factors.

### Blood Pressure

When we talk about blood pressure we are speaking of the pressure exerted by the blood against the wall of the blood vessel. Blood pressure measurements as used by doctors in caring for patients refer to arterial blood pressure. The output of the heart with each stroke (determined by the rate and force of the heartbeat), plus the resistance to the flow of the blood in the vessels results in the blood pressure. A simple relation-

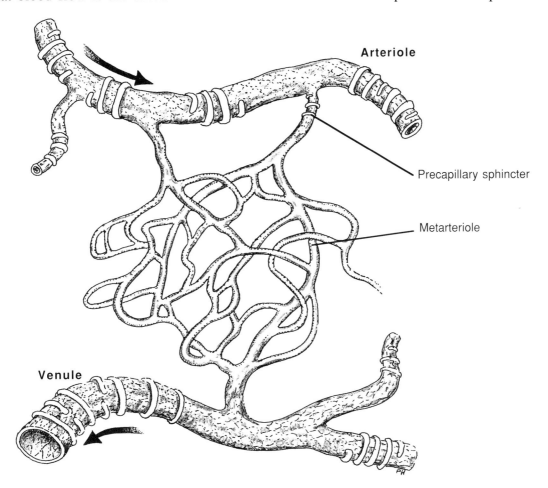

**Arteriole**

Precapillary sphincter

Metarteriole

**Venule**

**FIGURE 7-1** Structure of the capillaries. Note that the capillaries are a network of tiny vessels uniting the arteriole and the venule.

ship exists, blood pressure = cardiac output + resistance (we now have two definitions of resistance). Blood flow is always directly related to blood pressure. Increase the pressure and you will increase the flow, decrease the presssure and you will decrease the flow. Let me pause to show you why this is so important for you to understand as skin care specialist.

Three problems which you see most frequently in the skin care clinic are: **1. spider veins**, **2. varicose veins**, and **3. "cellulite"**. All three of these conditions relate in some manner to venous blood flow and venous blood pressure. In order to treat these conditions you must understand the underlying principles behind the pathology and treatment. The control of blood flow is the underlying principle.

Blood will always flow from a region of high pressure to a region of low pressure. In man the mean blood pressure in the aorta is about 100

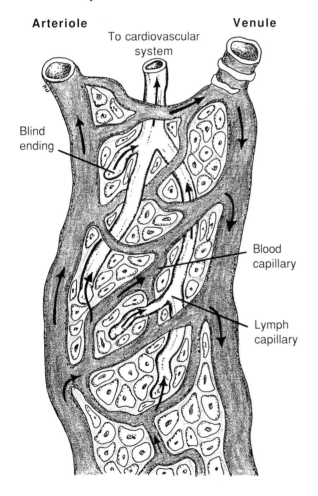

**Arteriole**

To cardiovascular system

**Venule**

Blind ending

Blood capillary

Lymph capillary

FIGURE 7-2 Comparison of lymph and blood capillaries. The lymph vessels have blind ends, whereas capillaries are joined to each other.

mm mercury (Hg), varying from 80 mm to 120 mm. As the blood flows to the smaller arteries the resistance increases and the blood pressure falls so that by the time it reaches the capillaries on the arterial side the blood pressure is only 30 mm Hg. At the venous end it is very low, only 10 mm Hg. As the blood returns to the heart the pressure continues to fall until on reaching the right atrium it is down to 0 mm Hg. (Obviously heart disease will affect the blood pressure).

### Resistance

Resistance is the opposing force to blood flow and is made up of three major components; 1. blood viscosity, 2. blood vessel length, and 3. blood vessel radius.

Viscosity means, roughly speaking, the thickness of the blood. The blood is made up of blood cells and dissolved materials. If you increase either one you will increase the viscosity, therefore, dehydration and polycythemia vera (a disease in which there is an increase in red cells) increase blood pressure. On the other hand, if you bleed or are anemic, the red cells are decreased and your pressure will decrease.

Blood vessel length relates directly to resistance to blood flow. The longer the vessel is the greater the resistance, and the lower the blood flow. This is why your feet are cold.

### Blood Vessel Radius

The size of the blood vessel in diameter is related to the resistance. Blood physiologists use the radius, or half the diameter as the measurement, and say that resistance of the blood vessel is inversely proportional to the fourth power of the radius of the blood vessel. This means that if you decrease the size (radius) of the blood vessel by one-half you will increase the resistance by 16 times. This is why the blood vessel diameter is so important.

Now we are ready to look at resistance as a whole and learn how this opposing force controls blood pressure.

### Peripheral Resistance and the Control Mechanisms

When we speak of peripheral resistance we are including all the factors that oppose blood

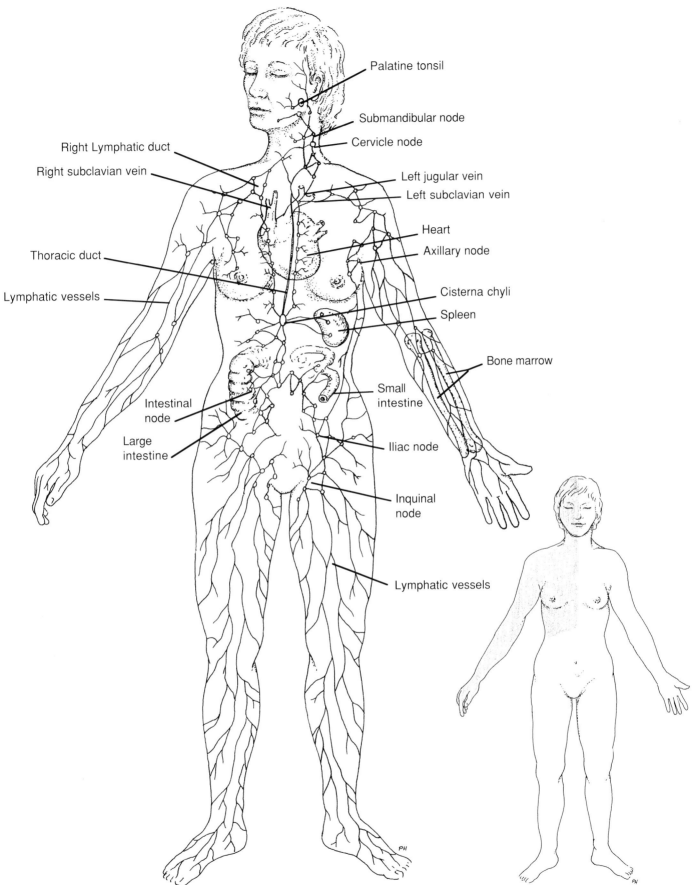

**FIGURE 7-3** Lymphatic drainage of the body. While the network of lymphatic vessels appears complex remember that the flow is into the groin, into the axilla and from the face to the neck. Inset indicates portion drainage of the right lymphatic duct while the remainder of the body travels through the thoracic duct.

Labels (clockwise from top):
- Palatine tonsil
- Submandibular node
- Cervicle node
- Left jugular vein
- Left subclavian vein
- Heart
- Axillary node
- Cisterna chyli
- Spleen
- Bone marrow
- Small intestine
- Iliac node
- Inquinal node
- Lymphatic vessels
- Large intestine
- Intestinal node
- Lymphatic vessels
- Thoracic duct
- Right subclavian vein
- Right Lymphatic duct

flow, but mainly, we are describing the arterioles and how the diameter of these vessels is controlled by various receptors and chemicals. Since blood flow is so essential to skin care, the time and effort spent understanding these factors will be well spent.

The major center for control of the blood vessel diameter is in the medulla of the brain and is called the vasomotor center. The nerves that control the muscles that open and close the arterioles are motor nerves. The **vasomotor center** constantly sends signals to the arterioles of the skin and the viscera of the abdomen. The viscera is mildly vasoconstrictive. This constriction maintains a constant vasomotor tone and is mediated by the sympathetic nervous system. When the number of impulses from the sympathetic nervous system decreases, the tone decreases and resistance falls. The sympathetic nervous system also increases heart rate and causes veins to constrict which work to increase blood pressure. Certain receptors feed into the vasomotor center to regulate the number of sym-

pathetic impulses that come down to the blood vessels. Here are the most important ones.

The **baroreceptors** are pressure receptors in the wall of the carotid sinus (located in the neck in the anterior triangle) and in the aorta. These receptors can send impulses to both increase and decrease blood pressure. See **Figure 7-4** for an example of this action.

**Chemoreceptors** are nerve endings that are sensitive to many chemicals in the body. The carotid body and the aortic body are sensitive to oxygen and carbon dioxide levels as well as to the hydrogen ions that regulate blood pH. Chemicals that regulate the blood pressure are epinephrine and norepinephrine which are produced by the medulla of the adrenal gland. These chemicals have a different effect on the arterioles depending on the anatomical site. In the skin and the abdomen they cause vasoconstriction while they dilate cardiac and skeletal muscle arterioles. This makes sense when you consider the fight-flight mechanisms. It also explains why we become pale and nauseated with fear or great

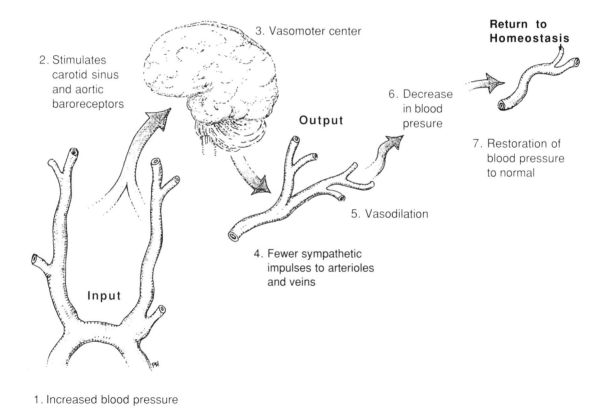

3. Vasomoter center

2. Stimulates carotid sinus and aortic baroreceptors

**Return to Homeostasis**

6. Decrease in blood presure

**Output**

7. Restoration of blood pressure to normal

5. Vasodilation

4. Fewer sympathetic impulses to arterioles and veins

**Input**

1. Increased blood pressure

**FIGURE 7-4** Baroreceptor action. The baroreceptors are sensitive to blood pressure and relay messages to the brain that control the flow of blood into the peripheral vessels (arms and legs). The brain is the priority organ for blood flow, it gets the most even if other organs must suffer.

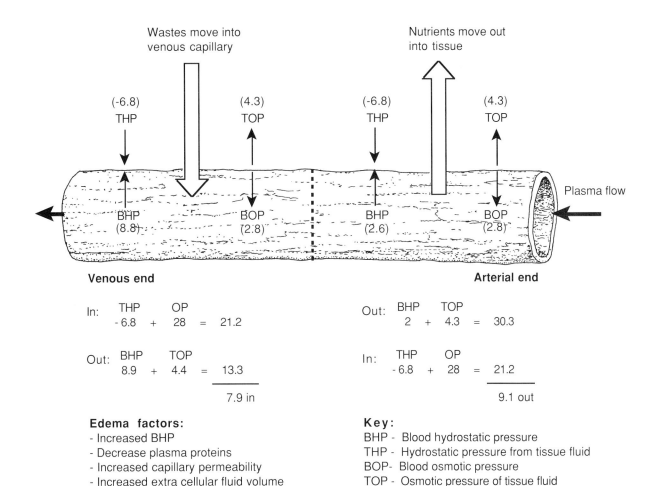

Wastes move into venous capillary

Nutrients move out into tissue

(-6.8) THP

(4.3) TOP

(-6.8) THP

(4.3) TOP

Plasma flow

BHP (8.8)

BOP (2.8)

BHP (2.6)

BOP (2.8)

**Venous end**

**Arterial end**

In: THP    OP
- 6.8  +  28  =  21.2

Out: BHP    TOP
2   +  4.3  =  30.3

Out: BHP    TOP
8.9  +  4.4  =  13.3
_____
7.9 in

In: THP    OP
- 6.8  +  28  =  21.2
_____
9.1 out

**Edema factors:**
- Increased BHP
- Decrease plasma proteins
- Increased capillary permeability
- Increased extra cellular fluid volume coupled with fluid retention

**Key:**
BHP - Blood hydrostatic pressure
THP - Hydrostatic pressure from tissue fluid
BOP - Blood osmotic pressure
TOP - Osmotic pressure of tissue fluid

**FIGURE 7-5** Pressure forces involved in normal capillary exchange. In this diagram, notice there are four forces that control the flow of fluid into and out of the capillaries and tissues, BHP, THP, BOP, and TOP. With edema (excessive tissue water) there is a change in one or more of these forces, altering the normal flow of fluid.

emotional shock.

One more item is local control. There is a regulatory system called autoregulation which provides the vasodilation needed to supply the oxygen and nutrients to the tissue. We know that potassium, lactic acid, and pH level are some of the agents that will cause local vasodilator action by this system.

### THE CAPILLARY EXCHANGE MECHANISM

Everything that we have learned so far is now coming to bear on the capillary exchange. It is this that should most concern the skin care specialist. Healing, infection, edema, and massage techniques are all related to capillary exhange and blood flow. Look at the diagram of a capillary where the arterial end joins the

venous end and observe the pressure relations.

As long as these relative pressures remain normal there is good exchange between the interstitial tissue and the capillaries. But what if the pressure in the veins increased? First, the inward flow of fluid would be reversed since the hydrostatic pressure is increased, and the veins would swell causing the velocity of blood flow to decrease, allowing more fluid to escape. Next, the arterioles are constricted, further decreasing arterial pressure and allowing proteins to escape, which decreases the blood osmotic pressure. We now have edema, which is an increase of interstitial fluid. See **Figure 7-5.**

Varicose veins arise from damaged venous valves and increased abdominal pressure. This often occurs in pregnancy. See **Figure 7-6.** Walking helps to return the venous blood to the heart by "milking" the veins with muscular contraction in the legs. Very little pressure on a vein will stop the flow. Constrictive underwear and tight jeans increase the incidence of varicose veins in young women. The solution is relatively simple - avoid bikinis and tight jeans, and take more walks!

## THE SKIN AND MASSAGE

You have studied massage techniques in your basic courses, so here we will only touch on the physiological implications of massage. Massage is one of the oldest therapeutic modalities in the history of medicine with written records going back 3000 years. The physiological basis for massage is the mechanical and reflex effects from the action.

The mechanical effects are: 1. assisted return of blood and lymph fluid when massage is given with the greatest force in the centripedal direction (to the center of the body), and 2. the effect on muscles to stretch fibers and mobilize fluid. (Note: Massage can not strengthen muscle fibers, only active exercise can do that.)

Reflex effects are produced by stimulation of receptors in the skin, particularly pressure and pleasure receptors. These effects cause increased blood flow by vasodilation and muscle relaxation. Mental tension is then reduced which has an effect on the central nervous system and the amount of adrenal medullary hormones excreted.

## Indications

Massage is indicated for any condition in which swelling and pain must be reduced and in which muscles must be mobilized. In skin care it is helpful in reducing lymphatic fluid in cellulite and in stimulating circulation in the feet, hands and face. There is no indication that massage will cause weight reduction and I do not advocate abdominal massage for this purpose. CONTRAINDICATIONS TO MASSAGE ARE INFECTIONS, TUMORS, IRRITATED OR INFECTED SKIN, THIN SKIN CONDITION, AND IN THE PRESENCE OF THROMBOPHLEBITIS (CLOTS MAY BECOME EMBOLI).

Therapeutic applications of pressure will be looked at more closely in the treatment of specific conditions chapters.

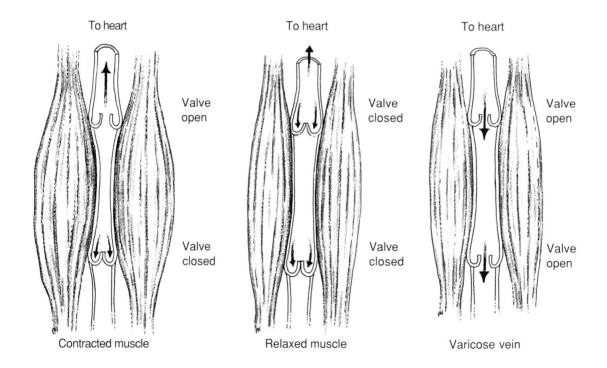

**FIGURE 7-6** Varicose veins. The muscles pump the blood up the legs by lateral pressure on the veins. The venous valves prevent backward flow down the legs. When excess pressure from venous constrictions prevents the flow of blood up the veins back pressure results and the venous valves give way. This produces dilated or varicose veins.

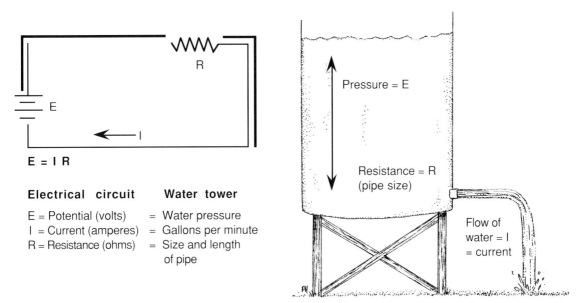

$$E = IR$$

| Electrical circuit | Water tower |
|---|---|
| E = Potential (volts) | = Water pressure |
| I = Current (amperes) | = Gallons per minute |
| R = Resistance (ohms) | = Size and length of pipe |

**FIGURE 7-7** Ohm's law. Remember that E=IR. You can calculate any of the three unknowns if you know two of them. Consider voltage as pressure in the drawing of the water tower; the resistance is the pipe size, and the current is the flow of water.

## ELECTRICITY IN SKIN CARE

A comprehensive knowledge of electricity and electronics is not necessary for the skin care specialist to be able to use this type of instrumentation. What is required, however, for safe and effective use of any electrical instrumentation is a basic knowledge of the elementary laws of electricity and the basic physical principles involved in the actual application of the these instruments. A knowledge of the construction and function of the particular instrument is also required.

In this section on electricity we shall discuss the basic concepts in electricity and look at some of the therapeutic applications of instrumentation. We shall discuss direct current, alternating current, epilation, cauterization and some new therapeutic uses of alternating current.

### Electricity - The Basics

Electricity can be either static or dynamic. When you rub a comb or other substance with a cloth or your hand you produce an attraction force. Substances that have this property are said to be able to gain an electric charge. Since electricity may be considered a fluid, when this charged electric fluid is stationary it is called **static electricity**. When the electric charge flows it is called **dynamic electricity**. When you add electrons to a substance it has a negative charge and when electrons are removed from a substance it has a positive charge. Since removing or adding electrons involves work we now have potential energy in the substance which is called the **electromotive force,** or more simply, **volts.** When this force is dynamic or flowing we have a transmission of energy called **current**. Remember, electricity may be generated by friction, heat or chemical reaction.

There is a relationship that exists between the various components of an electrical circuit. An electric current will only flow as long as there is a difference in potential energy between the two poles (the negative pole and the positive pole). It is necessary to make a loop or closed circuit to have the current cycle. Once the potential energy difference is no longer present the current will stop flowing (the dead battery syndrome). The amount of current flow is measured by a unit called the **ampere**. The ampere depends on the potential energy difference or driving force called the volt. The material connecting the two poles is the conductor which offers resistance to the flow of current. Look at **Figure 7-7** to see this relationship illustrated. The mathematical relationship of the three factors (called Ohm's law) is E = IR, where E is the electromotive force or volts, I is the current in amperes, and R is the resistance in ohms. For biological use, these quantities are all too large. We normally speak of milliamps and millivolts.

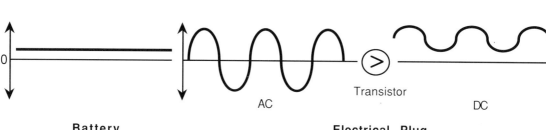

Types of current

Voltage

Alternating          ( Rectification)          Direct

Sources

Battery
Source of Direct Current
Smooth flow/Constant voltage

AC          Transistor          DC

Electrical Plug
Flow and intensity change

**FIGURE 7-8** Types of current and their sources. Alternating current changes direction with each half cycle. A rectified current is direct current produced from an alternating current. Transistors can be used as rectifiers.

Let's look at this a little more closely so you can see the relationship and feel comfortable with it. For example, an epilation instrument using 7 volts generated by a battery will produce a current in the skin of 0.5 to 1.3 milliamps (ma). This means that the skin has a resistance of 7 volts divided by 0.9 ma (0.0009 amperes) or over 7700 ohms. It is well established that skin has a high resistance to the flow of electrical current if it is dry. Wet skin is a far better conductor of electricity. The average resistance in the body is about 1000 ohms.

### Types of Current

There are two types of current used in skin care. One is direct current and the other is alternating current. Direct current is a constant flow of electrons in one direction only, whereas alternating current changes flow and intensity periodically. These two currents require different methods to generate the electron flow. A battery, for example, can generate direct current chemically, producing a smooth flow of current at a constant voltage. See the diagram in **Figure 7-8**. Direct current can be used to carry

certain chemicals into the skin.

### Physical Effects of Current Flow on Tissue

When electrical current flows in tissue there are three observable phenomena that occur: 1. heat is produced in all parts of the circuit, 2. there is a magnetic field produced, and 3. at times a chemical reaction takes place. Direct current is capable of moving ions that may produce a chemical reaction, while alternating current can not move ions for all practical purposes. Heat can be produced by both types of current and the relationship involves the current strength, the resistance, and the time that the current flows. This is called a **primary heating effect**. In the case of direct current, if a chemical reaction occurs there will be a secondary heating effect.

The body is a poor conductor of electricity, that is, it offers resistance to the flow of electricity. Now it stands to reason that those tissues that contain the most moisture are also the best conductors. Stratum corneum, which contains only about 10% moisture in the dry state, is a very poor conductor and offers a high resistance to the flow of electricity. Muscles and brain are the best conductors so it is easy to measure the electron flow in these structures and to stimulate them with electricity. Brain waves are measured by a system called **electroencephalography**, and muscle contraction can be measured with a system called **electromyography**. Electroshock therapy in psychiatry and electrical stimulation of muscle in physical medicine are well known therapies.

### Uses of Direct Current

You may be familiar with direct current as **galvanic current**, an old name. It finds use as a means to transfer medicaments into the skin, a method called **iontophoresis**. It is also used to heat electrocautery terminals.

### Iontophoresis

Iontophoresis is a delivery system that uses a direct current to carry certain medicaments into the skin. It is important to understand the polarity of direct current, since only direct current is applied to the body according to polarity. Polarity refers to the positive and negative poles, or contact points in the circuit. Current flows from the positive pole to the negative pole and the ions flow from the negative pole to the positive pole. Study **Figure 7-9** to see this relationship, keeping in mind that you have a loop system. A battery operated system that supplies direct current is marked on the electrodes as positive or negative. When using an instrument that plugs into an outlet, which is alternating current, you must make sure that the positive electrode is indeed positive. At one time alternating current connections were not made to assure polarity, but today the male plug is usually constructed in a manner that it will only fit the wall receptacle in one way, assuring correct polarity.

The body may be considered as a large container of electrolytes (salts that dissolve in water). Absolutely pure water is not a conductor of electricity, it requires some salts to conduct the current. When a direct current is applied to an electrolytic solution the positively charged ions will travel to the negative pole. Now herein lies a point of great confusion for students. The posi-

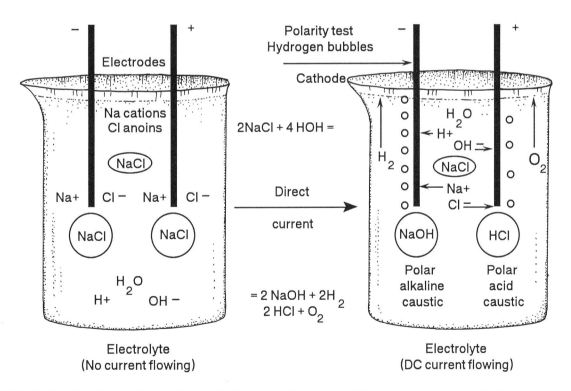

**FIGURE 7-9** Polarity. The positive electrode will attract negative ions and the negative electrode will attract positive ions. Since hydrogen is a positive ion, it will migrate to the cathode (the negative pole) and produce many bubbles of hydrogen gas. The process involves the decomposition of water which is $H_2O$ (or $H^+ OH^-$). At the negative electrode the hydrogen ion $H^+$ forms in molecular hydrogen as $H_2$ which is a gas, so it appears as a bubble.

## DIRECT CURRENT EFFECTS ON TISSUE

| EFFECTS | ANODE (POSITIVE) | CATHODE (NEGATIVE) |
|---|---|---|
| Sensation of heat | Mild | Mild |
| Vasomotor reaction | Stimulation | Stimulation |
| Ionic reaction | Metal and alkaloids repell | Acid and acid radical repelled |
| Pain sensation | Mild to severe | Mild |
| Nerve tissue reaction | Calming nerves | Stimulates or irritates nerves |
| Tissue tone | Hardens | Softens |

**TABLE 7-1** Note the great variation in effects from positive and negative poles.

tive pole is called the **anode** and it attracts negatively charged ions called **anions**. The negative pole is called the **cathode** and it attracts positive charged ions called **cations**. Try to remember that the names are the same but the charges are different; anode = positive pole, anion = negative charge which goes to the positive pole. There is a high percentage of sodium chloride salt (NaCl) in the body. When a direct current is applied to the body tissue it will cause NaCl to move in two directions. The sodium ions will travel to the negative pole(the cathode) along with the ionized hydrogen in the water to produce bubbles of gas and sodium hydroxide (NaOH) at the negative pole. At the positive pole (the anode), oxygen is produced along with hydrochloric acid (HCl). Note, in electrocauterization these are secondary reactions, but in epilation with direct current it is the primary method of destroying the hair shaft. In iontophoresis the ion migration forces the medication into the skin. See **Table 7-1** for clinical effects of direct current.

Iontophoresis is conducted either with pads wetted with a solution of the medicament, or the part to be treated is placed in a solution of the medicament. For example, copper sulfate is used to treat dermatophytosis pedis by soaking the feet in a solution of copper sulfate through which passes a direct current into the skin. See **Figure 7-10**. Electrodes are placed into contact with the normal unbroken skin and the current is gradually increased to avoid shock. If there

are any scars or inflamed skin, that area should be covered with petrolatum or some other water-in-oil type of emulsion, cold cream for example, to prevent the current from reaching that area. The treatment time is usually 10 to 15 minutes with a current of 5 to 15 milliamps (ma). You must be trained in this method before you attempt it. Make sure you are familiar with the equipment and the instructions. **Table 7-2** shows the various uses for iontophoresis. More will be developed in the future.

### Epilation Techniques - DC and AC Methods

Epilation by direct current involves placing the negative electrode into the hair follicle and applying a current of 0.5 to 1.5 ma. The production of sodium hydroxide at the site of the negative pole in the hair follicle will generate heat that will destroy the follicle. The action of the sodium hydroxide also aids in this destruction by softening the tissue and the hair. This allows easy removal of the needle. The most important thing to remember in direct current electrolysis of hair is that if you get the poles mixed up and connect the needle to the positive electrode several things will happen: 1. the skin will become hard, 2. the needle will stick, 3. you will tatoo the person's skin with metal from the needle, and 4. you will have a very unhappy patient.

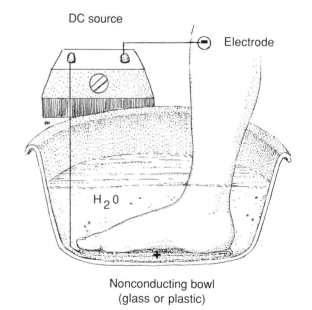

**FIGURE 7-10** Hyperhydrosis treatment. Direct current has an effect on the sweat ducts to reduce the flow of sweat.

INDICATIONS
Administration of corticosteroid, dexamethasone sodium phosphate, lidocaine hydrochloride, or various salts when it is advisable to:

1. Avoid pain from needle insertion or injection
2. To minimize infiltration of carrier fluids
3. To avoid damage caused by needle insertion when tissue is traumatized

CONTRAINDICATIONS
1. Patients with pacemakers
2. Electrically sensitive patients
3. Known sensitivity to the drug to be administered
4. Damaged or denuded skin, recent scar tissue
5. Treatment of orbital (eye) region
6. Across temporal region

**TABLE 7-2** Indications and Contraindications in Electrolysis.

In alternating current electrolysis high frequency AC is used to destroy the hair by heat. The resistance of the tissue to the passage of the alternating high frequency generates the heat that destroys the hair. Here we should mention that the needle is attached to the proper electrode; with the new instruments you cannot make a mistake.

Insertion of the needle into the hair follicle should be a smooth painless procedure. Insert the needle about 3-4 mm. As you reach the bottom you will find resistance, then stop. DO NOT APPLY CURRENT UNTIL YOU REACH THIS POINT. Application of current during insertion will produce pain and scarring. Easy removal of the hair after current application is a good sign that you have successfully destroyed the hair papilla. Coarse hairs may require more current than normal or fine hairs.

My advice to you is to learn one piece of equipment and to learn it well. Sterile needles and sterile technique, clean skin and clean needles are required for successful professional electrolysis. Current should be applied only as a short one second burst, or less, with 3 to 6 repeated bursts per hair. Do not epilate adjacent hair closer than 3 to 4 mm. The contact area must be with the tip of the needle to prevent scarring. Bits of tissue that stick to the needle must be removed to prevent current shorting to adjacent tissues. The number of hairs removed depends on the operator's skill and experience. Some expert operators are able to remove 50 to 100 hairs in 20 minutes or less. Finally, there may be as many as 30% of the hairs returning, which have to be removed again. After all, no one and no technique is perfect. Practice. Practice. Practice.

### Electrosurgical Techniques (Also called electrodiathermy)

Electrosurgery is the technique of converting high frequency electrical energy into heat to destroy tissue. The heat is generated as a consequence of the resistance of the skin to the passage of the high frequency alternating current. The heat generated will dessicate, coagulate, cut, or fulgurate the tissue. Fulguration refers to the destruction of tissue by electrical sparks (*fulgur* is Latin for lighting). There is no contact with the skin in fulguration. The high frequency alternating current used in electrosurgery can interfere with pacemakers or other electronic monitoring devices so be sure to ask about these devices before using the technique.

There are options to use with the electrical diathermy system. You may use a single or a dual electrode, damped or undamped wave forms and ranges of currents. The undamped wave is best for tissue cutting as it is only minimally destructive. The damped wave form is good for hemostasis and for tissue destruction. Using one electrode will concentrate the current

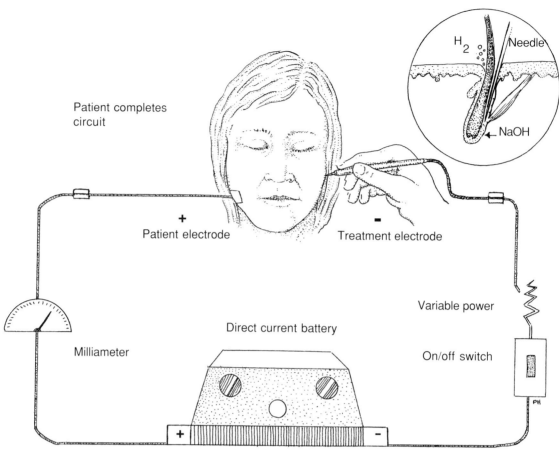

**FIGURE 7-11** Techniques in electrolysis and electrosurgery. Electrolysis. The negative electrode is inserted into the hair follicle. Hot sodium hydroxide is generated which destroys the hair follicle. The use of direct current in electrolysis is being replaced by high frequency instruments.

at one spot, while two electrodes spread the heat over a uniform area between the electrodes.

The electrical diagrams of these two types of units are presented in **Figures 7-11, 12**. If you are interested in the construction detail of these instruments the manufacturers will be happy to provide you with the information. I want only to go over the main elements in the circuits to familiarize you with the terms and functions of these elements. Coming out of the wall plug is an alternating current of 120 volts and 60 cycles (low frequency AC). Transformers raise the voltage at the first step and then pass the current to an oscillation circuit that greatly increases the frequency. You will hear this called a "spark gap" circuit. Next, the current goes to one of two types of coils depending on whether you select the single or dual electrodes.

The result is a damped high frequency high voltage AC current that will coagulate or dessicate tissue. In the undamped system a diode or triode tube is used in place of the spark

gap. This instrument is used mainly for cutting operations.

### The Effect of Electrosurgery on the Tissues

The application of moderate current from a single electrode to the skin will cause the dessication of cells. The water in the cells will then be evaporated and the cells will be shriveled and mummified. When two electrodes, or terminals are used the tissue is coagulated or cooked by boiling. The result is tissue that is without shape or design. The blood vessels will be thrombosed and a mild inflammatory reaction will ensue in a few days. Stronger currents will cause coagulation and even carbonization of the tissue, with resultant scarring of the tissue. The amount of scarring will relate to the intensity of the current and the anatomical location. Explosive vacuolization is the procedure in which the tissues appear to spread apart in front of the cutting edge due to steam generated

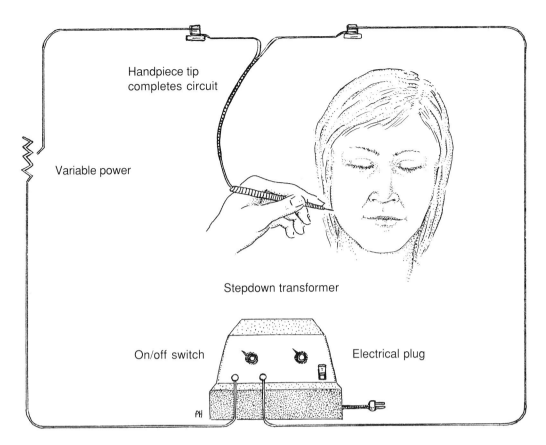

**FIGURE 7-11** (cont.) Techniques in electrolysis and electrosurgery. Electrosurgery. The tip is very hot and literally burns or chars tissue. Blood vessels are coagulated by this technique.

in the cells.

### Clinical Applications

**Electrofulguration** is a form of electro-dessication. The electrode, usually a needle or a ball type, is held above the lesion on the skin close enough to produce a spark. The spark is played over the lesion being treated. This is used for superficial lesions because the system will not penetrate very deeply. I like to use it for skin tags or filiform lesions.

**Electrodessication** employs highly damped current in a single electrode. The spark gap generator sytem is used to produce the current. The needle electrode must touch the skin. The depth and amount of destruction is controlled by the current intensity and the time of application. Warts are a good subject for this type of treatment.

**Electrocoagulation** occurs with either damped or undamped current of moderate intensity using biterminal electrodes. The concentrating electrode touches the skin at the site of the lesion and the dispersing electrode is held in the hand. This is usually a metal plate.

We shall discuss specific treatment methods employing these techniques when we discuss treatment in later chapters.

### Electrical Safety

Before using any piece of electrical equipment the student must be trained in the safety and use of the equipment. Most modern electrical equipment is manufactured to rather strict safety specifications but improper use will make any mechanical or electrical device hazardous or potentially lethal. It is important, therefore, to know the basic concepts in using equipment safely and training is, of course, the first step. Next, an understanding of the concepts of grounding, what is meant by the term electrical "ground", and the principles of equipment grounding will help the student to use this equipment safely.

### Definition of a Ground

A ground is a large conducting body that is

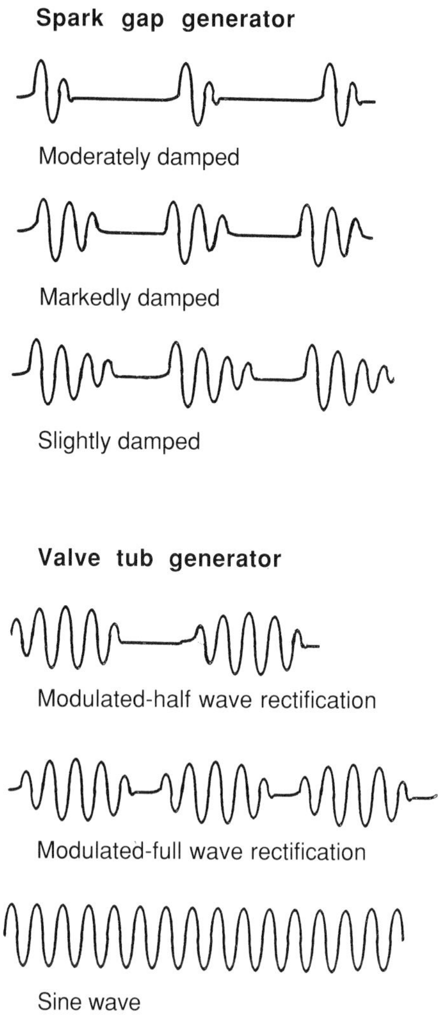

**Spark gap generator**

Moderately damped

Markedly damped

Slightly damped

**Valve tub generator**

Modulated-half wave rectification

Modulated-full wave rectification

Sine wave

**FIGURE 7-12** Damped and undamped current. The process of damping a sine wave changes the energy delivered by the high frequency current. Modification of the wave will either cut or coagulate tissue or do both.

used as a common return for electrical current and has a relative zero electrical potential. This may be the earth (from which comes the word ground) or the metal of a radio chassis, the metal skin of an airplane, or the frame of a car. The concept here is that anything which is grounded has a route for disposal of electrical current. Since current always takes the path of lowest resistance grounds are usually made of metal. Current will follow the ground pathway when a circuit is interrupted by a breakdown of equipment. Remember that the ground is not a part of the circuit pathway but only provides an alternate pathway if the normal circuit is somehow damaged or altered. Equipment that is earth grounded is connected to the earth by a wire which in turn is fastened to a copper rod driven into the ground. We need not go into the different types of grounding but you must be aware that not all equipment is earth grounded, so read the instructions and learn the equipment.

While equipment should be grounded, the patient should not be grounded. Why is this so important? If you are standing in water and touch any electrical equipment you can expect either a severe shock or death. The reason is your body is grounded and the current now will follow the pathway from the equipment through your body. Consider that an ordinary light bulb of 100 watts has one amp of current, which is ten times the fatal current for man (100 milliamps). Wet skin is more conductive than dry skin. Rings, bracelets, and watches are good conductors of electricity and should not be worn while working with electrical equipment.

In the case of high frequency low amperage equipment used in electrosurgery the patient should not touch a metal table or pipe. An unpleasant electric shock will occur, as the patient is then grounded. This is not a hazard if the equipment is working properly. See equipment diagrams for illustrations of grounds and "shorts."

## The Concept of Capacitance

Understanding the nature and action of electricity requires that you know the relationships that exists among the three basic quantities used to define an electrical circuit (that is, the volt, the ampere, and the ohm). Filling a bucket with water and filling a tub with water will result in two quantities or capacities of water held by these containers. You could say for the bucket that we have 4 gallons of water, and for the tub that we have 20 gallons of water. These are the capacities of the bucket and tub to hold water. With electrical measurements we have a similiar term called **capacitance**. Capacitance is the amount of charge stored between two conducting bodies for each volt of potential difference which exist between the two bodies. This property of electricity occurs when two conductive bodies are separated by a nonconducting material at a distance. Its quantity is related to the size of the conducting body. The human body has rather poor capacitance when insulated from

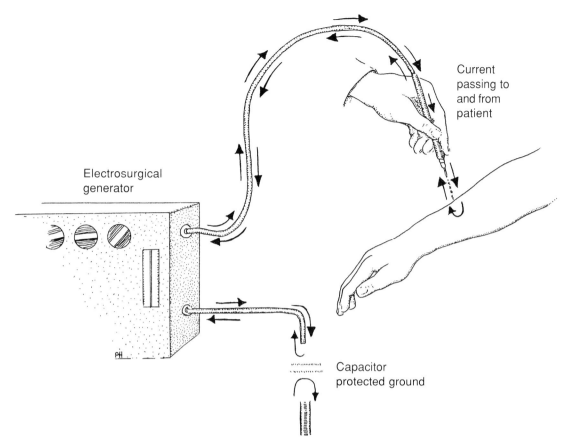

Current
passing to
and from
patient

Electrosurgical
generator

Capacitor
protected ground

FIGURE 7-13 Energy transfer to the patient. This unit is used to cut or coagulate tissue. It is high frequency current.

the environment. We must relate capacitance to both frequency and voltage. Low voltage and low frequency current in the human body produce very little capacitance. High frequency and high voltage will, however, produce increased capacitance.

As you handle an electrosurgical instrument of high frequency the energy will bounce back and forth between the patient and the instrument. The tiny point of contact with the patient's skin will produce the desired effect on the tissue by generating heat. As long as there is no patient grounding there is no shock. The energy transferred to the patient is either used up as heat or returned to the electrosurgical instrument.

Remember that only alternating current can produce capacitance. Direct current will not pass through a capacitor. See **Figure 7-13**.

## MUSCLE STIMULATION

Recently a great deal of publicity has been given to muscle stimulation as a means of improving facial muscle tone or strength. Unfortunately, I am afraid that much of the informa-

tion which has been spread about the usefulness of this method in skin care is incorrect. I shall review what is known about muscle tissue and the current medical methods used to stimulate muscles. Since this is very important to skin care we shall go into it with considerable detail.

## The Physiology of Muscle Contraction

When you tear a muscle apart and look at the fibers under a mircoscope at 1000 x, or 1000 times normal size, you see mainly red oblong cells with some nuclei. Under the electron microscope at a magnification of 35,000 x you see a new world of detail.

The basic unit of a muscle is the myofiber, or muscle fiber, which is 10 to 100 u, however, they may be as long as 12 inches or more. Around the muscle fiber is a membrane called the **sarcolemma** (*sarco* = flesh and *lemma* = sheath). The sarcolemma contains the sarcoplasm which is a quantity of cytoplasm containing nuclei and **myofibrils**. Also within the **sarcoplasm** is a host of other functional structures which includes the **sarcoplasmic reticulum** - a

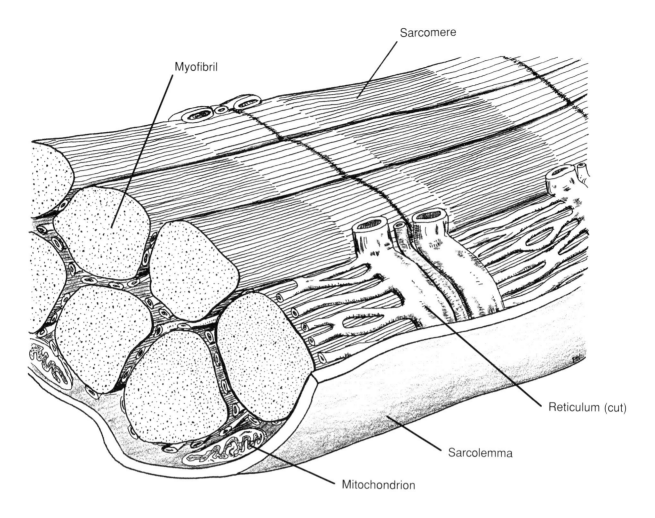

Myofibril

Sarcomere

Reticulum (cut)

Sarcolemma

Mitochondrion

**FIGURE 7-14** Histology of muscle tissue. Muscle fibers divide into myofibrils which divide into myofilaments. A sarcomere is a linear segment on a muscle myofilament that contains a Z line, an A band and another Z line.

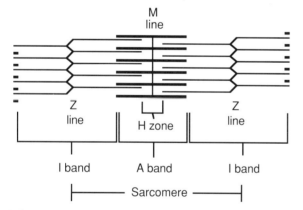

M
line

Z
line

H zone

Z
line

I band

A band

I band

Sarcomere

**FIGURE 7-14** (cont.) Closeup of the sarcomere. The sarcomere is a unit of the myofibril. The myofibril contains the myofilament which is the contraction unit. The thin lines represent actin in this diagram and the heavy thicker lines represent myosin.

network of tubes enclosed in membranes, sarcoplasmic reticulum dilated sacs called **terminal cisterns** and transverse tubules, or **T tubules.** These T tubules run transversely through the fibers and perpendicular to the sarcoplasmic

reticulum. A combination of a transverse tubule and two terminal cisterns is called a triad.

The muscle fibers are composed of smaller **myofibrils** that are 2 um in diameter. In a single muscle fiber there may be several hundred to several thousands of these fibrils. The myofibrils are composed of two smaller units, thin myofilament of 6 nm in diameter and a thick myofilament of 16 nm in diameter. As you read this description refer to the diagram in **Figure 7-14** and find the structures.

Now we shall go deeper into the structure. The **myofilaments** do not run the full length of the myofibril since they are arranged in compartments called **sarcomeres**. The sarcomeres are separated by dense zones called Z lines. Within a sarcomere unit we can distinguish a dark dense area called the **A band** (A for anisotropic), which represents the area of the thick myofilaments. The darkened area results from overlapping of the thick and thin myofilaments.

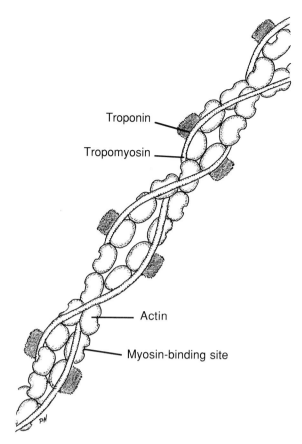

Troponin

Tropomyosin

Actin

Myosin-binding site

**FIGURE 7-15** Structure of myofilament. The myofilament is the basic muscle contraction unit. It functions almost like a "rachet" to contract the filament.

A light area composed only of thin myofilaments is called the **I band** (I for isotropic). There is a region in the center of the A band that contains only thick myofilament that is known as the **H zone** and in the center of the H zone is the **M line**. So we have bands, lines, and zones to remember. Now here comes the most important part.

The thin myofilaments are attached to the **Z lines** and project in both directions. They are composed mostly of a protein called **actin**. These actin molecules are arranged in two strands that entwine in a helical manner. See **Figure 7-15**. Each actin molecule contains a myosin-binding site which interacts with a cross bridge of a myosin molecule. The myosin molecule looks like a golf culb with the handle of the clubs called tails arranged parallel to each other to form the shaft of the thick filament. The heads of the clubs project outward from the shaft and are arranged spirally on the surface of the shaft. (You need two different views to appreciate this structure.) There are two other protein molecules in the thin myofilament, **tropomyosin** and **troponin** which

help to regulate muscle contraction. The tropomyosin is loosely attached to the actin helicals. The troponin is located at intervals on the tropomyosin molecule.

**Mechanism of Muscle Contraction**

During muscle contraction myosin cross bridges pull on the thin myofilaments causing them to slide inward toward the H zone. The sarcome shortens but the thick and thin myofilaments do not. The myosin cross bridges move like the oars of a boat on the surface of the thin myofilaments and pull the thick and thin myofilaments. The thick and thin myofilaments pass each other which causes the H zone to become narrow and the whole muscle fiber to contract. A completely beautiful biological mechanism.

The Muscle-Nerve Interaction - The Neuromuscular Junction

If you thought that was all there was to muscle contraction, "it ain't over yet." We need

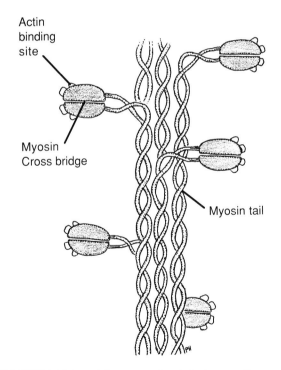

Actin binding site

Myosin Cross bridge

Myosin tail

**FIGURE 7-15** (cont.) Structure of actin in the myofilament. This is a good representation of the rachet action of the actin-myosin molecule. When the muscle contracts the thin filaments overlap. The myosin heads bind to sites on the actin and cross- bridge binding occurs. This results in a change in shape that pulls the filament toward the center of the sarcomere.

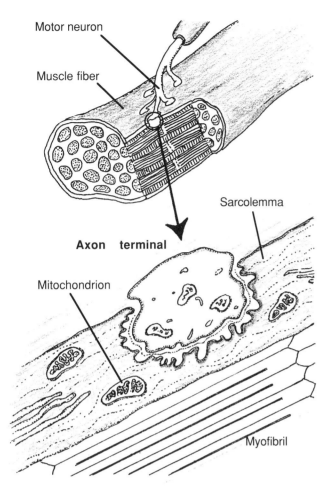

Motor neuron

Muscle fiber

Sarcolemma

**Axon terminal**

Mitochondrion

Myofibril

**FIGURE 7-16** The neuromuscular junction. The nerve joins the muscle fiber and sends chemical signals to the muscle.

a stimulus to make a muscle contract, and in the case of a muscle that stimulus is carried by a nerve fiber, called a neuron. Some of these neurons are as long as three feet, or 91 cm. Neurons that stimulate muscles are called motor neurons. The axon of the motor neuron enters the skeletal muscle and then branches into terminals that come into close approximation with the sarcolemma of the muscle fiber. This area is called the **motor end plate**. The motor end plate and the axon terminal of the motor neuron make up the **myoneural junction**. The distal ends of the axon terminals of the neuron now expand into bulblike structures called synaptic end bulbs. **Figure 7-16** shows a typical synaptic end bulb with synaptic vesicles that store neurotransmitter chemicals. The sarcolemma has invaginations (called synaptic gutters), that permit the flow of neurotransmitters to many more receptor binding sites in the sarcolemma.

On reaching an axon terminal a nerve potential initiates a sequence of events which liberates neurotransmitters from the synaptic vesicles. This neurotransmitter is **acetylcholine** (Ach). When free Ach crosses the synaptic cleft and binds with the receptors on the muscle fiber another series of events occurs. The permeability of the sarcolemma to sodium and potassium ions changes and leads to a muscle contraction.

There is a muscle contraction principle known as the all-or-none principle which states that there is a threshold stimulus needed to contract a muscle and that the muscles will contract fully only when this stimulus is applied. That is, there is no partial response by an individual muscle fiber. Below the threshold stimulus there is no contraction.

Contraction from nerve stimulation to relaxation:

1. The nerve impulse causes Ach release from synaptic vesicles.

2. Ach causes an action potential to spread over the surface of the sarcolemma and the transverse tubules.

3. The action potential enters the transverse tubules and the sarcoplasmic reticulum causing release of calcium ions into the sarcoplasm.

4. The calcium ions combine with the troponin which moves the tropomyosin-troponin complex which exposes the myosin-binding sites on the actin molecule.

5. Now ATPase splits ATP into ADP and P (phosphorus) which releases energy. It is this energy that activates the myosin cross-bridges to combine with the exposed myosin-binding sites on the actin. This action then pulls the thin fibers over the thick fibers towards the H zone.

6. The sarcomere shortens and the muscle contracts.

7. Now Ach is inactivated by acetylcholinesterase (AchE) and Ach no longer has an effect on the neuromuscular junction. (same as myoneural junction).

8. Without action potential being present the calcium ions are transported back into the sarcoplasm by calsequestrin and calcium ATP-ase using energy supplied by ATP breakdown.

9. Now all returns to the pre-excitement state. The tropomyosin-troponin complex reattaches to actin, myosin-binding sites are now covered on the actin and myosin cross-bridges separate from actin. ATP is resynthesized from

ADP and the thin myofilaments return to the relaxed position.

10. The sarcomeres now return to their resting length and the muscle fibers relax.

## More Anatomy on Muscle Tissue

We shall look now at the macroscopic and gross anatomy of the muscle, that is, going from the myofibril out to the fascia. The myofibrils are gathered into bundles called **myofibers**; there may be as many as several thousand myofibrils in a myofiber. Around the myofiber is the sarcolemma. The muscle fibers, or myofibers are grouped in bundles called **fascicles** (*fascia* = bandage). These fascicles are covered with a fibrous tissue called the **perimysium** (which means "around the muscle"). The whole thing looks very much like a multistrand electric wire. The individual myofibers in the fascicles are surrounded and separated by a fibrous connective tissue called the **endomysium** (meaning roughly "within the muscle"). So we have three coverings of fibrous tissue from the inside out: endomysium, perimysium, and the epimysium (*epi* = on, or upon). These three tissues all contain collagen and are contiguous with the other tissues that attach the muscle to bone and to other muscles. Within the muscle there is a blood supply usually accompanied by a nerve. These structures branch and supply the various fascicles and myofibers. Above the muscles that are visible to the naked eye is a fine structure called the superficial fascia which contains blood vessels, nerves and fatty tissue. Here water and excess fat from overeating are stored here. This area also serves as a buffer to mechanical insult. Between and around the muscles and the deeper body organs is the deep fascia. Now let us see how we can put all of this information together in a useful form.

## Application of Muscle Physiology

If you take the trouble to learn the above, what good will it do in skin care? Most likely a great deal of good. Let's take a look at some of these applications. Muscles are characterized by four main functions. These are: 1. excitability, 2. contractility, 3. extensibility, and 4. elasticity. We are interested in all of these functions but we need to know if it is possible to take a lax, flaccid muscle such as you see in aged skin and change it to a muscle with normal tone. Facial muscles in the aged are still supplied with nerves so they are innervated muscles. Let's look at this possibility.

## Muscle Tone

Muscle tone is a state of partial contraction in which some fibers are contracted and others are relaxed. This tone is generally a response to stretch receptor activation and can occur in a relaxed muscle. Our posture depends on this action. These receptors are called **muscle spindles** and they constantly monitor muscle tone and relay messages to the brain and spinal cord to make necessary adjustments. Now when a muscle loses tone it becomes flaccid. These are loose muscles which have a flat appearance rather than rounded. This can occur from disorders of the nervous system (flaccid paralysis), loss or reduction of tendon reflex, atrophy, or degeneration of the muscles. Flaccid muscles are also said to be hypotonic. Is it possible to change a flaccid muscle into an active normal muscle? Theoretically, the answer is yes. In practice, at this time, at least for the face, we must answer no. I can find no legitimate references to indicate this is possible in humans. There is some published work done on rabbits and rats, but for humans, the evidence is quite slim. Nevertheless, I shall cover the basic principles of muscle stimulation as practiced in physical medicine so that you will have a comparison.

## Mechanics of Muscle Contraction

We have discussed the anatomical and physiological mechanisms involved in the stimulation of muscle tissue and now we shall delve into the mechanics of contraction. When a muscle is stimulated, the fundamental reaction or response is called a twitch. It is the lowest recordable activity of muscle response. After the twitch there is a period of a few milliseconds before the tension in the muscle fibers begins to rise. This is called the latency period. During this period the slack is taken up in the elastic components of the muscle. The muscle continues contracting to develop a peak tension. This is the contraction time. Next, the muscle will release the peak tension and return to zero tension. This is called the relaxation time. Summing up we have three types of time components for a stimulated muscle: 1. latency period, 2. contraction time, and 3. relaxation time. The action potential (see **Figure 7-17**) which results from muscle stimulation will last only a millisecond or two, so it is possible to have several action potentials initiated before a twitch occurs. This process is called summation. The greater the frequency of stimulation the greater is the response in the tension up to a set maximum. When this maximum is reached the muscle will then be in tetany. What occurs in this process is the obvious loss of the relaxation period.

Muscles contract and do work. This work may be either static where there is no joint movement, or dynamic where there is mechanical work performed.

The **load** is the resistance offered to a muscle. The force a muscle must exert to overcome the load is the **muscle tension**. It is the relationship between the load and the tension that forms the basis of the classification of muscle contraction.

There are various types of muscle contractions that we should know.

**Isometric contraction** (an example of static contraction) occurs when muscle tension equals the load and there is no change in muscle length.

**Concentric contraction** occurs when the muscle tension equals the external load and the muscle shortens. (Example: biceps contract when you raise a glass).

**Eccentric contraction** occurs when the muscle tension equals the load and the muscle lengthens. (Example: The quadriceps lengthen when you descend the stairs).

**Isokinetic contraction** (*iso* = constant and *kinetic* = motion) occurs when a muscle is moved at a constant velocity. This is a combination of both concentric and eccentric contraction.

**Isoinertial contraction** (*iso* = constant and *inertial* = resistance) occurs when a constant load is presented to the muscle. It may involve both isometric and concentric contraction. (Example: lifting a box).

**Isotonic contraction** (*iso* = constant and *tonic* = force) refers to constant tension in a muscle through a range of motion. In reality, isotonic contraction does not exist in a true sense since the muscle tension will change as the joint

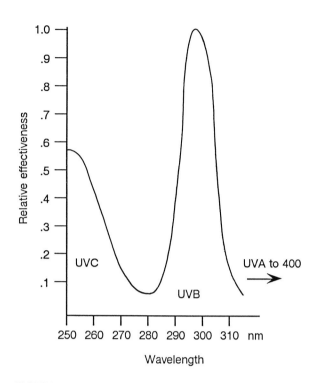

**FIGURE 7-17** Action spectrum of erythema (skin redness). The wavelength of light which is shown on the bottom of the graph indicates that the most effective wavelengths to produce erythema are between 290 and 305 nanometers.

moves when you take into account the leverage effect. See **Figure 7-18**.

Muscle contraction relates also to the type of fibers in the muscles. We distinguish **Type I fibers** or **SO fibers** which are slow twitch oxidative fibers since they work only in the presence of adequate oxygen.

**Type II fibers** can be Type IIA or Type IIB and are called **FOG** (Type IIA) for fast twitch oxidative-glycolytic or **FG** (Type IIB) for fast twitch glycolytic. The reference to glycolytic refers to the use of the Myerhoff pathway in glucose metabolism by the muscle cells. This metabolic pathway requires no oxygen. It is interesting to note that certain individuals with particular athletic leanings or aptitudes have muscle fiber types specific for the sport of their choice. For example, endurance type athletes have more Type I fibers, while sprinters and shot putter swho exert maximum effort over a short period have more Type II fibers.

### Muscle Atrophy - Effects of Disuse and Aging

Muscle atrophy or muscle wasting is caused

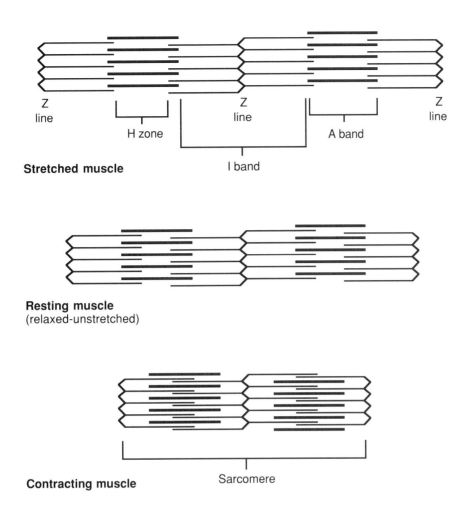

FIGURE 7-18 Muscle contraction. The Z lines are myosin tails that pull the attached filament together. In contraction the Z lines overlap.

by injury or by disuse. Muscles do not normally atrophy as a consequence of aging, but they do become weaker for a variety of reasons. We as skin care specialists are concerned mainly about how to improve muscle size and strength to prevent sagging in facial muscles. We must not neglect the muscles of the arms and abdomen which also present sagging problems with aging and disuse. The phenomenon of the couch potato is a curse to our modern civilization. The atrophy of muscles is centered on the muscle fibers which become smaller in diameter, and in turn decrease the tension of contraction.

### What can We Do to Increase Muscle Tone and Strength

Muscles must work to maintain their size and strength. The body has an economic law which says "those tissues that do not work will not be maintained". Unlike indulgent parents the body does not support unproductive dependents. Exercise is the main source of muscle activity be it walking, running, lifting, climbing steps, chopping wood, or dancing. Exercise increases the cross-sectional area of the muscle. A stretching action is beneficial to muscles prior to heavy use. Exercise is well known to benefit muscles in general but it is unknown if facial muscles benefit from exercise. I know of no controlled study that indicates facial exercises are beneficial but one frequently sees articles on the subject. My opinion is that in most cases it will do no harm and may help.

### Electrical Stimulation of Muscles

It is important to recognize that the facial

muscles are not the cause of aging changes in the face. We have discussed the real cause which is atrophy of elastic tissues in the papillary dermis. The muscles of the face are best exercised by chewing fresh fruit (such as an apple) and by normal facial expressions during the day. Much attention is being given to "facial muscle stimulators" but there is no objective evidence to support benefits from this form of treatment.

A great deal of time and effort has been spent to improve the muscles impaired in facial nerve paralysis (called Bell's Palsy). In this disorder the facial nerve is affected so that the motor nerves of the face are impaired. No amount of electrical stimulation has benefited this condition. See page 188 in <u>Manual of Physical Therapy</u> by Payton et al. I have not spent a great deal of time on this subject because it is one that is not founded in real science. The only possible benefit is the placebo effect, but the cost of the treatment in no ways justifies this expense.

## ELECTROMAGNETIC ENERGY

There are perhaps few subjects with more appeal and excitement than the study of electromagnetic energy. Just about everything we do is in some way related to electromagnetic energy. We need to be aware of the positive and negative effects of the sun and other sources of electromagnetic energy. The science that deals electromagnetic energy and life is called **photobiology**.

As skin care specialists we are mainly interested in the effect of light on the skin. A brief review of the physics of light and the interaction of light on the skin will be helpful in understanding the importance of light as both a positive and negative influence on skin health. Light may be phototoxic, causing injury to the skin. It may be used in phototherapy, in photohemotherapy, and may have an effect on the immune system. This last subject is now a new science called **photoimmunology**. All aspects of light and skin are important to the skin care specialist, however, it will assume an even greater importance in the future with new research findings.

### The Electromagnetic Spectrum

Light is an electromagnetic vibration that has two natures. Light is both a particle and a wave. In order to understand the action of light you must keep these two natures in mind. When light is reflected or refracted it is acting as a wave, but when it is absorbed or transformed into heat or chemical energy it behaves like a particle of energy. This particle of energy is called a quantum. Scientists have been trying to understand this for many years and only by accepting that light does have a dual nature can they make any sense of it at all. As we look into the physics of light you will see why this dual nature is a rational explanation for the behavior of light.

The electromagnetic spectrum represents a range of energy values based on the wavelength of the various waves contained in the spectrum. Visible light is only a tiny fraction of the electromagnetic spectrum which ranges from extremely tiny waves to extremely large waves. It was found that the wavelength of these various waves was related to the amount of energy in the wave. This remarkable finding was eventually to evolutionize science. For our purpose we need to know that light varies from high energy in the ultraviolet range to low energy in the infrared range.

The energy in a particle wave:
$$E = hv$$
where: $h$ = Plank's constant = $6.6 \times 10^{-27}$
$v$ = frequency

$$v = c/l$$
where: $c$ = velocity of light = $3 \times 10^{10}$ cm/sec
$l$ = wavelength
therefore: $E = h\,c/l$

Notice that the $l$ is on the bottom of the equation which means that the energy of the wave is inversely proportional to the wavelength. The larger the wave the smaller the energy. Since ultraviolet light is of smaller wavelength than infrared light it must have higher energy level.

We speak of the wavelength of light in terms of nanometers (nm). Nanometers are quite small, being only one billionth of a meter. (A nanometer is one-thousandth of a micron, which is one-thousandth of a millimeter, which is one-thousandth of a meter.) Ultraviolet light ranges down to 200 nanometers which is invisible. At 400 nanometers, light is visible as a blue color and at 800 nm it is quite red. Beyond 800 nm is the near infrared spectrum which is invisible. Think of light as little packets of energy in a wave form and you will have little difficulty understanding this concept. Let us now see how light interacts with living tissue.

### Biological Effects of Light

We know that light is absorbed by many materials much as a blotter absorbs water. When light passes through any material there are certain absorption laws or principles that determine how much light is absorbed. The absorbed light will interact with the material in certain ways which will have a specific effect on a particular material. Everyone is aware of how sunlight will fade the fabric on an upholstered chair, or the colors of an oriental rug. These are called photochemical reactions. The effect of the light on a particular substance, such as the tissues of the skin, is determined by the intensity of the light and the duration of one light irradiation. Together these two quantities make up the exposure, or dosage. It matters little if the dose is large over a short time, or small over a long time, the biological effect will be the same. The intensity is related to the wavelength and the energy. We need not go into the mathematics of the relationship except to say that intensity x time = a constant. When you look at the effects of light at different wavelengths on any given photochemical process you have created an **action spectrum.**

You will see the term action spectrum in the photobiology literature; **Figure 7-19** shows an action spectrum for erythema. These studies are important in understanding the nature of light, such as what effects particular energy levels will have on skin. For example, the action of ultraviolet at 308 nm is 1000 times more potent on skin then ultraviolet light at 350 nm. This is the real importance of understanding the action spectrum.

Light will react with the skin and produce effects depending on the dosage received. Sunlight coming through the atmosphere will be attenuated by the air, moisture, and dust. The amount of sunlight reaching the earth will be quite variable day to day.

Water absorbs light in the low ultraviolet range from 180 to 300 nm. The skin will reflect

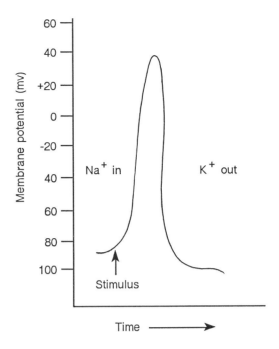

**FIGURE 7-19** Action potential. A contracted muscle generates a voltage called an action potential. It can be measured with electrical equipment and displayed graphically. The graph shows the voltage generated by the muscle contraction.

light and the stratum corneum will scatter light. White skin reflects about 45% and black skin about 17%. The longer rays (600 nm +) will penetrate the skin to the level of the subcutaneous tissue, giving the skin a red color. The stratum corneum and the epidermis absorb most of the shorter wavelengths from 280 to 310 nm. The very short waves in the range of 290 nm to 350 nanometers are absorbed in the first 60 nm, and the longer ultraviolet rays from 350nm to 450 nm are absorbed in the first 150 nm. The other parts of the spectrum from 450 to 1200 nm are passed into the dermis and absorbed by different components of the dermis. Remember that not all the energy of each wavelength is absorbed at a particular level but at least 37% of the incident energy is absorbed at these levels.

In the dermis, the reflected visible light provides the skin color which we see. The major absorption occurs with hemoglobin of the blood, bilirubin, melanin, and beta carotene. These substances reflect and absorb light and produce the skin color in this fashion. Two examples are the dark skins of blacks (from melanin) and the intense yellow skin of people who eat large amounts of carrots and other yellow vegetables (from carotene). In carrot induced yellow skin, the effect is most noticeable on the palms of the hands and soles of the feet because of the thick stratum corneum. These areas retain much of the carotene pigment. Between 600 nm and 1300 nm there is very low absorption in the dermis so that an "optical window" is produced in this region. This allows the use of selected infrared heat to penetrate deep into the tissue without damage to the upper layers. Water absorbs above 1300 nm to about 1600 nm and again at 1850 nm. This finding makes it possible to use highly specific wavelengths in the treatment of certain diseases.

Wood's lamp uses a spectrum in the UVA range of 310 to 400 nm. This lamp is used to diagnose various disorders of the skin due to fluorescence. The colors seen with the Wood's lamp are mainly epidermal in origin arising from the most superficial layers of the skin.

## Photochemical Effects of Ultraviolet Light

The most studied effect of ultraviolet light on the skin has been the effect on the DNA of the cell. Obviously, the importance of DNA in the repair and reproduction of the skin has spurred this research, but there are other effects as well. The RNA of the cell along with enzymes and cell membranes are also targets of UV irradiation. In the first few hours after exposure, both DNA and RNA synthesis is decreased and skin metabolism is markedly altered. Repair starts almost immediately with the DNA which is followed by recovery of the cell, or else the cell will undergo mutation or death. These changes occur mainly in the basal layer for it is here that cells divide and supply the upper layers. The repair process is accompanied with a protective action which, primarily, is increased melanin production. As the repair process continues there is increased proliferation of keratinocytes which results in peeling of the exposed skin. Repeated exposures of the sun or artificial UV light will produce skin cancer and premature aging of the skin.

This photoaging is distinct from chronological aging and is partially reversible. The tragedy is that it is totally preventable; only ignorance and obstinancy allow it to continue. We shall look further at this when we discuss clinical aging.

## Lasers and Light Therapy

Lasers are optical instruments that combine monochromatic light (single wavelength) with coherence (narrow beam). These two properties allow the laser to focus a very narrow beam of high intensity light onto a specific area of the body. Even single cells or parts of a cell may be selectively irradiated with laser light. The range of laser energy is tremendous, reaching above 10 billion watts. Lasers may be continuous or pulsed. The pulsed laser is most effective where a short burst of energy is needed. Lasers can be made that have a single wavelength only, or they may be tunable over several wavelengths using organic dyes. A laser is only one specific wavelength, even though an instrument may have the capability to be tuned to different wavelengths.

Lasers have found use in surgical procedures. Intense heat produced by the absorption of the laser energy destroys mainly the absorbing tissue and not the adjacent tissue. One of the main advantages in the use of lasers for surgical procedures is that the blood vessels are coagulated and bleeding is eliminated. The most commonly used laser for this purpose is the carbon dioxide laser with an infrared wavelength of 10,600 nm. In dermatology, the argon-ion laser with emission lines at 476, 488, and 514 nm is used to destroy port-wine stains, tattoos and hemangiomas. The choice of laser depends on the nature, size and depth of the lesion, patient age and other considerations. This is a particular skill that must be learned at the side of an expert in this field. In the future much more will be done with lasers in skin care.

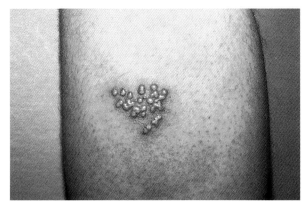

a. Herpes simplex type 1

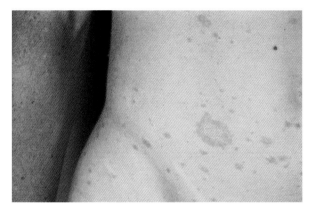

b. Pityriasis rosea

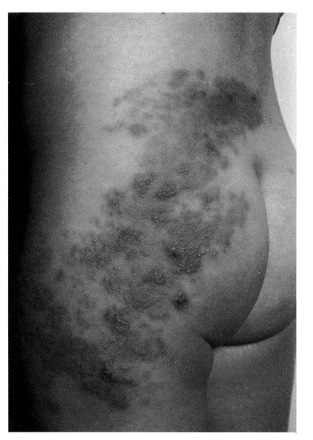

c. Herpes zoster (shingles)

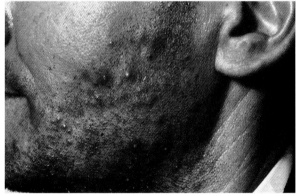

d. Folliculitis

**DISEASES OF THE SKIN**

**Viral Infections**

(Top half-page, a., b., and c.) Clusters of vesicles are seen in herpes simplex and herpes zoster. Herpes zoster always follows a nerve pathway, while herpes simplex does not. Note that the warts are quite variable. They may be flat or "vegetative".

**Bacterial Infections**

(Bottom, d. and e.) Bacterial infections manifest as redness and swelling of the skin. Pustules may be present or deep abscesses may occur. In this photograph of folliculitis, pustules and papules are visible.

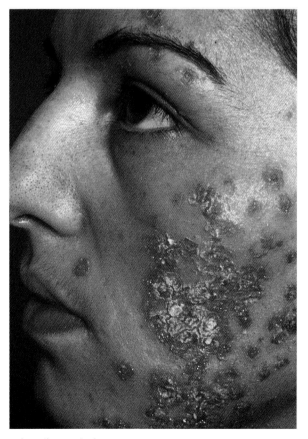

e. Impetigo contagiosa

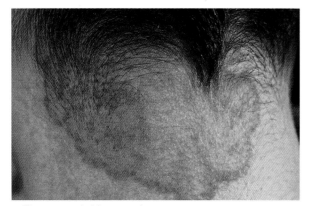

a. Tinea corporis (ring worm)

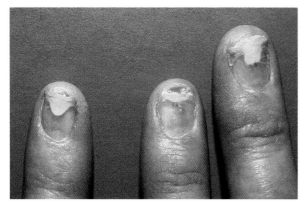

b. Onychia (from manicure sculpting)

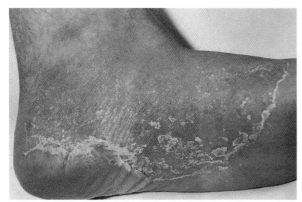

c. Tinea pedis (athlete's foot)

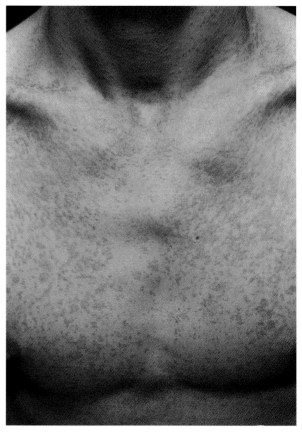

d. Tinea versicolor

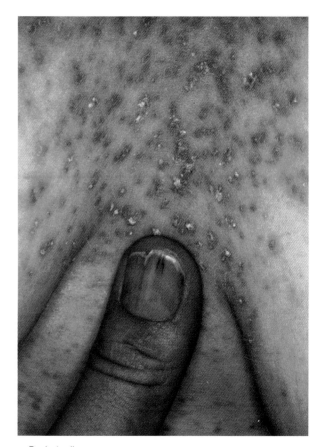

e. Darier's disease

### Fungal Infections

(This page) Fungal infections present in many ways and on almost any place on the body. In most cases there is redness and some scaling. You need to see these conditions "in the flesh" to be able to diagnose them correctly.

### Cancers of the Skin

(Opposite page) Even experts have trouble distinguishing malignant skin tumors. Biopsy is always indicated if there is reasonable doubt. Refer all questionable skin lesions to a physician. Study these photographs well as they are representative of the characteristics of malignant lesions.

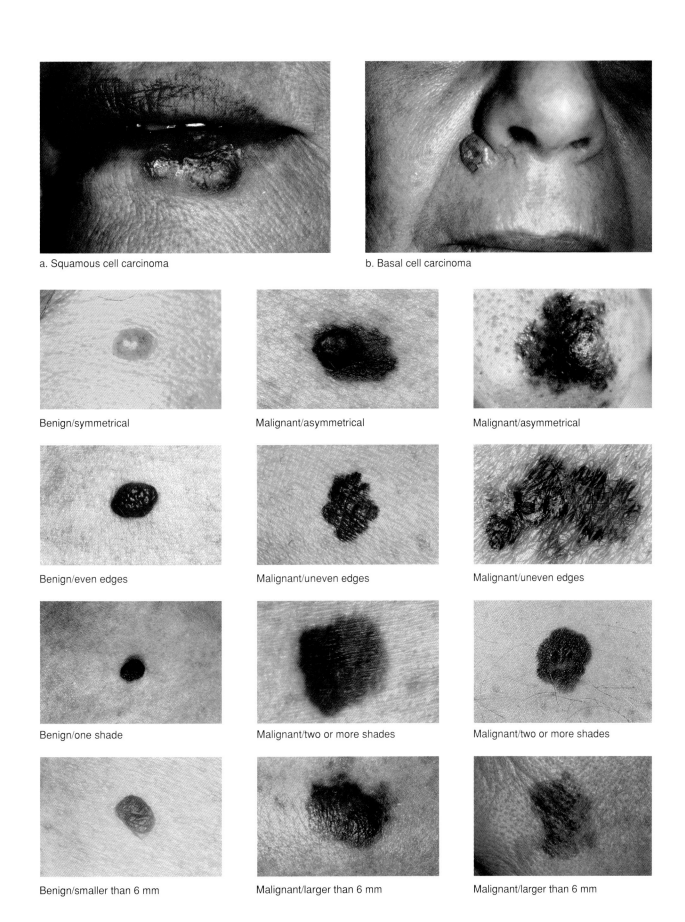

a. Squamous cell carcinoma

b. Basal cell carcinoma

Benign/symmetrical

Malignant/asymmetrical

Malignant/asymmetrical

Benign/even edges

Malignant/uneven edges

Malignant/uneven edges

Benign/one shade

Malignant/two or more shades

Malignant/two or more shades

Benign/smaller than 6 mm

Malignant/larger than 6 mm

Malignant/larger than 6 mm

**The ABCD's of Melanoma - Asymmetry, Border, Color, and Diameter** (Cancers of the skin photographs reprinted with permission of The Skin Cancer Foundation, New York, NY. Additional photographs courtesy of the American Academy of Dermatology.)

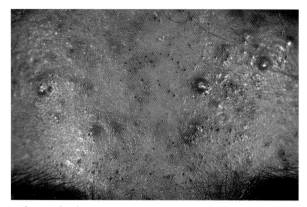

a. Acne vulgaris

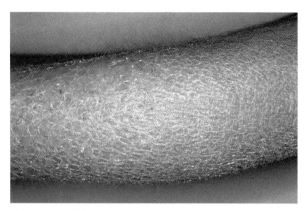

d. Ichthyosis (fish skin)

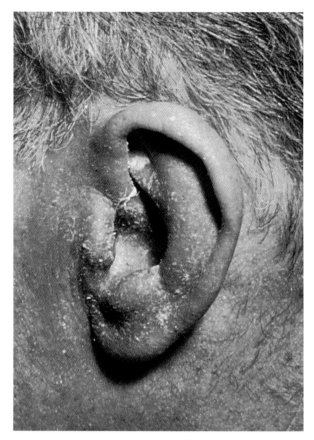

b. Seborrheic dermatitis

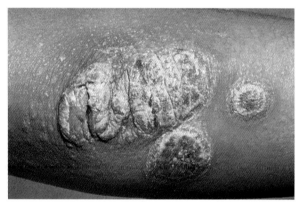

e. Psoriasis

### Disorders of the Sebaceous Glands

(This page, a., b., and c.) All sebaceous gland disorders are characterized by oily skin and redness of the skin. Some flaking is seen in rosacea and seborrheic dermatitis.

### Hyperproliferative Disorders

(Above, d. and e.) Hyperproliferative disorders usually have a thick stratum corneum and are scaly. Redness is frequently present.

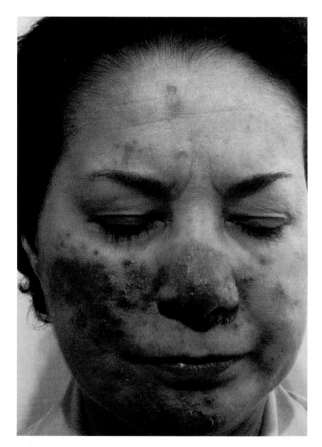

c. Acne rosacea

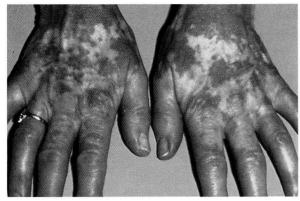

a. Vitiligo

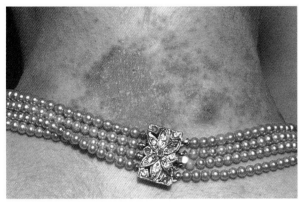

b. Contact dermatitis (from nickel)

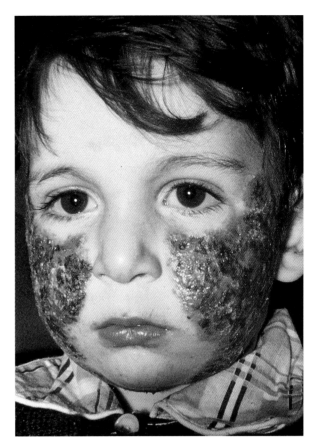

c. Atopic dermatitis (with secondary infection)

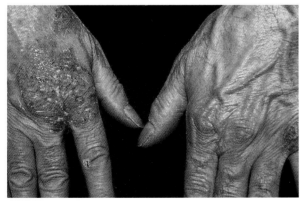

d. Nummular eczema

### Disorders of Pigmentation

(Top left, a.) Vitiligo and melasma (not shown) are at the opposite poles of the color spectrum: vitiligo - no pigment, melasma - excess pigment.

### Eczematous Dermatitis Disorders

(This page, b., c., d., and e.) Eczema and atopic dermatitis are similar in appearance at times. Scaling and redness are common along with scratch marks. Frequent sites for atopic dermatitis are the antecubital fossa, the popliteal fossa, and the face.

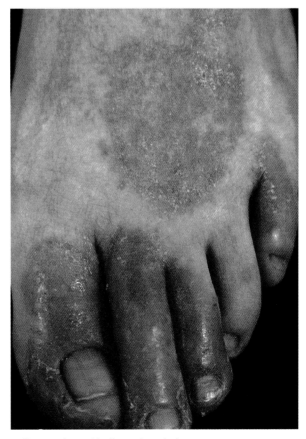

e. Contact dermatitis (from shoe dye)

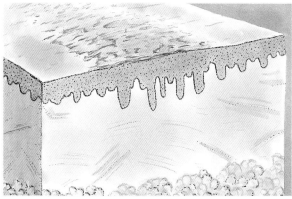

Lichenification

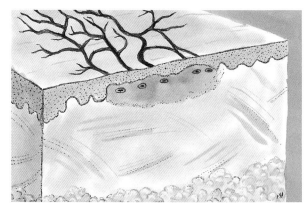

Telangiectasia

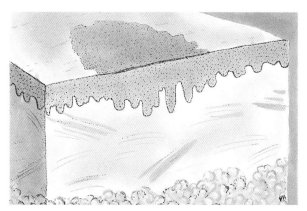

Macule

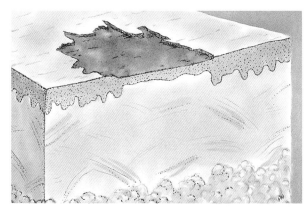

Erosion

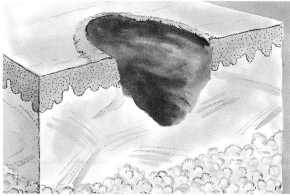

Ulcer

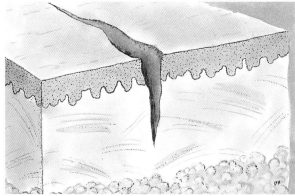

Fissure

### Common Lesions

#### Flat Lesions

**Lichenification** - Lichenification is a thicker lesion usually seen associated with chronic itching areas. The lesions are silver to purple and have small scales. They arise in areas of plaque.

**Telangiectasia** - Blood vessels are seen in a branching pattern. If you press a glass slide (microscope type) over the lesion it will blanche in most cases. Where the slide fails to produce blanching the lesion is most likely due to extravasated blood, like petechia.

**Macule** - The macule is not raised above the skin's surface. It may be any color, any size or any shape, and may arise from any component of the skin. The most common macular lesions are: 1.**Telangiectasias** on the nose and nail bed, 2.**Petechiae** are small purple spots resulting from blood that has gone into the

tissue from the blood vessels (called extravasation), and 3.**Ecchymoses** are large **purpuric** lesions such as bruises or a black-eye. 4. **Infarcts** are areas that result from occluded blood vessels They are irregularly shaped and range in color from grayish to dusky red.

#### Depressed Lesions

**Erosion** - Erosions that are not inflammed can occur from a number of causes, which may be traumatic, but usually results from vesiculation. Only the epidermis is involved and no scarring results as the erosion heals.

**Ulcer** - An ulcer is an inflammatory erosion of the skin that includes epidermis and dermis. It may contain pus or serum. The shape will vary from round to quite irregular. The aphthous ulcer in the mouth ("canker sore") is a typical ulcer. Ulcers may arise from a variety of skin disorders such as cancers, infarcts, nodules

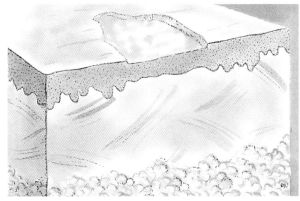

Depressed scar (striae)

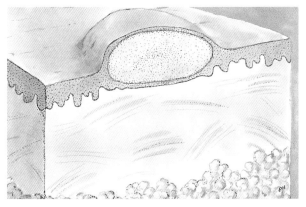

Pustule

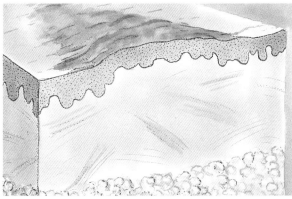

Wheal

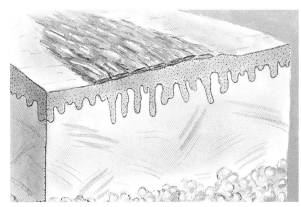

Plaque

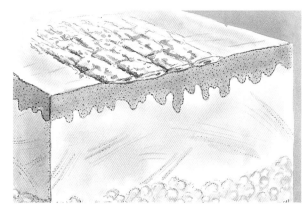

Scale

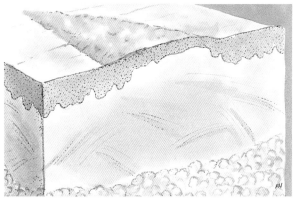

Elevated scar (as in a burn)

and venous stasis. Venous stasis is a condition in the skin caused by poor circulation and venous congestion. It occurs in the lower legs accompanied by increased pigmentation and edema.

**Fissure** - A fissure is a crack in the skin. It may be quite small or comparatively large. Fissures of the lips are common in wintertime with chapping. The hands, feet and perianal area are frequent sites of fissures.

**Depressed scar (Striae)** - Depressed scars show a surface defect and loss of dermal tissue components. They represent healing of ulceration in wounds. The normal skin lines and appendages (hair and sweat glands) are often lost in scar tissue.

Elevated Lesions

**Plaque** - Plaque is an elevated area of skin that may arise from confluence of papules. This is seen most often in psoriasis. Scratching plaque causes lichenification.

**Pustule** - Pustules are red raised lesions with pus at the apex. They are seen mainly in acne but also occur in psoriasis and impetigo. A furuncle is a large deep pustule arising from a hair follicle (folliculitis). When furuncles group or coalesce they form a carbuncle - a nasty painful and resistant infection.

**Scale** - Scale is a silvery, flaky lesion seen in hyperproliferative or inflammatory disorders. The most common disorder associated with scale is psoriasis but they occur also in fungal infections, pityriasis rosea and secondary syphilis. Solar keratosis produces lesion with dense gritty scales. Fish-like scales seen in ichthyosis are just stratum corneum cells that have failed to slough off.

**Wheal** - Wheals are pale, pink to red, lesions that are associated with allergy in skin irritation. They are soft to firm since they arise from intercellular fluid in the tissue. They may be as small as 3 to 4 millimeters or as large as10 to12 centimeters.

**Elevated Scar (as in a burn)** - Elevated scars usually are

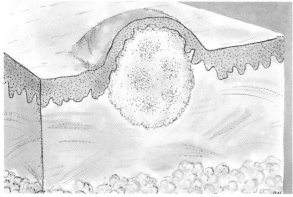

Nodule

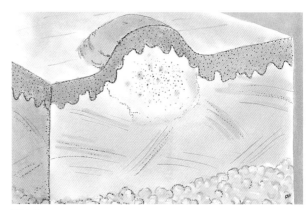

Papule

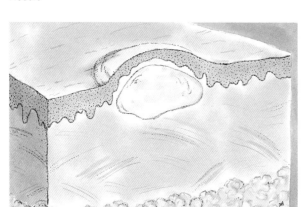

Cyst

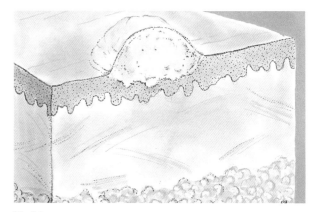

Vesicle

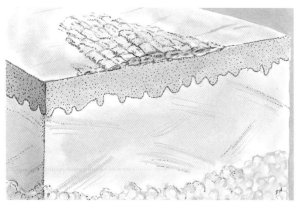

Crust

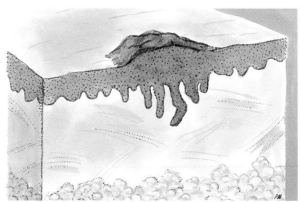

Mole

over-reactive scar. Keloids are an extreme example. They are very disfiguring and present a major problem to the cosmetic specialist.

**Nodule** - Nodules are hard lesions that are covered with the epidermis. They arise from a variety of causes. The dermatofibroma presents as a nodule. All nodules need careful medical evaluation for many are a sign of systemic disease.

**Papule** - Papules are red, firm lesions without pus. They may be another color but are always raised above the level of the skin's surface; they are less than 0.5 cm in diameter. They may be flat topped as seen in lichen planus, or vegetative as seen in a wart. Vegetations are small closely packed elevations in a lesion.

**Cyst** - Cysts are closed lesions usually covered with a sac or membrane. Sebaceous cysts are very common on the skin. They will vary in size from quite small to very large. Cysts may contain

fluid or semisolid matter. The most common cysts are epidermal keratinous types. Pilar cysts arise in the hair follicle and are lined with multilayered epithelium.

**Vesicle** - Vesicles are fluid filled lesions. The fluid is a clear straw-yellow. Big vesicles (over 0.5 cm) are called bullae. Vesicles are often covered only with the stratum corneum (subcorneal vesicle) in very thin epidermis (spongiosis); if they arise from the basement membrane they are called acantholytic vesicles. Vesicles may also arise from below the epidermis.

**Crust** - Crusts are composed of serum, blood, and stratum corneum cells. Pus also may be component at times. The classical lesion for crusts is the lesion seen in impetigo contagiosa.

**Mole** - Moles are either red brown or black. They vary in size from one millimeter to several centimeters. Consider every mole as a possibility for malignancy.

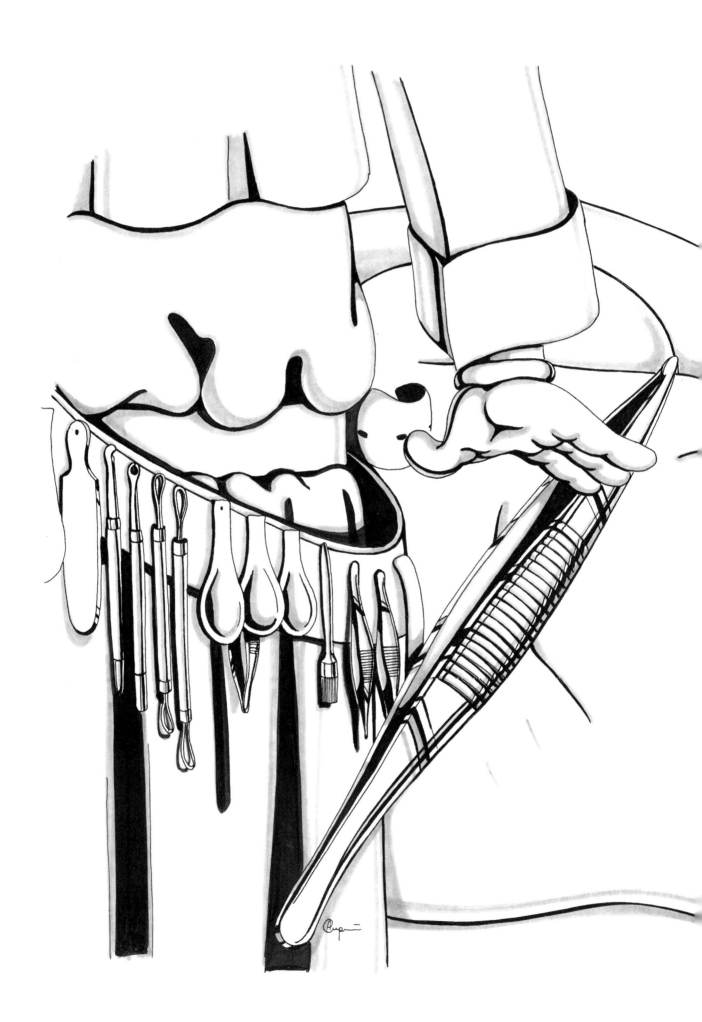

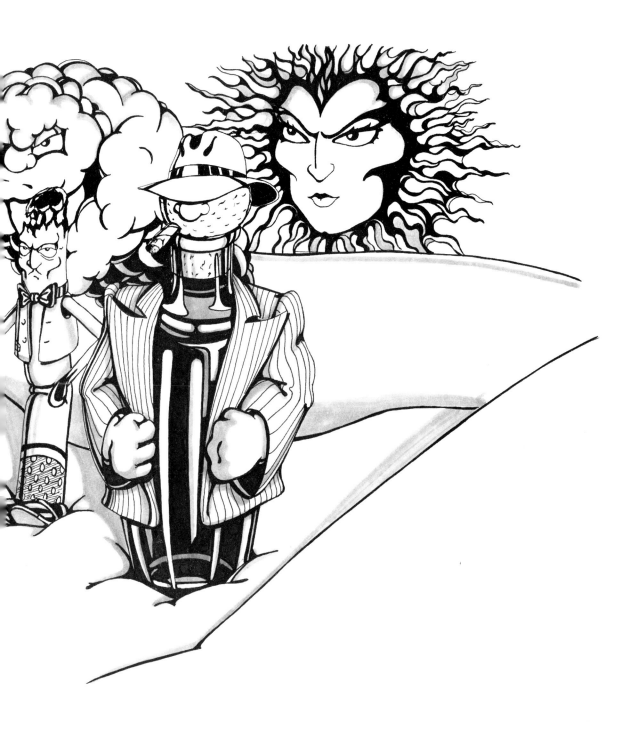

Somebody once said that to be really tough you've gotta walk softly and carry a big stick. Our work is a little more delicate than that, but the principle is the same. When this Wall presents challenges to our usual genius, we know we ought to call in the Artillery. But, even with that strength --we never, ever wanna lose our soft touch.

# Treatments, Methods, and Techniques

We now take up the subject of treatment. It is important for the student to learn early that specific treatments for specific diseases is still the ideal, but in many cases it is lacking. When we do not have a specific treatment for a particular disorder we use a term called "empirical" or "symptomatic" treatment. **Empirical** means only experimental, while symptomatic means even less; here you are treating only the symptoms of the disorder, the pain, itch, etc. It has been through empirical therapy that modern medicine has advanced. What separates us today from our colleagues in the past is that our empirical trials are now called clinical research which is rigorously controlled by the FDA (Food and Drug Administration). As we outline treatments, keep in mind that we shall not always have the best answer to the problem.

## ACNE - THE DISEASE AND METHODS OF TREATMENT

### Incidence and Other Aspects

**Physiological acne** occurs in about 80 to 90 percent of teenagers. It is characterized by the presence of a few comedones, while clinical acne is easily recognized by anyone remotely familiar with this condition. Most clinical cases appear around 14-19 (19 years of age in females and between 14 to 18 in males). There is some disagreement about the effects of the menstrual cycle and pregnancy on the severity of acne with evidence to support both an increase and a decrease of acne lesions due to hormonal changes. A person's diet seems to be unrelated to the presence of acne. The effects of chocolate, carbohydrates, lipids, proteins, minerals and vitamins all have been well studied and no correlation has been found. There are some reports that acne improves in the summer, but again, this is not substantiated by objective studies. There is a condition called "**acne Majorca**" characterized by closed comedones that occurs with the combination of sunscreen use and heavy exposure to ultraviolet light (sunlight). Finally, there is some evidence to suggest that acne may be aggravated by stress. While not without question, this relationship is worth pursuit. I believe everyone is familiar with the horrors of a "date goob", which occurs more frequently than chance alone can explain.

## Clinical Features

Let's review the basic types of lesions seen in acne and the overall clinical picture.

First, the skin appears greasy. Lesions will be seen on the face, back and chest (the most common sites). The open comedone, or black-head, is a lesion from 0.1 to 3 mm in size which takes several weeks or more to develop. The closed comedone is about the same size, is slightly raised, and may be felt. These lesions are frequently associated with inflammation since about 75% will go on to become inflamed, with the other 25% resolving spontaneously. Papules may arise from normal skin, from closed come-dones, or from blackheads. About 7% resolve into macules, which are flat, red areas. Most remain active or develop into pustules. A pustule may be superficial or deep. They contain white blood cells, polymorphonuclear cells, whose lysosomal enzymes may help resolve the lesions in five days. Deep pustules may take weeks to resolve. They are quite tender and red and often resolve by going through a papular stage. Nod-ules are deep, tender lesions that remain for many weeks (up to eight). Cysts are large lesions

several centimeters in size that contain creamy, yellow, thick pus. They are seen on the back, chest, face, and neck.

Next, let's look at acne scars. They may be formed by increased tissue formation or from tissue loss. The increased tissue scars are called keloids or hypertrophic scars. The tissue scars are either "ice-pick lesions", which may be soft or hard, or depressed fibrotic scars, which may be quite large. The difference between the two is one of size mainly, but ice-pick lesions may become depressed fibrotic scars.

Finally, let's review the four grades of acne which are based on the types and number of lesions present. **Grade I acne** is comedonal acne with less than 30 comedones present. **Grade II acne** consists of comedones and some pus-tules. **Grade III acne** consists of comedones, inflamed pustules and an occasional inflamed cyst. **Grade IV acne** consists of large pustules, cysts, connecting sinuses, inflamed nodules and scarring. This is called **acne conglobata**.

Before passing on to actual treatment it is important to state that the non-physician skin care specialist must limit their treatment to pa-tients with only Grade I and Grade II acne. Grade

III acne may be considered if cysts are not inflamed, and should be undertaken with a physician involved. Grade IV acne should only be treated by a physician.

**Treatment of Acne**

There are currently four basic principles which describe acne treatment: 1. correct the abnormal pattern of keratinization in the follicle, 2. decrease the activity of the sebaceous gland, 3. inhibit or decrease bacterial growth in the follicle, 4. produce an anti-inflammatory effect. Of these four, the first is the most important because abnormal keratinization is the fundamental pathology present.

<u>Cleansing</u>

Much is made of cleansing the skin in acne, yet little clinical evidence exists to support this action. While excess facial oil is present in acne, only mild cleansers are needed. I do not recommend the use of facial scrubs or abrasive sponges in acne. Almost any soap may be used, but one that leaves a little residue of germicidal action is beneficial.

<u>Topical Agents</u>

There are many keratolytic agents on the market today from which to choose. I have listed those that are OTC (over the counter) or non-prescription preparations. There are only four active agents that are permitted as OTC anti-acne products: benzoyl peroxide, sulfur, resorcinol, and salicylic acid. **Benzoyl peroxide** is most widely used by dermatologists. Understanding the active agents of the various commercial products will help you to choose a particular preparation.

Benzoyl peroxide acts in several ways. First, it is an antimicrobial agent being effective against Proprionibacterium (the most common acne causing bacteria) acnes. Second, it is an irritant, causing an increase in cell turnover, and a loosening of the keratin plugs. Being a powerful oxidizing agent may underlie both of these actions. There may be yet another effect on the keratin. This remains unknown. Benzoyl peroxide is used in a concentration of 2.5 to 10%, in either creams, lotions, gels, or ointments.

(Higher concentrations are available only by prescription.) The patient uses the preparation once or twice daily, using light massage over the affected areas. The eye area, lips, mouth and inside of the nose should be avoided, as stinging and burning can occur. Ultraviolet light should be avoided during the treatment period, particularly ultraviolet lamps. As with all medications there are some side reactions including sensitization, which occurs in 1-3% of users. You may see redness, dryness, peeling, and perhaps very mild swelling. These effects are the end result of benzoyl peroxide treatment and indicate a therapeutic effect. Excessive peeling, redness, or swelling indicates a reaction. In the case of a reaction, stop the product and remove any residue with warm and gentle cleansing. You may try the product again at a lower dose, after the reaction subsides. If it recurs you know you are most likely dealing with a sensitization and the product must be avoided.

**Sulfur** is used as precipitated sulfur or in a colloidal form, in concentrations from 2 to10%. The preparations are usually in lotion form and are applied as a thin film. The action is both bactericidal and keratolytic and is considered mild. Watch for reactions.

**Resorcinol** is still not recommended by itself as an anti-acne preparation but when combined with sulfur it appears to be effective. One of the problems with resorcinol is the discoloration of the skin produced by this chemical, particularly on darker skinned individuals. A brown scale is produced, but disappears when the product is stopped. It is used at 1 to 2% with sulfur from 2 to10% and comes in sticks, lotions, and creams. The usual precautions apply.

**Salicylic acid** is not considered effective by itself as an anti-acne agent. It is available in concentrations of 0.5 to 2% as a non-prescription product. At these concentrations it produces a mild keratolytic action which is superficial, but at 5% deeper keratolytic action is obtained. (5% salicylic acid requires a prescription.) Sometimes it is helpful to combine sulfur and salicylic acid with resorcinol. Low levels of salicylic acid appear most helpful in mild acne to shorten the inflammatory stage.

<u>Physical Agents</u>

**Ultraviolet light** has been used to treat acne

for many years. The action is not fully understood but is believed to be an irritant reaction causing a more rapid cell turnover. To be effective the dosage must be sufficient to produce erythema. I see little value in the use of ultraviolet light because it will also produce damage to other cells of the epidermis. The eyes must be protected from the ultraviolet rays so exercise care if you elect this treatment.

**Microsurgery** is useful in acne. The expression of blackheads with an extractor of the **Unna-type** (see **Figure 8-1**), or the **Shalita-type** will provide a cosmetic effect. Care in the use of comedone extractors is important since improper use will only aggravate the condition.

First, warm the skin with a wet towel, then place the hole of the instrument over the blackhead and with a gentle sliding pressure remove the plug. Do not use excessive pressure or struggle with a difficult or recalcitrant blackhead. It will only make the situation worse. After removal cleanse the area with 70% alcohol. Be careful in using the extractor about the nose or mouth, since it is possible to produce cellulitis by this method, though it is very rare.

Closed comedones or whiteheads have a tendency to become inflamed so it is best to remove them. Use a No. 25 gauge needle or other sharp instrument to enlarge the orifice, and then express the contents. Apply 70% alcohol afterwards. See **Figure 8-2**. In small pustules having a soft yellow top, the lesion may be opened with a sharp needle or scalpel. If you insert the needle at the base of the yellow area and cut in an upward manner you will cause less pain and avoid spreading the infection. Do not attempt to open cysts or large pustules. These should be referred to a physician for treatment. The client should be seen at least once a week during the

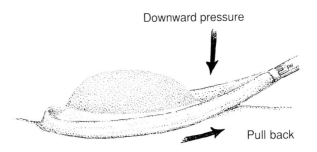

**FIGURE 8-2** Unna-type comedone extracting technique. First use a steamer on the face, or hot wet towel. Use a pressing motion. If it does not come out easily, do not force it!

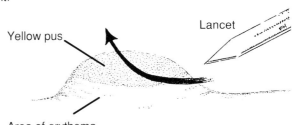

**FIGURE 8-2** (cont.) Lancet procedure. Insert lancet into yellow part of pustule and make a clear inward and upward incision. Milia can be opened in the same manner.

acute phase of the disease, and then monthly thereafter for a maintenance course of treatment. Remember that acne is a not curable at present, but it is treatable.

**Exolift**, a new acrylate polymer, is effective in removing blackheads. (See Appendix.)

## AGING SKIN - CLINICAL FEATURES, PREVENTION, AND TREATMENT

The treatment of aging skin is perhaps the greatest opportunity presented to the skin care specialist. It offers one of the most rewarding activities in this profession. Many studies have

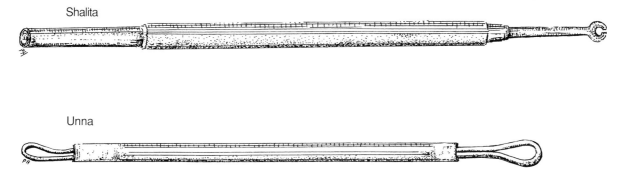

**FIGURE 8-1** Types of comedone extractors. One end of the Shalita extractor expresses comedones and the other end contains a lancet under cover. The Unna extractor has two different sizes of loops for different size comedones.

shown that attractiveness in the elderly is associated with both happiness and acceptance. Interestingly, the frequency of usage of cosmetic and skin care products is about the same in both attractive and unattractive elderly persons. The major difference in these two groups is the skill with which make-up and cosmetics are used. It is important, therefore, that the elderly be taught the proper use of cosmetics along with instruction in skin care treatment programs.

## Prevention - The Major Weapon Against the Ravages of Aging Skin

We see aging skin as being dull, mottled, yellow, marked with lesions of all types (pigmented and unpigmented), leather-like, and appearing dry and lax. Not a very attractive picture. These findings are mainly induced by overexposure to the sun, poor diet, and the excessive use of alcohol and tobacco.

Even in individuals of 25 years these signs are detectable, and as time passes they become much more noticeable. You must start this preventive program in the teen years to be truly effective, however, it is never too late to start. Outlined below is my recommendation for treating aging skin. As usual we start with the diagnostic signs of aging skin and the classification of the various types. I do not know of any absolute classification used by skin care specialists but this is a functional one.

Remember the major cause of wrinkling and sagging of aging skin is connective tissue, probably in the dermis. There are also epidermal changes that magnify the effects that make aging skin an unacceptable personal attribute.

## Distinquishing between Photoaging and Intrinsic Aging

We have discussed this before, but it is so important that we need to review it again. For ease of recognition and remembrance let us put this information in tabular form. See **Table 8-1**.

## Stage Two

### Physical Signs

Signs are loss of skin luster, areas of dilated veins on the nose, fine lines about the outer eyes,

## CHARACTERISTICS OF PHOTOAGING AND INTRINSIC AGING

| CHARACTERISTIC | INTRINSIC AGING | PHOTOAGING |
|---|---|---|
| Wrinkles | Noticeable lines | Marked wrinkles |
| Pigmented spots | Mild, yellowish skin | Dark, reddish to brown |
| Exposed areas | Mild to moderate changes | Marked changes |
| Blood vessels | Mild changes | Marked changes |
| Dermal changes | Papillary dermis | Collagen dissolution |
| Elastin changes | Less elastin | Elastosis |

**TABLE 8-1**

and some under eye puffiness. The hands may show early thinning and the neck will exhibit wrinkling, particularly immediately under the chin. This is more noticeable in women than in men since men show aging signs about 10 years later than women. However, men who are heavy smokers and drinkers may show these signs at the same age as women. Sunbathers will exhibit a dark leathery appearance which in the wintertime will take on a yellow hue. You will see these physical signs from 28 to about 35 years of age.

### General Measures

Insist that the client stop all abusive chemicals and avoid sun exposure. Carefully check diet and life habits and explore stress levels from occupation and personal relationships. Be supportive but not permissive. Design a treatment regimen that will include diet control, regular clinic visits, and active topical products in an outlined program. Here is the suggested program.

### Diet

Eliminate high sugar-containing foods. Add fruits and vegetables containing both fiber and vitamins C and A. Fats should not exceed 30% of the food intake and should include unsaturated fats. Total intake of food should be reduced to no more than 15 calories per pound per day, unless recommended otherwise by a physician.

### Topical Treatment

Start with a general facial cleansing, followed by a facial massage and a hydrating mask. There are many types but I prefer those with a clay base which contain natural ingredients of plant and flower extracts. My favorites are a combination of camomile, echinacea, and comfrey. (See Appendix on natural products).

Facial massage may be of benefit to improve lymphatic drainage and increase circulation, but it also stimulates fibroblast formation and helps to improve the tone and strength of the connective tissue. It is doubtful if there is any benefit to the underlying facial muscles.

### Active Continuous Treatment

The home regimen should consist of nightly facial care and body care. First, bathing at least three times weekly in a good low irritation, non-drying bath preparation containing an effective blooming bath oil. Avoid soaps of high pH and bath oils with mineral oil. Hard water is not usually a problem today but if the water is too hard you will need to add a water conditioner such as Calgon[R].

Facials at night consist of a cleansing followed by an emollient preparation containing the following actives: an antioxidant, a moisturizer, an immune stimulant, and effective vitamins which are vitamin A, vitamin E and panthenol. The morning treatment program is similar using a preparation containing vitamin C to replace vitamin A.

Any activity which involves sun exposure should include a protective hat, gloves, and a sun screen. Sunscreen should be applied generously and often. I do not recommend sunscreens above an SPF of 15. The chance of irritation rises with SPF, while the amount of added protection you receive from higher SPF is minimal.

### Stages Three and Four

### Physical Signs

In this stage of aging skin we see both qualitative and quantitative differences. The most notable change is the appearance of relaxed skin. (Sagging or drooping is more descriptive, though less kind.) The cheeks and mouth are the first areas to show this change, which is due to the degeneration of elastin fibers. The area of the nose and mouth show increase depth of the normal furrows and there is a marked increase in lines about the eyes. In addition, there are many skin lesions that are visible on both exposed and non-exposed skin. See **Figure 8-3**.

### Common Skin Lesions in the Elderly

Besides lax skin we see benign tumors, skin tags, nevi, lentigos, seborrheic keratosis, actinic keratosis, angiomas, telangiectasias, dry skin, premalignant and malignant conditions. You will find that over 65% of individuals over 65 will have at least one of these lesions and 50% may have two or more.

Look also for transparent skin. This is not the same as thin skin. Transparent skin is produced by a collagen defect and is associated with increased water content of the dermis (95% vs 65% for normal skin.) Transparent skin is linked to osteoporosis (thin bones).

### Initial Treatment

First, make sure the client has a personal physician and has been seen recently. It is important that there are no systemic diseases

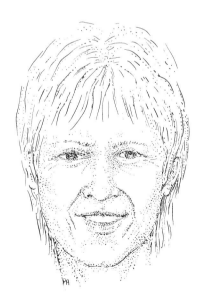

**FIGURE 8-3** Stage three aging face. The nasolabial fold is accentuated with some increase in the labial lines in the lower face. Crow's feet or lines at the outer corners of the eyes are becoming prominent. The lower lid starts to sag and may bulge.

manifested by skin conditions which may be overlooked by the skin care specialist. After your evaluation you must decide if a referral is needed for cosmetic surgery, or if the skin is in a condition that you can treat with confidence. Most conditions will frequently require some cosmetic surgery, including facial peels. Deep South Florida tans almost always leave a face that is furrowed beyond salvage by topical management alone.

Start with a preventive regimen. No more sun, reduction of alcohol, cessation of tobacco, nutritious diet high in vitamins A and C, and improve their concept of self with encouragement. This is the type of client that can benefit most from your care, but who is also the most resistant to lifestyle changes.

Develop a program of monthly visits for facial cleansing and massage. Total body massage coupled with an exercise program will greatly improve these client's feeling of well being.

Topical treatment should consist of the same products as listed above. Vitamin A acetate at 0.25 to 0.35% along with vitamin E acetate at 2% and panthenol at 2% provide an excellent treatment when combined in a moisturizing base. This product should be applied at night after gentle cleansing. Daytime treatment should include the above ingredients except for vitamin A which is replaced with vitamin C at 0.25% as ascorbyl palmitate.

This type of client will show no real improvement in line reduction or creases for about 6 to 8 months. The general appearance of the skin, the color and the texture, however, will improve after 30 days. Here you can not expect miracles but you can expect some changes that will be both obvious and pleasing to the client. Time, patience, persistance, confidence, and encouragement are important to the treatment of this client.

**Stage Five**

Physical Signs

The wrinkles, lines, and creases are more prominent due to further relaxation and deterioration of the elastin fibers. See **Figure 8-4**. The color of the skin varies from a sickly, yellow hue to a tawny, reddish-brown. Many lesions may be visible, particularly brown, flat and raised spots, patches that represent solar type disorders, and non-solar neoplastic disorders. Some of these include the following.

Proliferative types such as seborrheic warts, appear on the face, arms and trunk, and arise from the basal layer. Solar keratoses occur on the sun-exposed areas of the body. On the hands, they have a potential to transform into malignant squamous cell cancers. They are small, being less than 1 cm, well-defined, and usually red to pink plaques with adherent greasy scale.

Pigmented lesions include loss of pigment due to ultraviolet damage. Actinic lentigos are flat pigmented areas less than 1 cm in size and appear similar to freckles. They occasionally become malignant, at which time they are called lentigo maligna.

Dermal changes are associated with elastosis in the sun-exposed areas. The weather-beaten red neck with rhomboidal lines is common in outdoor types. The most striking form of elastosis is seen around the periorbital region of the eyes as yellowish, thick ridges with the skin thrown into folds and afflicted with large comedones and follicular cysts.

The mouth shows typical deep, furrowed

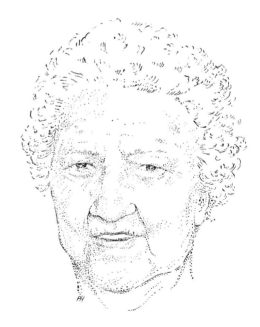

**FIGURE 8-4** Stage five aging face. The facial lines show greater prominence in the nasolabial fold, the forehead, the eyes, and about the mouth. The cheeks are seen to sag and the chin is more prominent. The upper eyelids begin to droop and bag.

lines running perpendicular to the orbicularis. The neck is also badly wrinkled, with "turkey-neck" folds becoming more prominent than that seen in Type II aging. If you examine the un-clothed client you will see additional signs of elastic degeneration manifested as wrinkles at the base of the buttocks.

### Treatment Referral

The first rule in the treatment is to refer the client for evaluation of all skin lesions by a physician. If the client does not have a primary physician, I suggest referral to a dermatologist. (See Chapter 11 on referrals.) Next, I suggest a referral to a cosmetic surgeon (plastic surgeon), as this will complete the team needed for the comprehensive treatment of these clients. Do not be shy about referrals; the best practitioners of medicine do a great deal of referring.

### Total Skin Care

While the client is primarily interested in facial appearance, do not neglect the other areas of the body. After the client has consulted with the physician, the next step is to prepare a treatment program with a physician if medical or surgical management is indicated. In many cases cosmetic surgery for eyelids, face lifts and neck repair will be recommended. With these clients, close relationship and cooperation with a physician will improve the care of the client both before and after the surgery. Here your skills in application of make-up over wounded skin will be gratefully received by the client.

At this stage a long term plan should be developed with the client being seen on a monthly basis. Careful follow-up after any surgical procedure will be required. Attention to diet and the general well-being of the client with consideration of his or her overall self-perception can add to the efficacy of your service.

## PIGMENTATION DISORDERS

All pigment disorders are due to defects in melanin production. Either there is excess melanin, too little melanin, or there is melanin in the wrong places. In any event, the skin care specialist will have contact with these problems. Different problems with skin pigment occur at various ages, with various races, and with certain types of occupations. Here again you must follow the rule that if you do not recognize the disorder, you must refer the client to a physician for expert diagnosis. I shall follow the classifications listed above with reference to age.

### Too Much Pigment - Most Common Disorders

**Freckles** (medical term =*ephelis*) are by far the most common disorder of pigmentation you will see. They appear at about age five years and appear as small brown spots resulting from tight clusters of pigment granules.

Freckles are normal since they are seen in so many people. Red headed individuals are most often blessed with these spots. They occur mostly on the face and other sun-exposed areas but can also be seen on the arms, chest and abdomen. The best treatment is avoidance of the sun as ultraviolet rays will make them darker. Most treatments to reduce the intensity of pigmentation are not warranted. The best treatment is to use a good foundation to mask them. I do not know that anyone has ever made a big deal about freckles; in fact, some people love freckles.

**Moles** are light to dark, circumscribed pigmented lesions smaller than a centimeter. They are called melanocytic nevi by dermatologists and are due to a proliferation of pigmented cells in the epidermis. In appearance they may be flat or elevated (macular or papular), and may be located anywhere over the body in a random fashion.

Moles may appear at any age, and occasionally are present at birth, but usually appear from about age one to age four years. Often moles will lose pigment and become flesh colored in adulthood.

The essential fact to remember is that all pigmented spots must be evaluated for melanoma. About 20% of melanomas arise in moles while the rest start in normal skin. The clinical signs to observe for melanoma are: 1. rapid growth reported by the patient, or observed, 2. color is not uniform, but speckled with different colors, 3. lateral spread into surrounding skin from the pigmented spot; this is often described as the appearance of ink spreading on a blotter, 4. inflammation in the surrounding skin, and 5. bleeding, crusting, and oozing of the lesion. **ANY OF THESE SIGNS REQUIRES REFERRAL TO A PHYSICIAN, PREFERABLY A DERMATOLOGIST.**

Moles are best covered with foundation or concealer. They do not usually require treatment. Surgical excision is required if there is a question of melanoma.

## Seborrheic Keratosis

### Definition and Description

Seborrheic keratosis is a benign proliferation of the epidermis. It is tan to dark-brown in color and appears as plaques or nodules with a rough surface. They occur in middle aged to older whites and are enhanced with sun exposure. The major distinquishing feature is the keratin top of the lesion which may be easily loosened with a fingernail. Melanoma and squamous cell cancers are fleshy growths and do not keratinize in the manner of seborrheic keratosis.

### Location

They are most commonly found on the trunk, but also occur on the face, scalp, and extremities.

### Treatment

Seborrheic keratosis is treated for cosmetic reasons only. The surface lesion is removed by the dermatologist with liquid nitrogen or with curettage.

## Vitiligo

### Definition and Description

Vitiligo (from Latin *vitium* = blemish) is an area of skin with complete lack of pigment. It appears as a white linear area or as widespread irregular areas. The disorder is probably autoimmune in origin.

### Location

It may occur in any area but most frequently in the eyes, around the mouth, around the genital area, and in any of the areas of flexion.

### Treatment

Medical management of vitiligo remains unsatisfactory. Only about 15 to 20% of cases can be repigmented. In 20% of the cases no response to therapy is obtained. Treatment is given with both topical and oral preparations. Cortisone and psoralens are used topically, and psoralen and trioxsalen are given orally. These treatments are best given by a dermatologist experienced with their use. After months of treatment if there is no response it is unlikely favorable results will occur with longer treatment.

The skin care specialist skilled in paramedical make-up will benefit these patients greatly. This is one area in which the dermatologist will refer patients to you!

## Melasma

### Definition and Description

Melasma is a hyperpigmented area. The color is light to dark brown and often mottled with irregular but sharp borders. The condition occurs most often with pregnancy, the use of oral contraceptives, or estrogen. It is rarely seen in males but it does occur at times.

### Location

Melasma most commonly covers the forehead, the malar eminences (cheekbones), and the lips.

### Treatment

After pregnancy the lesions usually clear. Stopping hormones will sometimes clear up the pigmentation. Avoiding sun exposure is also of benefit. Use of hydroquinone in non-pregnant females is helpful.

Use of hydroquinone should be at 3-4% in a cream or lotion base and is available by prescription. The over-the-counter 1-2% cream is only effective in very mild cases. Treatment may be from weeks to months depending on the darkness of the pigmentation. I have had no results with hydrogen peroxide. A new cream with azelaic acid is being tried and appears promising, though not available commercially.

## DISORDERS OF PROLIFERATION

### Psoriasis

Definition and Description

Widespread bright pink to red plaques with loose silvery scales.

About 1 to 2% of the population in America is afflicted with the condition known as psoriasis. This is a non-contagious, inheritable, proliferative disorder of the epidermis. The onset is usually in early or young adulthood. While not a trivial disorder, psoriasis is compatible with long life, with only rare cases of fatality from the disease. The cellular cause of psoriasis is unknown, though it is known to be genetic in origin. There is abnormal or rapid cellular growth of the epidermis which results in loosely adherent scales (stratum corneum cells). Associated with the rapid epidermal growth is some inflammation of the dermis.

Location

Psoriasis may occur anywhere on the body but most commonly over joints such as the elbows and the knees, trunk, buttocks and the palms and the soles. The hair and nails are also involved at times, as is the vagina and the penis.

Clinical Variations

The most important form of psoriasis for the skin care specialist to recognize for referral is severe, wide spread psoriasis as it may indicate a systemic disease. Here are a few other types.

**Guttate or drop-like psoriasis** is seen as many small scattered lesions. Pustular type is seen as bright red areas with scattered painful pustules. These pustules are not infected but rather are sterile, that is, no bacteria may be cultured from them. This type is most frequently associated with fever or other signs of illness.

**Erythroderma type** is characterized by bright, red erythema (redness) over most of the skin. It is not a good sign and the client should be referred to a physician.

General Principles of Treatment

Psoriasis presently cannot be cured, but it can be treated so that it will disappear from view (medical term = go into remission). Here we shall talk only about the treatment of mild to moderate psoriasis. All treatments of psoriasis are directed at reducing the proliferation of the epidermis and reducing the thickness of the stratum corneum. The choice of agents is rather limited because of safety. Physicians use ultraviolet light (UVB) along with tar or drugs called psoralens and UVA. Cortisone is also a favorite as well as certain antimetabolites used in cancer treatment.

Treatment by the skin care specialist is best done jointly with a physician.

Some recommended topical treatments are composed of the following agents: 1. salicylic acid 3 to 6%, 2. Whitefield's ointment, 6% salicylic acid and 12% benzoic acid (also half Whitefield's, 3% and 6% respectively), 3. urea creams as 5 to 10%, 4. commercial preparations (Aquacare and Carmol), 5. lactic acid at 5 to 20% in a cream or lotion; this is a potent keratolytic so it must be used carefully, 6. tars such as coal tars have been used for years; the better ones (less of a bad odor) are Pragmatar[R], Estar[R,] and Psorigel[R].

All of the above items are over-the-counter so they do not need a prescription. Follow the directions with the product being used. Do not overtreat. You must be familiar with this condition before you begin a treatment program otherwise you will not understand what to expect as the treatment progresses. Most treatment programs for psoriasis are done in an intermittent manner. Prolonged use of any agent will cause tolerance or irritation, both of which are undesirable.

Physical Modalities in Therapy

The treatment of psoriasis, is an opportunity to use gentle massage with certain essential oils. Use only calming oils such as lavender or rose, or kochia oil (from the seeds of *Kochia scoparia*) twice a day. Kochia oil is difficult to find but is available in some health food stores. Use light massage, somewhat heavier than lymphatic drainage, as this stimulates the sympathetic nervous system as well as the immune system.

Electrotherapy using stimulation is recommended by some skin care specialists but my experience is limited to the use of low voltage AC current at a frequency of 1400 to 4000 hertz. Using the Electroderma$^R$ instrument as mentioned above for daily treatments of 20-30 minutes is beneficial in many cases, either alone or when combined with other treatments.

Baths of all types have been used, particularly herbal and essential oil baths. The main function of a therapeutic bath is not to hydrate the stratum corneum but to loosen scales and apply a general treatment in low dosage to a wide area. Use this preparation sparingly because of expense and potency. Calming oils, such as rose, lavendar, and camomile (16 drops in a bath of warm water) with one scant tablespoon of clay (bentonite, kaolin, or rose) along with one tablespoon of a very mild surfactant such as a baby bath is frequently beneficial.

A light diet, antioxidants such as vitamin E, and reduction in stress will assist in improving psoriasis.

### ICTHYOSIS (Fish Skin, the "Alligator Man" in the circus)

Description

Icthyosis comes in many forms, from mild to extremely severe. The basic problem is a failure to slough off the stratum coreum so that it builds up to a very thick horny layer. Unlike psoriasis, it is not red and the scales are dry. The disease is worse in the winter and worse on the legs. This is a genetic disease having no known cure at this time; many treatments have been tried with varying success. This is a disfiguring condition but is not often disabling.

Treatment

The treatment is very much like the treatment of psoriasis except harsh agents are not used. Bland vegetable oils and various keratolytic agents are used.

### DISORDERS AFFECTING MAINLY THE FACE

The most common conditions that affect the face are seborrheic dermatitis, impetigo, folliculitis, furuncles, contact dermatitis, atopic dermatitis, rosacea, angiomas, urticaria and drug reactions. Subclassification by cause is as follows: 1. infectious - impetigo, folliculitis, and furuncles; 2. allergic - contact dermatitis, atopic dermatitis, urticaria (hives), and drug eruptions; 3. sebaceous gland dysfunction - rosacea, seborrheic dermatitis, and milia; 4. neoplastic benign - angiomas.

We shall look at each of these groups and discuss general treatment. Again, I must emphasize here that if you are unfamiliar with these conditions and have no experience with them you are obligated to refer the client to an expert physcian. In this way you will learn more about each case and most likely you will be able to handle the next case you see.

### The Infectious Group

These conditions are all due to bacterial infections in the skin. We distinquish two types of bacterial skin infection: 1. primary or spontaneous infection where the skin is unbroken, and 2. secondary infections, or pyodermas, occuring with broken or damaged skin. Impetigo is a primary infection.

Impetigo

Impetigo is a common, contagious, superficial infection of the skin caused by Streptococcus and secondarily by Staphylococcus. It is seen mainly in children, in hot climates, and in crowded and poor socioeconomic conditions. The lesion is most frequently seen on the face as an oozing erosion or as a thin blister which grows in one to three days into a crust that has a honey-color, granular appearance. Lesions may be itchy, tender, or asymptomatic. The lesions spread rapidly by scratching and rubbing with the fingers.

Most uncomplicated early cases may be treated locally. Soap and water three times a day with careful cleansing to remove crusts, followed by application of an antibiotic cream or lotion is very effective. The treatment can be carried out by the mother at home. Make sure the child's hands are washed at the same time as the facial treatment is given, as the fingers are the major source of spread of the infection.

Appearance of widespread infection requires immediate medical referral. While most cases of impetigo are easily treated, some cases result in kidney disease called glomerulonephritis due to the Streptococcus.

### Folliculitis and Furuncles

These lesions are due mainly to superficial Staphylococcus infection which occurs in the hair follicle. A furuncle is a deep infection in one or more hair follicles. Furuncles are tender, red, swollen areas also known as "boils".

The time-honored method of treatment is hot, wet soaks, or compresses, which help to "point" the boil to a head. Incision and drainage is then used by the physician. Refer all folliculitis and furuncle clients to a physician for treatment, as sometimes systemic antibiotic therapy is indicated.

**Pseudofolliculitis barbae**, also known as "barber's itch", or "beard bumps" is a condition that results from ingrown hairs in the beard area. It occurs mainly in Blacks because of the coiled hair shaft. This action results in inflammation due to a foreign body reaction and bacteria. The problem can best be treated by avoiding shaving. Careful teasing of the ingrown hairs with a wooden probe under a magnifying lens (3-5x) helps the condition. Sometimes the use of mild depilatories instead of shaving is helpful.

### The Allergic Group

The skin care specialist must understand that this group of disorders is immunological in origin. The cause of the allergy should always be identified in these cases if possible. First, a careful history must be taken about possible exposures to various agents. Remember that most cosmetic products are associated with irritation reactions rather than allergic reactions. Allergic reactions that involve the eyes tend to be more severe than on other parts of the face. This is due to the thinness of the eyelids.

By definition an allergic reaction cannot occur with the first use of a product. Two to six weeks are required for most products but constant use can yield a reaction in ten days.

### Contact Dermatitis

Poision ivy dermatitis or Rhus plant dermatitis which includes poison oak, ivy, sumac, and mango rind is the most common allergic reaction seen during the summer (see **Figure 8-4**.). It may occur anywhere on the body but fre-

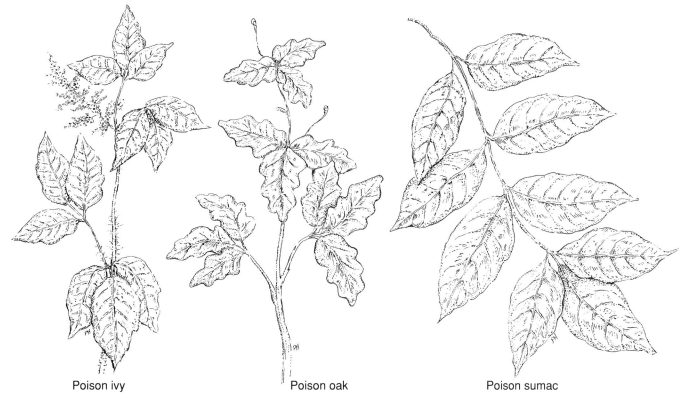

Poison ivy          Poison oak          Poison sumac

**FIGURE 8-4** Poison leaves. Take a few minutes to recognize these plants, it may save you weeks of discomfort. Remember that the allergens from these plants can be carried in the air, or spread by smoke when the plants are burned.

quently appears on the face. The rash will appear from 1-4 days after exposure starting as small blisters and spreading with itching and redness. The spread of the reaction does not occur from the blister fluid as is believed by many people. The Rhus antigen which causes the reaction is fixed to the skin within 15 minutes, and may be washed off with soap and water during that period. After 15 minutes washing is of no use, except to remove unbound excess antigen; the reaction will, however, occur from the residual bound antigen.

Early mild poison ivy will respond to soaks, baths or compresses three times daily for 10-20 minutes each. Astringents such as Burow's powder are helpful. Burow's powder is aluminum acetate and is available in a pharmacy. Add one tablet to a pint of water to make a 1:40 solution.

In case of severe reactions with widespread involvement, systemic steroids are needed, so referral is mandatory in these cases. Hives (urticaria) can be particularly severe at times so I recommend referral for hives as well.

Other allergic materials include rubber, nickel (from jewelry), leather, and many topical medicaments, particularly the "caine family", such as benzocaine. Once the offending agent is identified all future use of the product must be avoided. In the case of nickel dermatitis from jewelry the allergic potential can be eliminated or reduced by coating the jewelry with urethane varnish, available at most hardware counters or paint stores.

## Atopic Dermatitis - Atopic Eczema

Atopic dermatitis is an inherited disease. It is seen mostly in individuals with hay fever or asthma but it is itself not an allergy. Sensitive skin individuals are most often afflicted from childhood. The condition can be brought on by scratching, rubbing, soaps, detergents, dry weather or even rough clothing. The rash is varied and may be red, edematous, weeping or dry, lichenified, or hyperpigmented.

Prevent scratching and irritation of the skin. Adequate bathing with mild superfatted soaps and subsequent lubrication of the skin with a mild oil or cream is helpful. Many creams are on the market, but a vegetable oil may also be used. Avoid wool and polyester clothing, stick to cotton clothing. Also avoid environments with heat and moisture as rashes may develop.

Topical treatment consists of a mild steroid 0.05 - 1% hydrocortisone.

## Irritation Contact Dermatitis (non-allergic type)

Many products will produce irritation on first use in some individuals. These are not allergic reactions but irritation reactions and this type is far more common than allergic reaction dermatitis. These conditions occur on the face and hands and are associated with many products. Some of the more common ones are industrial lubricants and solvents, household cleansers, and cosmetic products. The treatment and course of the reaction is the same as in allergic dermatitis. It is important to find the offending product to advise the client to avoid any future use of it.

## Sebaceous Gland Problems

### Seborrheic Dermatitis

Seborrheic dermatitis is distinguished as a scaly, greasy, pink to red disorder with a tendency to involve the brows, lashes of the eyes, the nose at the labial folds, the mouth, and the ear inside and outside. The condition is most common in fair skinned individuals and less common in dark skinned individuals.

The recommended treatment is hydrocortisone 0.05 - 1% twice a day. In severe cases a more potent steroid is used, but this should be done only by a physician and only for short periods.

### Rosacea

Rosacea is a disorder that occurs mostly in middle aged males of fair complexion. It also occurs in females, but less often. It is a red and scaly disorder with telangiectatic masses and red, pimple-like papules and pustules. When the sebaceous glands enlarge along with enlargement of the nose the condition is called **rhinophyma**. Hot spicy foods, alcohol, and heat make the condition worse.

Avoid strong steroids. Use mild cortisone 0.05 - 1% or water based benzoyl peroxide 2-5% twice a day. Work with a physician on these cases as they are slow to respond and take a great deal of encouragement and patience.

## Milia

Milia are small, superficial keratin plugs that block the pilosebaceous ducts. They are best removed by tiny incisions and expression with a comedone extractor.

## Benign Neoplastic Angiomas

Actinic or solar damage results from excessive exposure to the sun. There are many manifestations that include the dryness, scaling, epidermal atrophy, pigmentation changes, wrinkling, dermal atrophy, and telangiectasia.

Telangiectasia are composed of dilated capillaries usually on the nose and the cheeks. Spider-angioma are red dots with dilated capillaries that radiate out from the center. They are seen most commonly on the face and the backs of the hands. With pregnancy, estrogen therapy, and chronic liver disease they are more frequent and numerous.

These conditions should be referred to a physician if they are severe. Cosmetic covering with appropriate creams can help in mild cases, and the use of vitamin C preparations can also be of benefit when applied topically three times a day.

## SCARS - THE FIBROBLAST GONE AWRY

All scars result from a biological response to heal an inflammatory process. Whether it be a simple infected pimple or a post-operative wound, there will be some scar formation. Scars are the physical manifestation of action by the fibroblast cell to repair or heal a wound or inflammatory reaction.

Not all wounds will result in visible scarring, but deep in the wound there will be some fibrous tissue seen when examined under a microscope. Scars and the treatment of scars will be a concern to the skin care specialist, so we need to go into some detail about how they form and how they can be treated. We shall go into more detail on this subject when we study wound healing and wound treatment, but for now a little explanation is needed.

## The Mechanism of Scar Formation in the Skin - The Response of the Fibroblast

Wounds and other inflammatory reactions go through stages of resolution in which various cells are called into play. White cells, called granulocytes, first enter the picture along with macrophages to clean up the wound and fight off bacteria. Next, the fibroblasts move in to prepare a network for the keratinocytes to migrate across in order to seal the wound. In many wounds this will take place within 3 to 7 days. At this stage the fibroblasts will begin to form collagen and elastin to close the dermis and start to strengthen the wound. This process begins at the bottom of the wound and continues until the wound is completely healed. Now, a rather unknown process occurs which involves the formation of a different kind of dermis than existed before. This is the process called **fibrosis**. First, the architectural nature of the dermis is lost. The collagen bundles are disorganized and there are few blood vessels in the wound with fewer elastin fibers. The greater the fibrosis the less the number of elastin fibers.

As this process continues, the area of the scar will at first appear red and raised above the skin surface. As time passes, up to one year in some cases, the scar will become pale and begin to fall below the skin surface resulting in a depression; however, not all scars will go through this stage and no one can predict which ones will and which ones will not. Stretch mark scars, for instance, always become depressed, while burn scars often stay elevated. Here are some modes of treatment.

## Cosmetic Treatment

Scars can be covered with foundation make-up, concealer or special para-medical make-up. (See Chapter 12). This often is all the treatment that is needed if the scar is small and not disfiguring. Special training in this area is often needed to produce a maximum result.

## Treatment With Vitamin E

There is fairly good evidence that vitamin E when applied topically will reduce even an old scar. It is best to use the vitamin E after the scar is formed as there does not seem to be a preventative action by vitamin E in scar formation. Apply tocopheryl acetate cream 2 to 5% twice a day over the scar, rubbing in the long axis of the scar. Results will take several months to appear, but remember since it takes a long time for the scar to form it will take a long time for it to undergo revision.

### Alternating Electrical Current

Science has found that the application of low voltage and low amperage alternating current of various frequencies will have a beneficial effect on scar tissue. Frequencies between 1500 cycles per second and 6000 cycles per second are effective ranges to ease scars, even those of long duration. (Remember, a cycle per second is called a hertz, but when we speak of frequencies over a thousand hertz we use the term kilohertz, kHz.) I have worked with only one instrument in this area and I am sure there are other types and brands. I do not recommend any instruments that do not have a fixed frequency or that have many controls to vary the current or wave form. Electrobiology is a complex science and requires a great deal of knowledge to understand what is happening. Unless you are prepared to undertake a course in electrophysiology, it is best to stick to the simple-to-use instruments.

The Electroderma$^R$ instrument from EMR, Santa Monica, California, is an effective instrument that requires a minimum of training and is easy to use. It may be used to treat almost any scar from acne scars to burn scars and stretch marks. The action of this instrument appears to be on the fibroblast to stimulate the formation of new replacement collagen. This requires the action of collagenase to remove old collagen and the laying down of new collagen.

How this is actually done is unknown but it appears that the weak electromagnetic fields generated by the instrument will produce more cellular transport of normal active metabolites and help to increase enzyme activity. This is a new science, quite complex but very exciting and well worth the effort to study it.

Again you will need at least 30 to 40 treatments to effect a result.

The number of treatments relates to the frequency and time of treatments. A course of 30 treatments of 20 minutes each at a frequency of three times a week will produce a good result in most cases. The greater the damage the longer it will take to effect a cure. Follow the directions given with the course of instruction and after you gain experience you can vary the treatment time and frequency. I have varied treatment time from 20 minutes to 45 minutes and have varied frequency from 3 times a week to 5 times a week. The condition of the client determines the treatment choice.

### Surgical Treatment

Some scars may require surgical removal. These are usually large scars that interfere with daily functioning, are infected, or are quite disfiguring. Burn scars and acne scars are the most common type. Keloids often respond to surgical treatment. Referral to a dermatologist or a cosmetic surgeon will be necessary. Ask the client to have his family doctor make the referral, or if you refer the client send a note to the family doctor to inform her/him of the referral. (See Chapter 11.)

## BAGGY EYES - A TOUGH PROBLEM

Baggy eyes are known by a number of names which convey the sad plight of the unfortunate client with this condition (puffy eyes, suborbital edema, morning eyes, etc.). The cause may not be the same in all cases, so you need to think about the age and the general condition of the client. First, let us look at the mechanism behind this condition and then work out a treatment system. There are a number of medical conditions associated with puffy or baggy eyes: sinus infections, allergies, thyroid disease, and kidney disease. It is not necessary that all clients be referred to a physician for evaluation of puffy or baggy eyes, but you should consider this if there is any question as to the cause.

### Anatomy and Physiology of the Eyelids

You recall from our discussion of the anatomy of the eyelid in Chapter 2 that this structure is very thin. The orbicularis oculi are not very strong muscles and it is unfortunate that globs of fat rest under them. The fat is obviously for protection of the eyeball from the trauma of rubbing and stroking, but it also can produce an unattractive bulge. Next, we need to consider the lymphatic drainage of the eyelids and the implications of this system. Many of the problems that cause baggy eyes relate to the lymphatic system.

The lymphatic system is an alternative system to the blood. Fluid and cells from the tissue spaces diffuse into the lymphatic vessels as long as the pressure within the lymphatic is lower than the tissue pressure. Here is one reason why these bags form. When the pressure in the lymphatic vessels is increased the fluid will flow out into the tissue and cause edema or puffy skin. Standing on your feet all day is an example of this; your feet will swell as the day goes on and your shoes will become tighter. Simply putting your feet up higher than your hips will drain the feet and provide relief.

There are three factors that enter into the baggy eye problem: age, hormones, and stress. All of these factors are related to the lymphatic system in some manner.

AGE produces a change in the tissues that relates to the strength and resiliency of the collagen and elastin. Sagging occurs around the age of 30 years in women and about age 40 in men, due to hormonal differences in the tissues. The effect of alcohol and tobacco on these tissues is well known and contributes to the problem.

HORMONES are related to sex and the age of the person as noted above. With testosterone there is a stronger connective tissue as opposed to the effect of estrogen, which produces a softer tissue.

STRESS has a tremendous effect on the tissue but it is unknown how and to what extent stress plays a role in general aging and aging of the face in particular. We know, for instance, that the pressor hormones of the adrenal gland, epinephrine and norepinephrine, have profound effects on the blood pressure, on certain metabolic pathways, and on the brain. All of these factors contribute to the sagging and destruction of skin tone.

### Treatment

There are a few treatments for baggy eyes and they may be divided into topical products, manual methods, and surgical methods. Surgical methods will be covered later.

TOPICAL PRODUCTS have been used for thousands of years dating back to the ancient Egyptians. An old remedy is tea bags placed on the eyes at night. The effect is most likely due to astringency of the tannin and the slight pressure of the tea bag on the lymphatic system around the eye.

Vitamin C, both orally and topically, has an effect on the collagen and perhaps on the elastin. There are some commercial preparations but many are unstable. A cream with 0.25 to 0.50% vitamin C palmitate is quite effective in some cases.

Vitamin A is effective if applied at the right concentration. Use vitamin A palmitate at a level of 0.5% in a cream base or an anhydrous base and apply at night. Vitamin A appears to penetrate the skin rather slowly so it is not very effective in a mask if used for only twenty minutes. Combining both vitamin A and vitamin C in the same compound may be irritating at the high levels suggested here, so I recommend you use them alone.

Manual methods involve manual lymphatic drainage or lymphatic massage. The method developed and described by Dr. Emil Vodder is a contribution to skin care treatment that cannot be overestimated. The technique takes two weeks to learn but many months to master. Essentially the Vodder method uses very light pressure applied to the skin in specific maneuvers to promote drainage of the lymphatic fluid from the skin. I can not do justice to the technique in this chapter but I believe every skin care specialist should learn this technique. The book Introduction to Dr. Vodder's Manual Lymph Drainage by H. and G. Wittlinger (Karl Haug Publisher, Heidelberg) is a good start, but not a replacement for actual hands-on instruction.

One of the areas not discussed in detail in the Vodder method is the lower eyelid as a specific site of lymphatic drainage. In this area the lymphatic vessels of the inner one-third of the lower lid drain toward the nose while the outer two-thirds drain outward and downward. (See diagram in **Figure 8-5**.) Again very, very light maneuvers are used for these drainage areas.

Surgical corrections will be discussed later but there are two new procedures being tried of which you should be aware. Fat suction of the lower lid and melting of the fat in the lower lid with heat are now available in certain medical centers. I have had no experience with these new

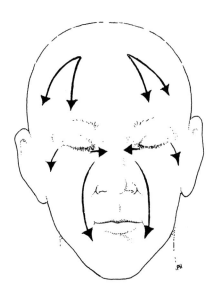

**FIGURE 8-5** Lymphatic drainage of the face. Note that the inner one-third of the lower eyelid drains medially toward the nose. Remember that lymphatic drainage is accomplished with very light pressure.

techniques and therefore can not evaluate them directly or indirectly. Let us watch and wait to see how they are accepted.

Another treatment recommended for sagging eyelids is acid peels. These again are only for use by dermatologists trained in the procedure or by cosmetic surgeons. We shall discuss many of these medical and surgical procedures when we discuss the referral options.

## FACE PEELS

The following description is **not** intended to serve as instructions for doing a face peel for the novice. This description is intended to serve as an introduction to this procedure. **ONLY THOSE INDIVIDUALS TRAINED BY AN EXPERIENCED PERSON IN A HANDS-ON PROGRAM SHOULD PERFORM THIS PROCEDURE.**

### Use of the Jenner Face Peel

The peeling compound used is made up of the following materials:

| | |
|---|---|
| Salicylic acid | 14% |
| Resorcinol | 14% |
| Lactic Acid (85% solution) | 14% |
| Alcohol | 58% |

This material may be purchased from SAV in New York or made up by a pharmacist.

Pretreatment and Precautions

1. Client should not be on Retin A for at least 6 weeks.
2. Clients should be free of pustules and have no fever blisters.
3. Earrings and contact lens should be removed.
4. Client should read and sign informed consent.
5. Have client use a sunscreen daily for at least a week prior to the treatment day.
6. Remove all make-up and cleanse the face thoroughly.
7. Have the materials ready and include a small shot glass or 50 ml beaker.
8. You will need peeling solution and cotton tipped applicators and a small fan. The fan should be placed to blow over client's face.
9. Patch test for 72 hours with the material under a bandaid. Use about 0.5 grams of peeling solution. (This is approximately 10 drops.)

Treatment Technique

1. Have the client undress and put on gown. Cover the hair in the usual manner.
2. With the client reclining in a semi-sitting position start to apply the peeling liquid. Pour a small quantity into a shot glass and dip the cotton tipped applicators into this material. Do not dip from the original bottle. Roll the applicator against the inside of the glass to remove excess material.
3. Apply the material to the forehead in light strokes. With sufficient material the skin will take on a frost like appearance in a short time. Go slowly as it will take 40 to 45 minutes to apply the material. Go over the area lightly until frosting occurs.
4. Apply the material into the eyebrows but do not go closer than 1/4 inch to the eyes. Do not touch the upper or lower lids.
5. When client experiences a burning or tingling sensation turn on the fan.
6. Continue to apply the peeling material down the cheeks, across the nose and up to the vermillon border of the lips. Not on the lips. Carry the coverage down to

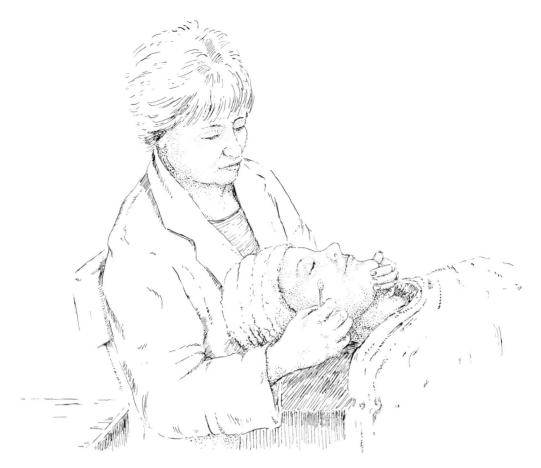

the chin and slightly under the chin. Do not go below the mandible of the lower jaw.

Post-treatment Appearance and Client Instructions

**Day One** - Instruct client not to wash face for 24 hours and not to use make-up; skin will appear  red and frosty all day. Use fan to play air over the face to reduce discomfort.

**Day Two** - Skin becomes tight and drawn. Rinse skin with cool water 2-3 times a day. Face may be washed and moisturizers, lipstick and eyeliner may beused. Discomfort is less.

**Day Three** - Skin is tighter and appears crinkly, may start to peel slightly. Discomfort may increase. Moisturizers may be used.

**Day Four** - Peeling begins, usually about the lips. Itching is noticed along with tightness. Mist face with water to reduce discomfort. A mild exfoliant may be used to help lift skin. Continue to use moisturizers.

**Days Five to Seven** - Peeling continues through these days and is complete by day 7 in most cases. Continue to use exfoliant and moisturizers. Skin comes off in large sheets; do not force or pull off peeling skin.

General instructions

Keep client away from sun and heat. If the face becomes red and swollen after treatment this represents a reaction, either primary irritation or allergy. This will occur in some clients. Pretesting clients before treatment with a patch test for 72 hours is mandatory.

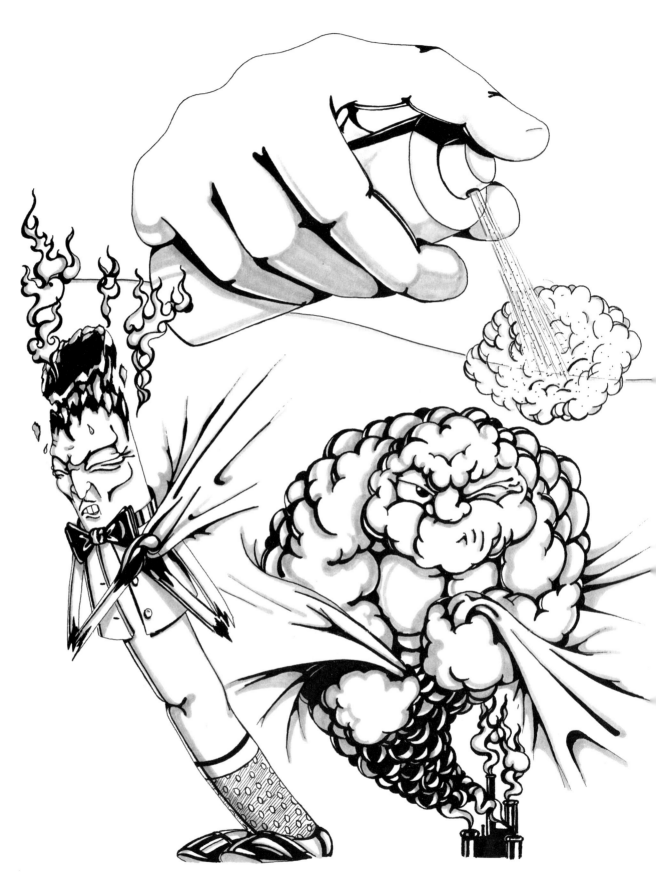

This place has a lot of territories, and sometimes trouble may be festering before we can see it, even in places a lesser Intelligence wouldn't think to look. A smooth operator like Yours Truly slides onto the scene

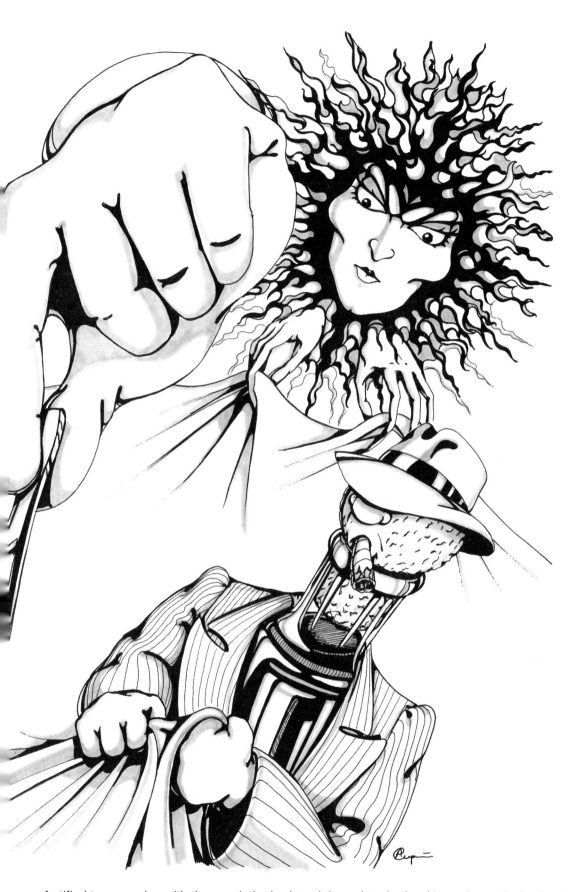

fortified to recognize with the good, the bad, and the ugly, whether it's staring us in the face yet or not.

# Treatment of the Neck, Hands, Feet, and Breasts

We shall cover a number of skin conditions in this chapter that are associated with the four regions outlined in the chapter title. In each of these there are specific problems which are unique to the region, while at the same time they share common skin problems afflicting many other regions of the body. For instance, the feet are frequently infected with a fungus that is called "athlete's foot", but many of the regions of the body can also become infected with any fungi. Some fungal organisms have a tendency to infect certain body parts because of the optimal growth conditions in that part. Thick stratum corneum favors "stringy" fungi (like athlete's foot), while moist, wet conditions favor small bud-like fungi, an example of which are the yeast fungi. Having a knowledge of the existing conditions such as the warmth, moisture, and thickness of the keratin layers of each region will help you to make a correct diagnosis and to choose the most effective treatment. In these treatment programs we shall look at physical modalities, such as massage, heat, effective products, and common sense methods. Keep in mind that all of these are suggested treatments which may be modified in order to meet with

specific conditions.

## THE NECK

The neck is an often neglected area of anatomy for examination. It extends from the bottom of the mandible (lower jaw) to the borders of the clavicles (collar bones) in the anterior portion, and to the top of the scapulae in the posterior portion. It is cylindrical in shape. In women the thyroid cartilage is not as prominent as it is in men so it serves as a convenient land mark. (See **Figure 9-1**) Most of the inflammatory conditions that affect the face can also involve the neck, chief among these is acne.

### Acne

Acne involves mainly the posterior neck often extending down the back and onto the shoulders. This involvement is mainly with Grade 3 or 4 acne, that is, comedones, inflamed pustules and cysts or nodules. These clients need referral to a physician for treatment. The general treatment of acne in the absence of cysts, outlined in Chapter 8, can be applied.

### Viscoelastic Problems (Wrinkles, Sags, and Turkey Neck)

I believe the major problems that you will see in the neck will be related to poor elastin. The offending muscle is the **platysma muscle**, the thin flat muscle covering the front of the neck. The sagging muscles and fat in the neck can

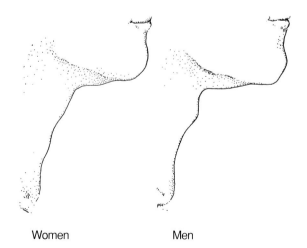

Women                    Men

**FIGURE 9-1** Thyroid comparison between men and women. The thyroid gland covers the cricoid cartilage or Adam's Apple in the front of the neck. The cricoid cartilage is more prominent in men than in women.

cause some disfigurement. These conditions respond well to cosmetic surgery and will be discussed in Chapter 11. For minor relaxation problems you can try the following treatments. Clients under 45 years of age and with mild to moderate viscoelastic problems are the best choices.

**Diet** should be rich in vitamin C (500 to 1000 mg daily), vitamin E (400 mg daily), and vitamin A (5,000 units). Avoid simple sugars and excessive unsaturated fats.

**Exercise**, while quite controversial in wrinkle repair, may help in the neck. Head lifts, done by touching the chin to the chest, followed by extension of the head, that is, by raising the chin very high (the Mussolini look) 10 to 20 times a day along with isometric exercises, such as pressing the hands together, is helpful.

**Electrostimulation** with alternating current may be helpful but I have not worked in this particular area. The theory behind alternating currrent stimulation indicates that it may be of benefit. This is an area undergoing research, but at present I feel there is insufficient data to substantiate any claims.

**Topical treatment** may be of benefit, particularly the following formula: vitamin C in 1-2% concentration with vitamin A palmitate at 0.5% and vitamin E at 2%. The addition of an immune stimulant such as beta 1, 3 glucan at 2.5 milligrams per ounce will be of additional benefit. Some of these preparations are on the market now but more will be available by the time this book is published.

**Environmental protection** from the sun, wind, and heat is also important if your client is serious about treatment. Keep the neck covered in the winter with a warm scarf and wear a sunscreen year round, especially in the summer.

## Lesions

The neck is a frequent site for skin tags, or **papillomas**. These are easily removed with electrodesiccation. They are usually quite small and respond to a spark at the base of the lesion. If you are skilled in this treatment and have the equipment I see no reason why you can not perform this function. Obviously, a physician can easily remove papillomas. Moles and inflammatory lesions, lumps or cysts should always be referred to a physician.

### Recognizing Thyroid Disorders

The thyroid gland sits between the manubrium and the thyroid cartilage (Adam's Apple) in the neck. The two sides of the gland are joined by the section called the isthmus. With the neck extended you can easily feel the thyroid gland. If the gland is prominent enough to see, it is usually too large and the client should be referred to a physician. People with overactive thyroids are usually nervous and tired, are more comfortable in cool rooms, and may have an excited appearance. On the other hand, people with underactive thyroid glands are slightly overweight, pasty-faced, sluggish, are more comfortable in a warm room, and may have thin eyebrows, paticularly in the outer third. If you have the slightest question about the thryoid gland you must refer the client to a physician. We now pass from the neck to the breasts and the chest.

## THE BREASTS AND CHEST

There are many myths about the chest, but as you have learned in the section on anatomy the breasts are essentially milk-producing glands. Only a small part of the breast is glandular, the rest is fat and connective tissue. The characteristic shape of the breast is due to the retention of fat within a confined area that is supported by Cooper's ligaments. Around the nipple there are sebaceous glands and beyond the pigmented area of the nipple, called the areola, there are hair follicles as well. As a young female develops, her breasts will go from hard to soft and from pointed to rounded. The breasts swell during pregnancy and remain large during lactation and nursing. During this period the nipples will darken about the areola and the surface veins will be more noticeable. These changes are normal and will reverse themselves after pregnancy and lactation cease.

## Treatment of the Skin of the Breast

The two most common problems seen on the skin of the breasts are acne and excess hair about the nipples. Acne lesions may be simple comedones, pustules, or rarely, cysts. These lesions are viewed as acne and are treated in the same manner.

**Hair** around the nipple is best removed by shaving or waxing. These are usually dark terminal hairs that may be quite long. Shaving is less traumatic and can be done by the client as needed. I do not recommend epilation by electrolysis on the breast, however, a skilled operator can obtain satisfactory results. For most cases shaving and waxing are adequate methods.

The hirsute breast (hair all over the breast), presents another problem. As in all cases of excessive hair on the body in women, this may signal an endocrine or hormonal problem and should be referred to a physician for a professional opinion. **(See Appendix.)**

**Sagging breasts** present a real problem in that there are no known topical or physical treatments that can help to restore sagging breasts. The only known method is surgical. Implants into the space behind the milk glands will produce a shapely breast if done well. While there are few complications of this treatment it must be done by an expert cosmetic surgeon. Some breasts will only droop slightly and may be helped with a lifting type bra. As long as there is adequate fat in the breast tissue there will be shape and form. The flat breast is mostly devoid of fatty tissue and is a flaccid, shapeless mass. This condition can only be helped with breast inserts and reshaping the breasts. Poor tissue, however, could result in some postoperative sagging. Two other treatments must be mentioned as they are often a topic of conversation by clients. These are silicone injections and fat injections into the breast.

Silicone injections into the breasts have been disastrous in most cases. The complications are migration of the silicone and inflammatory reactions severe enough to require breast removal. **Under no circumstances should silicone injections be used in the breasts.** The use of fat cell transplantation does not seem to be a practical method at this time to augment breasts. In this method fat cells are taken from other areas of the body (such as the buttocks) and injected into the breasts. The problem is that sometimes the fat cells do not "take". **I would not recommend fat cell injection treatment at this time.**

### Other Conditions Affecting the Breasts

**Inverted nipples** are fairly common in women, more rare in men. This is a normal variation of the nipple position and needs no treatment. Often on sexual arousal the nipple will become erect and evert spontaneously. In nursing, this eversion is easily done by the mother and infant.

**Fissures and cracks** of the nipples are seen often during nursing. It is a condition brought on by wet nipples and sucking-trauma. Usually, just washing and drying the nipple after nursing is all that is needed. The milk residue, the baby's saliva, and the sucking-trauma set up the conditions for infection of the nipple. Cleansing is important in nursing care.

**Inflammatory reaction** and **hyperproliferative disorders** also affect the breast. **Contact dermatitis, allergic dermatitis, psoriasis,** and **various eczemas** also affect the breast. These are treated the same as on any other part of the body.

One of the common conditions seen in women with pendulous breasts is known as **intertrigo** or **intertriginous dermatitis**. This is a condition affecting both the breast and the chest wall that results from poor personal hygiene. The tissue under the breasts becomes macerated due to accumulation of moisture and bacteria or yeast. Generally there is a very unpleasant odor emanating from the breast which is more intense when the breast is raised from the chest wall. Simple, daily cleansing will prevent this condition, but once started, an antibacterial or antifungal agent is needed for treatment. Bacitracin ointment usually works well. In the case of yeast (monilia), Nystatin cream is effective. Nystatin is only available by prescription.

**Lumps, bumps and cysts** all require referral to a physician. The smallest lump could be a problem so **you must refer all cases in which there is any lump, bump or cyst. Cystic mastitis** is a very common benign condition but it must be diagnosed by a physician. The reader must remember that **breast cancer is the leading cause of death in women. Every abnormal finding requires referral**.

### Complications of Plastic Surgery of the Breasts

This section is included in this chapter because more and more breast surgery is being performed today and will only increase in the future. Fortunately, better training received by cosmetic surgeons is reducing the complications. Here are the major complications.

Predisposing factors

These include **age**, at each extreme of life. **Prepuberty** breasts are only a bud behind the nipple and any surgery, infection, or tumor may damage the bud resulting in unequal growth or no growth at all. In **advanced age**, breast tissue normally becomes ptotic (sagging) so correction is more difficult.

**Obesity** results in great variation in the fat content of the breasts. It is best that any overweight client have a weight reduction program to stabilize the fat content of the breast before augmentation or reduction of the breast is planned.

**Quality of blood supply and previous scarring** will affect the eventual result. Scarring is more common on the anterior chest particularly in the area **between the breasts**.

**Improper placement of the incision** can cause scarring. Proper placement of incisions is seen in **Figure 9-2**. Incisions should be made in

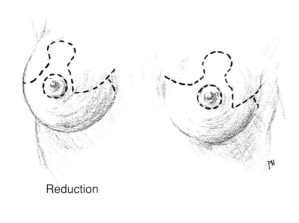

Reduction

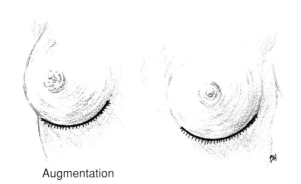

Augmentation

**FIGURE 9-2** Breast incision placement. Reduction incisions are more prominent and tend to produce more visible scarring, while augmentation incisions follow more natural curves and are virtually invisible.

relaxed skin.

## Post-Operative Complications

**Hematoma** is a collection of blood beneath the skin which forms in the cavities of the breast tissue called "dead space". If adequate control of bleeding is not maintained, breasts are not bandaged properly, or supported immediately after surgery  hematomas can form. The hematoma will delay healing and predispose to infection.

**Foreign body reactions** occur from the implant at times in breast reconstruction. **Capsule formation** is a form of foreign body reaction in which a biological reaction walls off the implant. This is normal in all implant surgery, but in some patients there will be a contracture of the capsule which results in a hard, globe-like breast. Sometimes these capsules can be stretched by pressure exercises and by having the patient lie on her breast. In some cases, surgery must be performed again to correct the capsule formation; fortunately, this is uncommon. Vitamin E

has been used to reduce capsule formation.

**Ptosis** or sagging of the breasts occurs with poor connective tissue and is a frequent complication after pregnancy. The breasts sag and the nipples lie below the inframammary fold (see **Figure 9-3**). The condition results in a ball-in-sock deformity. Sometimes this condition occurs years after the initial implant surgery.  To correct ptosis a procedure known as **mastopexy** is performed. This procedure shortens the breast skin and reshapes the breast.

## Breast Reduction Complications

Two of the major problems seen with breast reductions are scars and poor shaping. Often the **nipples are misplaced** and the scars do not fade. Reduction with implants may produce slippage of the implant to the side of the chest or the breast may slide off of the implant. (See **Figure 9-4**.) All of these conditions require additional surgery for correction. The role of the skin care

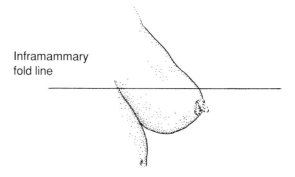

Inframammary fold line

**FIGURE 9-3** Sagging breasts. The inframammary fold is the area where the underside of the breast first meets the chest wall. If the nipple falls below this line the breast is classified as sagging.

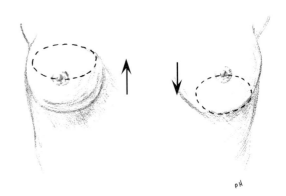

**FIGURE 9-4** Breast implant slippage. While breast implant slippage is rare it can occur with either an upward or downward displacement.

specialist with these clients is to help reduce anxiety, help prevent scarring of the incision, and promote healing with good skin care after surgery. We shall cover this care in Chapter 12.

## THE HAND

Hands are not only one of the most sensitive parts of the body they are also the most visible. Before 1945 women wore gloves when they went outside and it was quite rare to see a lady without gloves at any social function. Gloves were a part of the dress code of men and women. In both summer and winter, gloves were in fashion. The result of this habit was hands that showed no sun damage. Today all of this is gone with the new dress code freedom. Somehow, we forget that with every new gained freedom there is a price to pay. The price is great areas of the skin showing damage in later years. How much later? Well, 18 to 20 year olds will exhibit some of the sun exposure damage that was incurred as a 10 to 12 year old child. Figure about 10 years for moderate damage to appear and about 20 years for severe damage to appear. The major problem seen with the hands are thinning, veining, pigmentations, and joint deformities. (Disorders of the nails will be covered in a separate section of this chapter.)

### Thinning and Veining of the Hands

The back or dorsum of the hands thins with age as a result of fatty tissue loss. The space between the interossei muscles of the metacarpals show apparent widening but this is in fact atrophy of the tissues. The veins become more prominent probably as a result of tone loss in the muscle layer of the vein, or a combination of tone loss and back pressure of the vascular system. Look at the back of your hands with the hand in your lap. In about 3 minutes or less the veins will swell regardless of your age. Next, lift your hand to a level above your heart which is on line with your shoulders; in less than a minute your veins will empty and remain flat. In the older individual from age 50 years onward the veins are large, and more markedly so if sun damage is present.

The thin skin allows the light to penetrate the skin and reflect back as blue light from the underlying veins. If the skin is well hydrated and

"plump" it will reflect more light at the surface of the skin which decreases the vein color. In cases of anemia, where the skin exhibits a very pale color, the veins will be more prominent. There are two main factors to contend with in treating thinning skin of the hands. One is the loss of thickness of the dermis and fatty layer. The other is the change in the vascular system tone. To these two we must add the color changes in the dermis produced by free radical products, by debris from metabolic processes (the skin is a vast dumping ground for unwanted refuse in the body), and finally, the marked changes produced by sun exposure. We shall examine these factors and see what can be done to improve the appearance of the hands.

Many skin care specialists have been taught that old skin has less water, but this is not true. If simple moisturizers would be of benefit to thin hands we would no longer have this problem. Thinning hands have a complex mechanism, not yet fully understood, but it deserves full attention.

### Surgical Techniques

As of today I know of no satifactory, effective or, safe method of restoring or improving the thinned skin hand. Various injection methods have been tried including **paraffin** (with disastrous results), liquid **silicone** with poor results (silicone can only be used in microinjection), and **fat tissue** injection from other sites in the same patient with some success. I do not feel that fat tissue injection is a highly viable means as the fat is rapidly metabolized in the dorsum of the hand. Keep an open mind however, as this could be effective in the future.

### Physical Treatments

The use of physical methods offers some hope for the treatment of thinning hands, even though it is not curative. The aim in this treatment is first to **prevent further damage** and second **to restore the tissues to normal**.

**Preventive measures** include avoidance of all solvent materials such as soap, alcohol, and detergents. **AVOID ALL SUN EXPOSURE** by wearing gloves and protective clothing. Do not smoke and do not drink beyond 2 ounces of alcohol a day. Avoid coffee and other caffeine drinks.

**Positive measures** include a balanced diet, high vitamin C (1000 mg daily), high vitamin E (500 mg to 1000 mg daily), niacin (100 mg 3 times a day), and at least six glasses of water a day.

Topical Treatments

We have no miracle agents that work in all cases. Badly damaged poor skin will generally yield poorer results than less damaged skin. Here are some preparations that should help. Some of these are available currently and the others will be available at the time this book is published.

Formula #1 for moderate thinning of hands. Vitamin A and vitamin E cream with a sunscreen. Currently available. Apply three times a day.

Formula #2 for moderate to severe thinning of hands. Vitamin A palmitate 0.5% with vitamin E acetate 2% and ascorbic acid at 5%. Use only at night and observe for irritation. This product is designed to increase fibroblast growth and may produce some reactions. It is not necessary to discontinue the treatment, only reduce the amount applied. Currently, this formulation is not available as a complete product.

Formula #3 for moderate to severe thinning of the hands. The same formula as Formula #2 with the addition of certain essential oils that promote growth. These may include special extract of Echinacea root and others.

Formula #4 for moderate to severe thinning of the hands. Retin A, available by prescription, only has been tried for thin hands with some success. I suggest starting with 0.05% applied only at night, and do not use in combination with any other agent except a mild vitamin A-free moisturizer. This treatment must be done with a physician.

Formula #5 for moderate to severe thinning of the hands. This formula consists of the following ingredients, some of which are proprietary: vitamin A acetate at 0.3%, vitamin E acetate at 2%, an alpha hydroxy acid at 6%, special extract of Echinacea, behenyl alcohol, essential oils and beta 1,3 glucan in a microemulsion base. Apply twice a day.

New formulations are being tested by many companies, and hopefully, effective products will be on the market soon.

**Pigmentation Problems of the Hands**

**Aging spots or actinic keratosis (also called senile keratosis)** is a pigmented lesion resulting from repeated exposure to the sun. They are most common in farmers, sportsmen, and sunbathers. Blondes and redheads are more severely affected than dark-haired or dark-skinned individuals. The typical lesion is a small area of red scaling which, over time, becomes elevated and obtains a grayish top surface. While most of these lesions are not dangerous they may become squamous cell epitheliomas which are dangerous. I recommend that you send these clients to a dermatologist for evaluation before treatment.

Simple hypopigmentation agents will help to hide and sometimes clear these lesions. Currently, 2.5% hydroquinone is used as a bleaching agent in a cream base, with or without a sunscreening agent.

There are other pigmented lesions of the hands that occur, including vitiligo and melanoma. These conditions should be referred first for diagnosis to a physician. Remember also that infections of the hands and fingers are common. I have listed below some of the more common conditions that affect the hands.

**Common Dermatological Conditions Affecting the Hands**

Contact dermatitis in the spaces between the fingers and on the back of the hands.
Fungal infections, including yeast organisms
Superficial bacterial infections
Neurodermatitis
Atopic dermatitis
Paroychia, an infection at the base of the nail
Scabies, located on the palm and interdigital spaces.
Ichthyosis ("fish skin")
Photogenic reactions including sunburn, keratosis and tumors.
Psoriasis
Ganglion (a new term, from the Greek *ganglia* - a knot) is a lump on the back of the hand due to a nerve sheath tumor)
Warts

## Joint Deformities and Other Lesions of the Hands

The most frequently seen joint deformities are due to some type of **arthritis** of the hands. There are two types of arthritis which affect the finger joints. **Osteoarthritis** is the most common type and it manifests as swelling of the distal interphalangeal joints (last joint in the fingers). It is painful at times and causes a rosary-like deformity of the fingers. The other type of arthritis is **rheumatoid** arthritis which occurs mainly in the proximal interphalangeal joints (the first joint in the finger after the knuckle) causing the fingers to appear as fusiform or cigar-shaped. Rheumatoid arthritis is usually more painful then osteoarthritis and is associated with more swelling and redness. Most clients will be on some type of therapy from their physician so be aware of what these conditions are and how they will affect your overall treatment. Remember that most arthritic conditions benefit from heat and slight motion. Hand massage will benefit most clients. Watch for periods of acute pain and swelling of the joints, for at these times any motion can be very painful.

**Synovial cysts** on the finger joints can occur at times, though they are not common. They appear as soft, squishy, ball-like masses on the joints. Most of the time they will recede if left alone, but they can be aspirated or excised by a physician if they get too large. Most of the ones I have seen are about the size of a small grape or smaller. They are frequently associated with arthritis or are a fore-runner of arthritis. Injections of cortisone is of benefit to these lesions.

**Xanthomas** are yellow masses that appear in the palms and on the back of the hands and fingers. They indicate a severe lipid disorder and require thorough investigation by a physician. When they occur on the eyelids they are called **xanthelasma**, though this is an old term.

**Ganglion** is a cystic condition occurring as a protrusion from a tendon sheath or joint capsule. They are soft, fluctuate, and non-tender.

Finally, the hands are into everything and are a frequent site of contact dermatitis, infection, and trauma. Mechanical, thermal, and chemical trauma are constantly present on the hands along with daily sun exposure.

These conditions set up a state of hyperreactivity to other milder insults. The hands are frequently wet with sweat and slightly abraded which makes them more susceptible to infection. Most disorders of the hands are disabling because of the pivotal role the hands play in daily care. It is essential that a continuous education program in this area be maintained.

## THE FOOT

### Some Basic Information on the Feet

The future skin care specialist will function in many areas of medicine as well as in the beauty business. The advent of health spas and newer types of nursing homes will require better trained skin care specialists to serve these areas. The feet of most people are a most neglected part of the anatomy, mainly because they are difficult to reach and to see. The feet serve us well. Despite the horrors of tight shoes, high heels, and sweaty sneakers the feet of most people somehow continue to serve with minimun complaints. This section will look at basic knowledge about the feet and explore common foot problems that you will see over the course of your professional life.

Structure and Function

The foot serves as **a base, a lever, and a shock absorber**. While standing, the foot serves as a base of support for the body. Consider that the foot not only bears the weight of the body but it must also bear the opposing force from the ground. It is remarkable that of all the muscle tension needed to balance the standing human-body very little of that tension is transmitted to the foot. The foot does not require muscle activity from within or without to sustain it in quiet standing. The weight of the body is borne by the back of the foot (the hindfoot) and the front of the foot (the forefoot).

The bones that carry this burden are the **calcaneous** of the hindfoot and the **metatarsal** heads of the forefoot. When walking, the foot becomes a lever in which the body is propelled forward over the fulcrum of the metatarsal heads. (See **Figure 9-5**.) We need not go into the various actions of all the bones and muscles that make up the act of walking (though it is a fascinating study in itself). What you need to know is that as the heel strikes the ground, it is

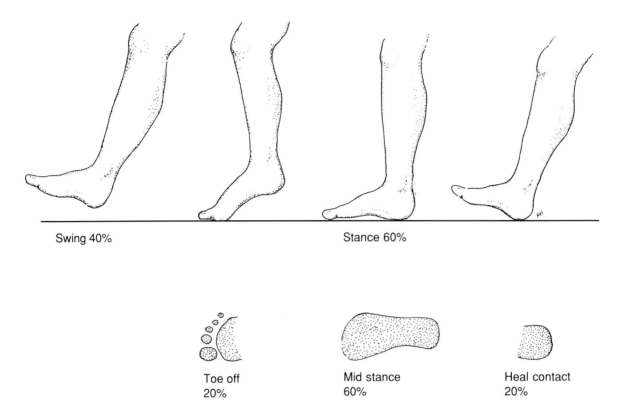

Swing 40%    Stance 60%

Toe off
20%

Mid stance
60%

Heal contact
20%

**FIGURE 9-5** The walking cycle. The heel hits the ground first, then the full weight of the body on the surface of the foot. The toes provide spring to the gait. Bottom half of diagram shows percentage of foot contact.

carrying the full load of the body and in the toe-off (or step) the forefoot is subject to maximal stress. These two facts will help you to understand the following discussions.

**Examination of the Feet**

History

The client should be seated higher than the examiner in a position of comfort. With the knee bent (or flexed) there is less strain on the leg and foot. If the client complains of pain in the foot it is important to determine: 1. the site of pain, 2. when and how it occurred, 3. the nature of the pain (sharp, dull, severe, or mild), 4. if the pain is influenced by walking, running, elevation, or standing, 5. if the pain is constant or intermittent, and finally, 6. if the client has any systemic disease such as diabetes, arthritis, or neurological disorders.

Examination

Observe the skin for signs of color change, for texture change, and for temperature change.

Is the skin wet or dry? Is there hair present on the foot and, if so, is it coarse or fine? Look for cracks, fissures, eczema, psoriasis, and callused areas. Observe the nails for ridges, cracks, and thickening. Look for overgrowth and ingrowing as well as curved growth. Check also for pigmented disorders. Look for swelling in the ankles and the toes. Determine the consistency of the swelling. Is it hard, firm, fluctuate, or soft? Is the swelling red, hot, or cold?

Next, check for abnormalities of the blood vessels. The best method is observation and feel. Blue skin, dusky red skin, and pale skin all have significance in determination of blood flow. Is the skin warm to touch? You can feel the pulse of the foot at the **dorsal pedis** by running your finger up the top of the foot from the base of the big toe and second toe toward the point where the foot curves up to the leg. Feel medial to the tendon and you will find the pulse in a normal foot. Severe lack of blood to the foot yields a weak or absent pulse.

There are other tests and examinations on the foot which are done by a physician that involve testing for neurological disorders or muscle disorders. For our purpose make sure the client has feeling in the feet by simply touching various areas with your fingers or your nails. A great deal of information can be gained from examining the footwear but this is a task for a specialist in this area, such as a chiropodist or an orthropedic surgeon. Remember that we are studying the foot as part of our study of skin. Although skin is skin, each area of the body presents different tasks to the skin that covers it. Weight bearing skin is different from the skin on the eyelid. Both share a common origin and a common basic function even though anatomically they are quite different.

### Disorders Affecting the Skin of the Foot

We can divide the conditions affecting the foot into five broad classifications: 1. conditions due to mechanical stress, 2. conditions due to infection or virus, 3. functional disorders of the sweat glands, 4. system deficiency state due to vascular, neurological or metabolic disorders, and 5. primary dermatological disorders such as psoriasis and eczema.

We shall examine each of these conditions and what we can offer as treatment.

Conditions Due to Mechanical Stress

Hyperkeratosis results from excess pressure or friction on the stratum corneum. This process causes the epidermis to respond in a hyperproliferative manner resulting in an increased production of corneocytes. The net result is a thick stratum corneum. The most common lesions are corns and calluses. A **callus** is a diffuse area of relatively even hyperkeratosis. A **corn** is a an area of callus that has been molded into a nucleus. There are four types of corns: **hard, soft, vascular,** and **neurovascular**.

**Hard corns** result from concentrated pressure on specific areas of the foot and toes.They may occur on the dorsal surface of the interphalangeal joints (i-p joints) of toes or on the plantar surfaces beneath the metatarsal heads or the i-p joints of the big toe.

**Soft corns** occur only between the toes, most often between the 4th an 5th toes but also between the other toes. These corns appear as ring structures with an extremely thin center, they are usually moist and often macerated because of the moisture from sweat.

**Vascular and Neurovascular Corns** result from long standing lesions. They are deep and may show nerve endings or capillary vessels about the callus.

Treatment of all corns is aimed at restoring the skin to normal by combination of surgery, medications, and mechanical treatment. The most important step in treatment is the relief of the mechanical stress which produced the lesion. In most cases referring the client to a chiropodist (same as a podiatrist) is the best move. The skin care specialist must know how to recognize these lesions but the treatment is best left to the experts. Small or minor corns should be treated as potentially serious in anyone with a metabolic disorder. In the absence of a systemic disorder minor corns can be treated. A change of shoes reduces pressure and the use of padding protects the lesion from pressure. Do not attempt surgery or recommend keratolytic agents for corns.

Conditions Due to Infections

**Bacterial infections** of the foot are usually minor and trivial thanks to antibiotic therapy. The skin of the foot has a large number of bacteria, yeast, and fungi. The moist condition of the foot in a shoe supports bacterial growth but the thick stratum corneum acts as a good deterrent to penetration of the bacteria. The most common infection is called **erythrasma** and is due to bacteria called Corynebacterium minutissimum. The site is usually between the toes with the lesion occurring as a well circumscribed scaly brownish patch. It occurs in other sites of the body wherever there is a skin fold (this is called **intertriginous dermatitis**). The treatment is rather easy. Broad spectrum antiseptics or keratolytic agents may be used. If in doubt, check the lesion with an ultraviolet lamp. The organism is highly visible under a Wood's light giving a coral red fluorescence.

**Intertrigo** is a term that refers to any condition that arises in a skin fold in the presence of heat and friction. Bacteria are the primary causative agents but yeast may be present as secondary invaders. The space between the toes is this type of site on the foot. Treatment is done by separating and drying the toes with absorbant material such as cotton. Sometimes mild antiseptics, such as peroxide, are used, or antibiotics, such as bacitracin ointment.

**Staphylococcus pyogenes** - The most common infective organism causing severe or pyogenic infections on the foot is called **Staphylococcus pyogenes**. Typically it will infect corns, scratches, abrasions, and surgical wounds. The infected area is red, swollen and tender, and pus may be present. On the dorsal surface of the foot these infections are often associated with hair follicles. Hard corns appear to be the most common infected site.

Treatment involves cleaning the area around the wound as well as the wound itself. Surgical drainage by a professional is followed by irrigation with 0.5% chlorhexidine, or simple sterile saline. The foot can be soaked in a warm hypertonic saline bath at 43 degrees Centigrade for ten to fifteen minutes. Make sure to cleanse the foot after the bath to prevent the spread of infection, then dry, and apply a sterile dressing with an antiseptic chlorhexidine cream (trade name Hibitaine), or an iodine ointment such as Betadine (10% povidone iodine).

Remember, in these conditions mechanical factors are important so the skin care specialist must be able to suggest methods of preventing pressure from further interfering with the healing process. Most deformed feet in the elderly client will require some measure such as cutting a hole in a shoe or special padding.

**Streptococcal infections** - We shall learn more about the different types of skin bacteria when we study wound healing but we need to cover one more type of bacterial organism that infects the skin of the foot. The nasty part of "Strep" infections is that they spread rapidly, unlike "Staph" infections which produce boils and abscesses. The spread is believed to be due to particular enzymes that the bacteria has. They are able to clear a pathway through the tissues allowing the bacteria to multiply and spread. Typically these "Strep" infections cover wide areas. Here are a few.

**Cellulitis** is a localized but spreading infection in the connective tissue of the skin characterized by heat, redness, and diffuse edema. **Make sure you do not confuse this term with "cellulite" which is a French term for a purely cosmetic condition of the fatty tissue**.

**Lymphangitis** is an infection of the lymphatic vessels that ascend the leg. Usually you will find a red line running up the leg from the area of infection. When I was a child this condition was called "blood poison", as it was an ominous sign before the days of antibiotics. The course of the red line usually follows the **saphenous** vein.

**Lymphadenitis** is a condition of infected lymph glands or nodes. They are tender and swollen and often occur along the path of the saphenous vein. If the infection passes beyond the lymph nodes the infection enters the blood stream and a serious systemic infection occurs. This is rare today since most cases of cellulitis will be treated with antibiotic and not pass beyond this stage. **Treatment is always by a physician. Do not attempt to treat these conditions**.

Plantar warts are really tough challenges. They are painful and troublesome and are often severe enough to disable a client. They are also contagious as they are viral infections of the skin. You can best help the client if you understand the nature of these warts.

First, remember that they are warts and not a callus. Warts are caused by a human papovavirus called HPV of which there are 15 known types. These viruses are able to cause benign tumors in both man and animals. The type associated with palmar warts is called HPV 1, while those associated with plantar warts are types HPV 2 and HPV 4.

Secondly, warts affect mainly children and young adults. If you examine the wart with a 10X lens you will see the typical appearance of a papilloma, that is, a dome-like shape with multiple parts.

Third, swimmers and sports inclined individuals are most often infected as the virus enters through tiny cracks in the moist skin.

Fourth, the warts frequently resolve without treatment in six to eight months. The decision to treat depends on the degree of discomfort and pain.

Treatment is at best left to a podiatrist or physician. It is well known in the medical circle that if you have many different treatments for a disorder you have not found the correct one. This is surely the case with plantar warts. They have been frozen, dried, fried, and excised, all of which works for some people. I always treat them by excising the top of the lesion with a fine scissors in a cone-like fashion, being careful not to cut so deeply that pain is produced. The aim is to relieve pain so the client may walk. They return in a week or two for the same procedure. In most cases the treatment will require about 4 visits before the wart is completely excised. This method forces the wart to move downward to the surface, which reduces the capillary blood supply and starves the wart. The vessels actually clot. Only if you cut too deeply will you see any blood with this method.

**Tinea pedis** - Most common fungal infections occur on the foot. The shoes of civilization are the main offender. The most often infected people are those who live in groups, military men, college lads, and miners. The fungi causing the most common of these infections are long in name but here they are: **Trichophyton rubrum, Trichophyton interdigitale, and Epidermophyton floccosum**. These organisms cause maceration and desquammation between the toes and acute vesiculation (tiny blisters) on the soles, usually on one side of the foot.

Treatment has improved. Many over-the-counter (OTC) drugs are available. They include **tolnaftate** and **miconazole nitrate** used twice daily. These products have various trade names but you can simply ask the pharmacist for the product by its chemical name.

**Scabies** is a tiny mite just visible to the naked eye; the organism is called Sarcoptes scabiei. It is usually transmitted by prolonged person to person contact. The mite burrows under the skin into the superficial layers. It infects the hands and the wrist most commonly, but is also seen in the sides of the feet and the soles, and frequently in young children. The elbows, the breasts, the buttock, the axillae, and the male genitalia are also sites of infection. Treatment entails the meticulous application of a scabicide. There are two effective agents on the market. **Gamma benzene hexachloride** and **benzyl benzoate** are available in several forms. Itching may continue for weeks after treatment even after the scabies mite is gone. Careful identification of other human contacts and treatment of these individuals is also necessary.

**Syphilis** is still with us and the palms of the hands and the soles of the feet are frequently involved in secondary syphilis. The lesions appear as bluish-red spots that develop into infiltrated papules. The epidermis, which is thickened sheds and leaves a ring of scaling at the site, but pustules may be present as well. The manifestations of secondary syphilis are multiple so question any rash or lesion that you do not clearly recognize. **Treatment is referral to a physician**.

**AIDS** is now a real problem that requires an awareness of the disease. The manifestations may take years to develop and the signs are variable and difficult to catalogue. Awareness of the possibility of infection and the habit of taking precautions to prevent infection is your best protection. **Treatment is referral to a physician.**

## DISORDERS OF THE SWEAT GLANDS

Many conditions that involve disorders of the sweat gland are described with the word **hidrosis**, meaning "sweat." The three conditions that are most frequently seen are hyperhidrosis, bromhidrosis, and anhidrosis.

**Hyperhidrosis** describes excess sweat production. It affects young males more than women but both sexes are afflicted. Sweating may occur to the point of saturation of clothing and shoes. Treatment consists of reducing sweat with **anticholinergic** drugs or with antiperspirants. The use of aluminium chloride hexahydrate in alcohol is sometimes beneficial. A 3% solution of formalin as a foot bath is also helpful. Formalin is a 10% solution of formaldehyde, so dilute this solution further. Take 3 milliters of formalin and add 97 milliliters of water. An effective anticholinergic is glycopyrrohonium bromide. This must be used with iontophoresis as the delivery system, and is used by physicians.

**Bromhydrosis** (also called bromohyperhidrosis), describes malodorous feet. The malodor is caused by a combination of keratin and sweat and their decomposition by bacteria. Most of the individuals with this condition have tried talc and other home remedies so these are not worth advising. Again, the use of 3% formalin soaks or boric acid foot baths are effective.

**Anhidrosis**, the absence of sweating, is a serious condition. The causes of anhidrosis may be from primary disorders in the brain, spinal cord, or peripheral nerves. In the sweat glands there may be primary atrophy of the gland, or congenital absence of the gland. The gland may be plugged with keratin or closed by prickly heat causing a dysfunctional condition. Treatment involves finding the cause - **these cases must be referred to a physician**.

**Erthyema pernio** is a condition that is an abnormal vascular reaction to cold. It is seen only in the winter time, and occurs when the feet are warmed after being cold. It occurs at any age but mainly affects children. Itching and pain with erythema starts on the dorsum of the toes, heels, and lower leg. It may also be seen on the fingers, nose, and toes. While it is not generally serious it may sometimes result in ulceration and necrosis of tissue. Treatment is directed at relieving symptoms. Prevention is the best therapy but warm and gentle care is usually sufficient in most cases. The condition may last as long as two to three weeks.

There are many other conditions that affect the feet not mentioned in this chapter. Any condition that can affect skin in other areas may affect the feet also. The skin care specialist must view this chapter as only an introduction to foot problems. Many good texts are available and are listed at the end of this chapter.

## THE NAILS

### Anatomy

The nail consists of five parts: the nail plate,

the nail bed, the matrix root, and the nail fold. (See **Figure 9-6**.) The **nail plate** is composed of closely packed keratin cells much more dense than the stratum corneum. It owes its flexibility to the presence of phospholipids in its structure. The nail plate grows out of the **nail matrix** which is the germinative part of the skin. The nail plate develops in three layers from the nail matrix. The nail root is the posterior portion of the plate, which lies above the matrix and below the nail fold. The **nail fold** forms the roof, floor and sides of the nail. The **nail bed** on which the nail plate rests is a highly vascular area which gives the color to the finger nail.

The growth of the nail continues throughout life, being greatest in childhood and decreasing over time. In advanced age the nail becomes harder, loses color, and acquires longitudinal ridges.

Cutting of nails should always be done so that the nail projects over the nail bed. The nail should be cut so that it conforms to the shape of the digit, or straight across. Rough edges should be removed by filing.

### Some Common Nail Conditions

The skin care specialist can help the client maintain his or her nails in good condition and

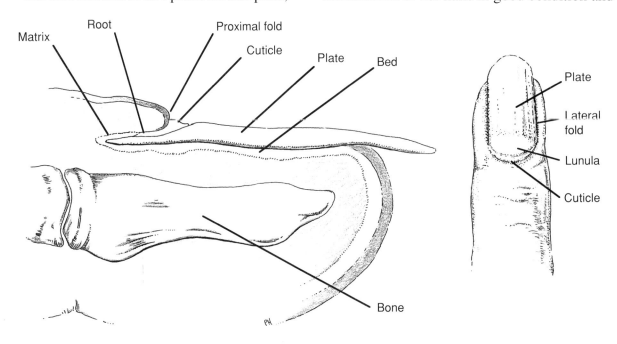

**FIGURE 9-6** Nail anatomy. Remember that the nail is keratin protein and grows in a manner similar to the epidermis. The nail in humans provides support to the soft ends of the fingers and toes. In some animals nails serve as both offensive weapons, (e.g. tigers and bears) and food gathering instruments.

most abnormal conditions are best treated by podiatrists or physicians. The following conditions are listed mainly for recognition purposes, though some are treatable by the skin care specialist.

**Involution** is a condition of the nail in which the lateral edges grow in towards the nail bed. This may be mild or so severe that the nail edges meet in the center. Involution may be congenital (from birth), or may be acquired from improper shoes, or malnutrition. In mild cases the only treatment necessary is to cut the nail properly as described above. More severe cases must be referred.

**Ingrown toe nail** (**Onychocryptosis**) is a condition in which a splinter or sliver of nail has penetrated the subcutaneous tissue. The condition occurs most commonly in adolescent males but also occurs in women, with the big toe (hallux) being the favored site. The skin is red, shiny, and tense, and slight pressure on the tip of the toe at the site of the inflammation produces intense pain. The three main causes are hyperhidrosis, poorly fitted shoes, and improper nail cutting. All these are fairly common in teenage lads.

Treatment is best left to physicians or a podiatrist, however, if the case is mild you may be able to assist the client. Have the client soak the foot in warm water with 2 tablespoons of salt to 2 quarts of water for 15 to 30 minutes. Dry the foot and then carefully examine the red area by cleaning the space between the nail and lateral fold with a cotton tipped applicator. If you can do so without great pain to the client gently probe the anterior nail to locate the sliver. This can usually be bent upward with fine forceps and then cut off with a fine pointed sissors. Antibiotic ointment such as bacitracin applied three times daily after saline soaks will clear the infection.

If you can not remove the sliver place a small wedge of cotton under the nail between the fold and the nail bed. This will sometimes give relief until definitive therapy can be obtained. Most cases of ingrown toe nails that I treated required partial excision of the nail under local anesthesia. This is an operative procedure which only physicians and podiatrists may do, but it is often required to correct this condition.

**Paronychia** is a condition characterized by an inflammation of the tissues around the nail plate. **Onychia** is an inflammation of the matrix and the nail bed and often occurs with paronychia. Paronychia is characterized by a red swollen tissue at the side or back of the nail and often pus is present. It is very painful.

The causes of paronychia are many, from simple stubbing of the toe to chronic yeast infections. Consider this condition seriously until you know the cause. Treatment is simply hot hypertonic saline soaks and application of antiseptics three times a day. If pus is present the client must be referred for incision and drainage. In children this is often very traumatic, and incision and drainage is usually avoided unless there is no other way. Using hot saline soaks and covering with a generous coating of bacitracin will frequently macerate the infection site enough to produce a spontaneous drainage.

**Beau's Lines** are ridges or grooves that appear transversely on the nail plate at the base and move forward. They reflect some temporary retardation of growth.

### Some Rare Conditions with Unusual Names (Impress your Friends)

**Onychorrhexis** is "brittle nail" seen with arthritis and anemia.

**Koilonychia or spoon nail** is seen on the hands more than on the feet and is hereditary or a sequelae of a serious illness.

**Onychomycosis** is a fungal infection of the nails, tough to treat but will respond to long term antifungal systemic therapy.

**Onychogryposis** (Ram's horn or Osler's Toe) is a gross deformity of the nail characterized by an enlarged and curved toe nail usually on the big toe but could be on all toes. **Treatment is surgical or palliative by trimming**.

**Onychauxis** is an increased thickness of the nail starting from the base to free edge. It results usually from some trauma to the matrix, fungal infection of the nail or neglect of nail care. If several toes or all the toes are involved suspect some systemic disorder and refer the client.

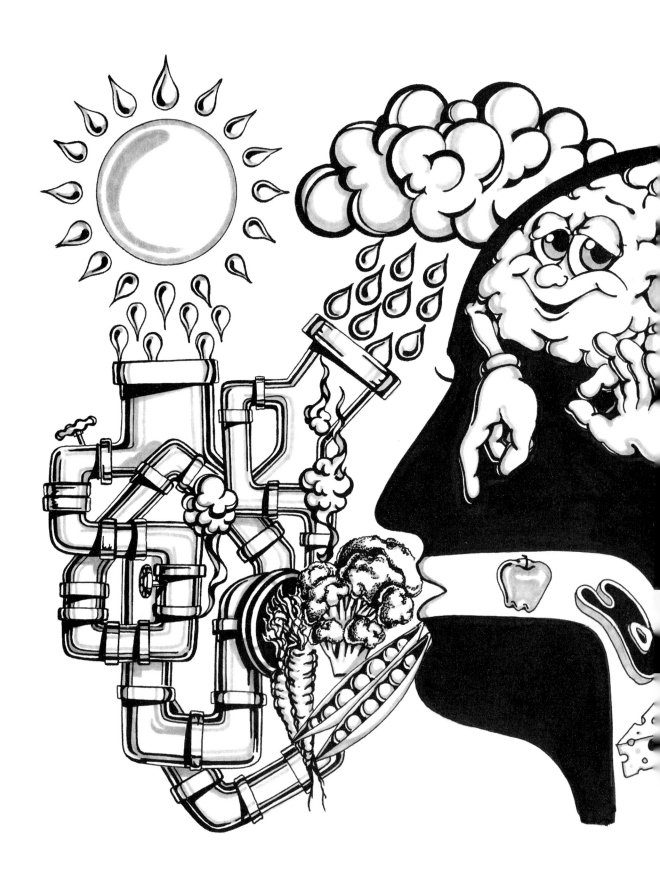

As part of our strategy to whip the enemy, we Topical Agents incorporate some powerful helpers in doing the job. Like we call in the VITA-MEN E & A TEAM to mop up those Free Radicals. We may employ

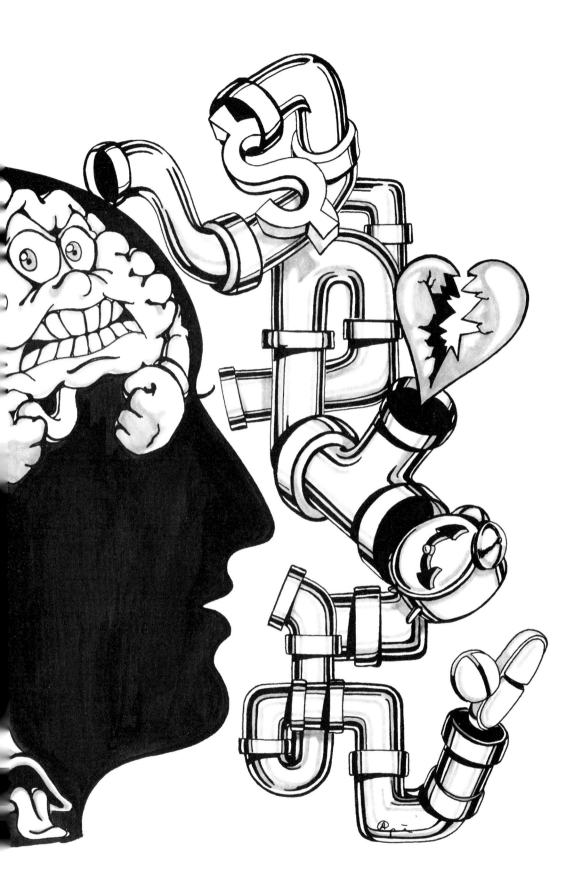

Magic Bullets to unzap UltraViolet's wicked trickery. And sometimes our best offense when things start to heat up is the coolest defense against meltdown -- just chill out and relax..................

# Stress Management and Nutrition

"You are what you eat." This statement has been around for many years and is quoted by many writers and lecturers on nutrition. It is, however, only partly true, for man is much more than the sum total of what he consumes. This is not to say that our choice of food does not have a profound effect on our life and well being. It most assuredly does! There are many other factors, though, that combine to make us what we are, including our environment, friends, reading, religion, parents, etc. While food is important, it is only a part of our total life needs. In this chapter we shall cover the importance of proper diet, the biochemistry of nutrition, and some practical material on diets and how they affect the skin. I have included a section on **stress and the skin**.

## WHAT IS NUTRITION?

**Nutrition** is the science or study of the nourishment of humans or other creatures. The word nutrition is derived from the Latin word *nutrire* meaning to feed. Another Latin word *nutrix* meaning nurse is derived from the same root word. Nourishment comes to us through the French language and is a variation of the word nutrition. The study of nutrition is essentially the study of how to feed humans and other animals. Human study involves a knowledge of the basic anatomy and physiology of the human body as well as some knowledge of human biochemistry. In this chapter we shall discuss first the three basic nutrients, **carbohydrates, proteins, and fats**. Next we will discuss the **vitamins** and their role in nutrition with particular reference to the skin. We shall follow next with a discussion of **minerals** and **trace elements**.

## Why Do We Need to Eat ?

We eat to stay alive, even though we enjoy it immensely. Food supplies us with energy and the building materials for growth and repair of our bodies. All the energy we use on earth comes from the sun and is locked into the chemical bonds of plants through a process called **photosynthesis** as diagrammed in **Figure 10-1**. The energy is stored in the form of high energy bonds within the three basic foods (carbohydrates, proteins, and fats). As we eat plant foods, we break down the plant chemicals (mostly starches and sugars) and release the stored energy. The body then uses the energy to keep us warm and to make other chemical compounds that are needed for our growth and repair. The total process of breaking down foods and building up body components is known as **metabolism** and is an important part of nutritional study.

## AN OVERVIEW OF THE NUTRITIONAL PROCESS IN THE BODY

The body contains about 1% carbohydrate, 15-20% fat, 10-15% protein, and about 70% water. The rest of the body is made up of minerals such as calcium and phosphorus. Other minerals, present in small amounts, are called trace elements and are essential to complete the list. Our diet must reflect an intake of these important materials. We call these essential materials **nutrients** and we divide them into six categories: carbohydrates, proteins, fats, vitamins, major minerals, and trace elements.

After consumption of food, **digestion and absorption** of the nutrients are required. Large molecules such as proteins and starches are broken down into smaller blocks such as sugars,

amino acids, and fatty acids. All foods, except vitamins and minerals, must go through this process to be used by the body.

Digestion begins in the mouth with the formation of saliva. The action of certain enzymes in the saliva begins the breakdown of the complex sugars which will be completed in the small intestine. Proteins begin to breakdown in the stomach which has hydrochloric acid and the enzyme, pepsin. This process is again completed in the small intestine where the pancreatic enzymes trypsin and chymotrypsin reduce them to amino acids. Fats are first attacked in the duodenum after they leave the stomach. That is why a fatty meal stays with us longer than a sugar meal.

Fats require bile salts and lipase to be metabolized. These are supplied by the liver and the pancreas. Non-nutrients are not acted upon by the digestive system of the body but are passed along and either absorbed into the blood stream or excreted in the bowel or urine.

The fluids secreted into the gastrointestinal system function not only to break-up the large food molecules but also to provide protection for the body against bacteria and foreign mate-

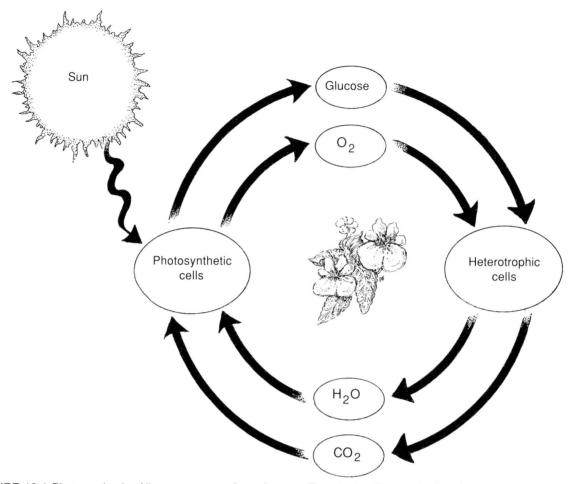

**FIGURE 10-1** Photosynthesis. All energy comes from the sun. The plant cell converts the photons from the sun into glucose using water and carbon dioxide. We use the energy in glucose by breaking down the molecule and releasing the energy.

rials that may act as antigens. Proteins are one of the most antigenic of all natural materials. The low pH of the stomach (which is about pH 1) destroys most bacteria, though some escape and serve a symbiotic function in the middle and lower intestine.

The great bulk of these secretions are reabsorbed and recycled. Bile, for instance, is lost at a rate of only 1% a day. High fiber diets may cause somewhat more to be lost. High fiber diets may also cause cholesterol to be lost.

Most absorption of nutrients will occur in the duodenum and the small intestine. The lower, large intestine is filled with many types of bacteria which are responsible for providing substantial amounts of vitamins to the body and for maintaining ammonia and nitrogen balance.

The use of antibiotics can markedly upset this delicate balance and cause adverse effects on the total nutrition. Treatment with antibiotics for seven to ten days can result in destroying a large number of these bacteria. There is

no direct evidence that yogurt or similar foods will repopulate the gut after antibiotic therapy.

Absorption of the nutrients occurs through the intestinal wall by simple diffusion. Water soluble molecules under 12,000 molecular weight (12 kd) will pass easily through the intestinal wall.

Some proteins are absorbed as whole molecules (which we shall discuss later) but most large molecules are broken down. After passing into the intestine the nutrients enter the blood or lymph. From the blood stream they are distributed throughout the body. Fats enter the lymphatic system and pass into the blood stream through the thoracic duct. Most of the nutrients are filtered and acted upon by the liver. They are either used immediately or stored with some biochemical changes. When nutrients are stored they generally are stored as a complex molecule such as glycogen, protein, or triglyceride.

Remember that there is a constant turnover in the body's composition. Energy is required for the replacement of tissue building blocks. Even the building blocks themselves are derived from the food we eat.

Materials which are not utilized by the body are excreted as water, carbon dioxide, urea, and ammonia. Most of the water is reabsorbed in the large intestine leaving little but bacteria and indigestible fiber in the feces.

## CARBOHYDRATES

**Carbohydrate** means literally carbon and water. The composition of these compounds is relatively simple. They can serve as a primary energy source for the body. When carbohydates are utilized they produce two by-products, carbon dioxide and water. Oxygen is used in the process of breaking down carbohydrates and releasing the energy. This process is called oxidation. In the United States carbohydrates provide about 50% of a person's caloric needs. In other areas of the world they are 80 to 100% of the food intake.

### Types of Carbohydrates

Carbohydrates may be divided into three groups: **monosaccharides, disaccharides, and polysaccharides**.

**Monosaccharides** are simple sugars that are sweet to the taste and require no further digestion before being absorbed directly into the blood stream from the small intestine. They include **glucose, fructose**, and **galactose**. Glucose is found in corn syrup, honey, molasses, sweet fruits, and some vegetables. Fructose is a fruit sugar and is sometimes called levulose. Galactose is not a natural sugar but is a product of milk digestion.

**Disaccharides** or double sugars are also sweet to the taste but must be broken down to simple sugars in order to be absorbed. They include **sucrose, maltose**, and **lactose**. You will recognize sucrose as common table sugar and the major sugar in molasses and maple syrup. Maltose is an intermediate sugar produced from starch metabolism and is not found naturally. It is not very sweet. Lactose is found in milk. It, too, is not very sweet. It is not found in plants and can cause gastrointestinal distress in people who have little lactase enzyme.

**Polysaccharides** are also known as complex carbohydrates. They are composed of three or more simple sugars and include starch, dextrins, cellulose, and glycogen. Starch is found in greater amounts in grains and lesser amounts in vegetables.

**Figure 10-2** shows a longitudinal section of a wheat grain and displays the various parts of the grain. The center of the grain is called the endosperm and contains most of the starch. White flour comes from this part. The outer coat is tough and is called the bran. Fiber comes from this part. The **germ** is a rich source of vitamin B complex and vitamin E. Whole wheat flour contains all three components.

**Dextrins** are intermediates of starch digestion. They form spontaneously when bread is toasted. **Glycogen** is a form of complex sugar which is stored in the body of animals as an energy reserve. We have a 12 to 48 hour supply of energy stored as glycogen in the muscles and the liver. **Cellulose** is the fibrous part of the plant that makes up the framework. It absorbs water and aids in providing bulk to the stool. It can not be digested by humans.

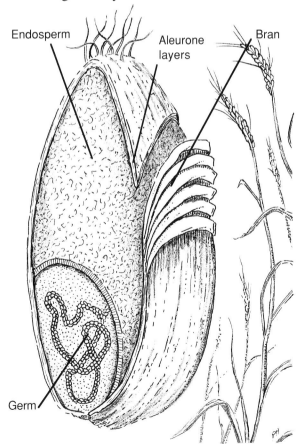

**FIGURE 10-2** Structure of wheat. Wheat is a very old grain. Note that the germ contains the DNA needed to reproduce the plant.

## FATS AND NUTRITION

### Definition

Strictly speaking, fats are only part of a larger group of compounds called **lipids**. Lipids are oily, greasy, and water insoluble compounds. The nutrient fats are divided into **true fats or triglycerides, phospholipids, and sterols**.

### Classification

**Triglycerides** are composed of glycerol and fatty acids. Fatty acids are composed of long chain hydrocarbons with at least two oxygen molecules. When three fatty acids are linked to a glycerol molecule we have a true triglyceride or fat. Two fatty acids attached to a glycerol molecule produces a **diglyceride**. One fatty acid attached to glycerol produces a **monoglyceride**.

Triglycerides are high energy sources. They contain 9 kilocalories (kcal) per gram of fat as compared to 4 kcal for both carbohydrates and protein. The shape of the fat molecule makes it ideal for storage. The bulk of the fats are stored in cells called **adipocytes.** These adipocytes are 99% fat. It is interesting that the total number of adipocytes in the body is determined in childhood. Overfeeding will produce a greater number of these cells. Triglycerides serve also to protect the internal organs, such as the heart and kidneys, and the breasts.

**Fatty acids** may be **saturated** or **unsaturated** depending on the number of hydrogen atoms present in the molecule. Unsaturated fats are essential in our diet, particularly linoleic acid which is a $C_{18}$ fatty acid with two double bonds and linolenic acid, a $C_{18}$ fatty acid with three double bonds. These fatty acids are called essential fatty acids because the body cannot make them from other fats or raw materials. Most of the body fatty acids are from $C_{12}$ lauric acid, $C_{14}$ myristic acid, $C_{16}$ palmitic acid and $C_{18}$ stearic acid.

**Mono-unsaturated fats** contain only one unsaturated site, examples being olive oil and avocado oil. A polyunsaturated fat contains two or more unsaturated sites, examples being corn oil and peanut oil. The question of a high intake of polyunsaturated fatty acids as protection against heart disease is still controversial. There are some studies that show a diet high in unsaturated fat from fish oils will offer some protection against coronary heart disease.

**Cholesterol** is a sterol molecule that forms the basis of many hormones in the body as well as other compounds such as the bile acids. It is a multiple ring structure as seen in **Figure 10-3**. Cholesterol comes into our diet through animal foods and is not found in plant foods. Our body will make cholesterol if the intake is too low. We need about 1.1 grams of cholesterol a day. We take in about 200 to 300 milligrams in our diet and the rest is made by the liver. If you take in more cholesterol your body will make less, however, reducing cholesterol intake drastically has only a 10 to 15% effect on the reduction of serum cholesterol levels.

Gallbladder disease frequently arises from the formation of cholesterol stones in the bil-

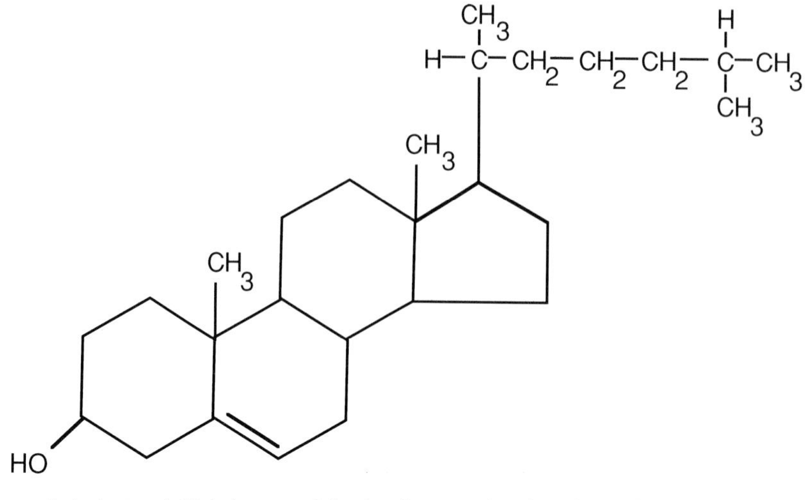

**FIGURE 10-3** Structure of cholesterol. This is one of the fundamental molecules of life. All cortisone, sex hormones, and bile acids are based on this structure. Cholesterol is a lipid material and does not dissolve in water.

iary tract. The specific cause of gallbladder disease is not fully known, but the recommendation of dietary restriction of fats in the presence of gallbladder disease is good advice. Individuals with high fat intake and menopausal females are at high risk for gallbladder disease.

The **phospholipids** contain a phosphate group in the molecule and thus have detergent or emulsification action. We find phospholipids in many foods in the form of lecithin (also called phosphatidyl choline). We get phospholipids from egg yolk. This is why egg yolk is used to make many recipes with fats. The phospholipids make up the major part of the cell membrane.

### PROTEINS

### Definition

**Proteins** are the basic building materials of the cells. Only protein can be used to build and repair the body structures. An adequate supply of protein is needed for normal growth and development and to maintain the body in good health. So important is protein that the very name means "of first importance".

Like the fats and carbohydrates, proteins are composed of carbon, oxygen and hydrogen, but in addition they contain nitrogen and often sulfur. Proteins function as components of enzymes and hormones. They can serve as an energy source if fats and carbohydrates are not sufficient. Proteins are made up of **amino acids** which are composed of carbon, hydrogen, oxygen, nitrogen ,and, at times, sulfur. There are nine essential amino acids of the twenty-two amino acids used by the body. These nine amino acids must be supplied to the body since they cannot be synthesized by the body's cells. We listed the amino acids in the biochemistry discussion earlier. The essential amino acids are: histidine, isoleucine, leucine, lysine, methionine, phenylalanine, threonine, tryptophan, and valine.

There is some evidence that the liver can synthesize histidine so there may be only eight essential amino acids.

### Function of Amino Acids and Proteins

The greatest use of amino acids is for the synthesis of new special compounds. The amino acids are digestive products of ingested proteins. They are formed into peptides, small compounds of two of more amino acids. The peptides are arranged into polypeptides which contain several peptides. Polypeptides are formed into proteins. The amino acids are used to form neurotransmitter hormones as well as other hormones and enzymes. The building blocks of the body such as elastin, collagen, and muscle tissue all contain proteins.

### Protein Requirements

Adults need about 1 gm of protein per kg of body weight. For an average person this means 60 to 70 grams of protein per day. In infancy, childhood, and pregnancy the need is much greater. **Figure 10-4** shows the use of protein by the various body systems. It also shows how the protein is lost.

### VITAMINS

**Vitamins** are organic molecules that are necessary in the diets of higher animals for normal metabolic functions. By definition vitamins cannot be synthetized by the body. We divide vitamins into two major classifications based on their solubility in water.

### Water Soluble Vitamins

Vitamin C - ascorbic acid
Vitamin B complex - niacin ($B_3$), pyridoxine ($B_6$), riboflavin ($B_2$),  pantothenate, thiamine ($B_1$), biotin, folic acid, cobalamin ($B_{12}$).
Several of these vitamins are components of coenzymes.

### Water Insoluble or Fat Soluble Vitamins

Vitamin E (tocopherol)
Vitamin K (phylloquinone)
Vitamin D (calciferol)
Vitamin A (retinol)

### Biological Functions of the Vitamins

**Table 10-1** will provide you with a quick

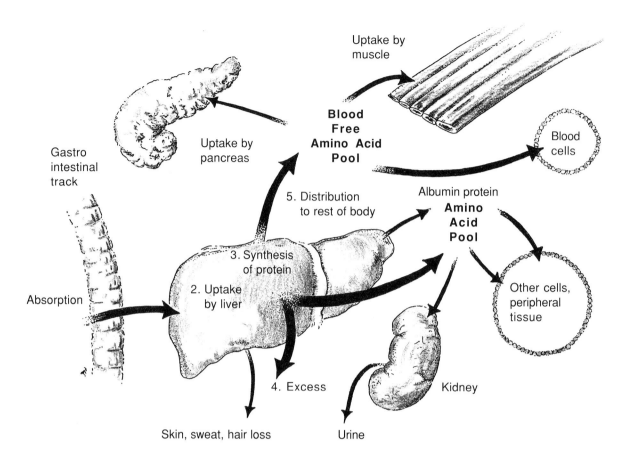

**FIGURE 10-4** Protein use by various parts of the body. All food which we take into our bodies is metabolized by various organs. Some is saved, some utilized, and some excreted immediately.

reference for the names, actions, sources, and the diseases associated with a deficiency of each of the vitamins.

Remember, as a rule, fat soluble vitamins can be stored and water soluble vitamins cannot be stored.

**Thiamine** (vitamin $B_1$), along with the other B vitamins, is important as a coenzyme in intermediary metabolism. Specifically, it is used in decarboxylation reactions and transketolase reactions. You will see these reactions in **Figure 10-5** along with the actions of the other vitamins. We need between 1 mg and 1.5 mg of thiamine a day. Good food sources of thiamine are seeds, nuts, wheat germ, legumes, and lean meats.

A deficiency of thiamine, rare in civilized countries, can lead to a condition known as **beri-beri** which is characterized by neuritis (called peripheral neuropathy) which manifests itself as tingling, burning, numbness, and weakness of the extremities. Excessive use of coffee or tea may cause a need to increase thiamine intake.

**Riboflavin** (vitamin $B_2$) is an important con-

stituent of two coenzymes that link the Krebs cycle to the electron transport system. They are strong oxidizing agents. You can see their function in **Figure 10-5**. Keep in mind that riboflavin deficiencies are not rare in our society. We need about 1.5 to 1.6 mg a day. Pregnant and lactating women require more, up to 2 mg a day. Milk, meats, eggs, and seeds are good sources of riboflavin. The structure of riboflavin is shown in **Figure 10-6.**

A deficiency of riboflavin is seen as angular stomatitis and seborrheic dermatitis in the scrotum and nose.

**Niacin,** also called nicotinic acid or vitamin $B_3$, is also a component of the coenzymes that function in the intermediary metabolism and in the electron transport system. Niacin is very important in many enzyme reactions involved in fatty acid metabolism. We need about 13 to 20 mg/day of niacin. Good food sources are meats, fish, milk, eggs, wheat flour, and corn.

A deficiency of niacin leads to the disease known as **pellagra**, which is characterized by the 4 D's: dermatitis, diarrhea, dementia, and

# SUMMARY OF SKIN DISEASES CAUSED BY VITAMIN DEFICIENCIES

| WATER SOLUBLE VITAMINS | SKIN SIGN | MUCOUS MEMBRANES |
| --- | --- | --- |
| Thiamine (B1) | None | Small blister like lesions on buccal surface |
| Riboflavin (B2) | Eyes red, naso labial dermatitis | Glossitis, cheilitis, angular stomatitis |
| Niacin (B3) | Pellagra, itchy rash on hands and blisters, scaling, skin with fissures | Glossitis, stomatitis ulceration of mouth |
| Pyridoxine | Seborrheic dermatitis-appearing facial lesions, perleche | Glossitis and magenta colored tongue |
| Cyanocobalamin (B12) | Hyperpigmentation of feet and hands, lemon-yellow palor | Glossitis with marked smooth atrophy of tongue, stomatitis and ulcers of oral cavity |
| Ascorbic Acid (Vitamin C) | Scurvy, keratosis of arms then generalized hemorrhagic lesion and bruising | Gingivitis, ulcers, bleeding gums |
| Folic Acid (Folacin) | Anemic palor | Cheilosis, glossitis, pharyngitis, perirectal ulcerations |
| Pantothenic acid | None known | None known |
| Biotin | Exfoliative dermatitis, dry flaky skin, seborrheic-like dermatitis | Papillary atrophy of tongue |
| **FAT SOLUBLE VITAMINS** | | |
| D | Rickets, no skin lesions | None known |
| A (Retinol) | Dry skin, xerosis of eyes, hyperkeratosis, follicular keratosis | Keratinization of salivary glands |
| E (Tocopherol) | None known | None known |
| K | Large cutaneous hemorrhages, and ecchymoses | None known |

**TABLE 10-1** This table is for reference use. Look at it occasionally to refresh your memory. The use of junk food and irregular lifestyle can produce subtle vitamin deficiences. Adapted from Nutritional Biochemistry and Metabolism by Maria C. Linder, Ph. D., Elsevier Science Publishing, Co., 1985.

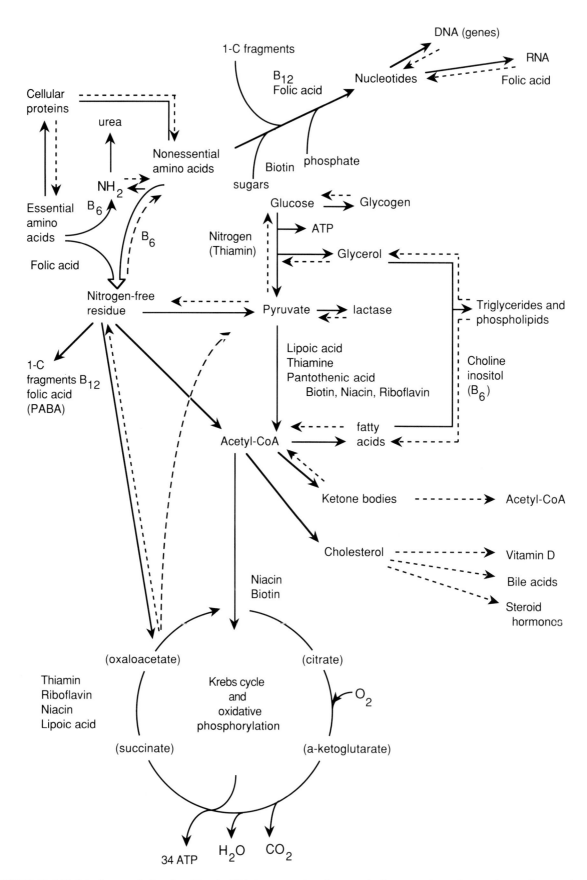

**FIGURE 10-5** Metabolism and vitamins. Granted this is a complex diagram ,but you can have fun tracing various pathways in and out of this system. The diagram shows the interrelationship of many substances and pathways in the body.

death. India and Africa still have many cases of pellagra. The dermatitis is usually around the orifices of the body - mouth, vagina, and rectum. An erythematous skin with scaling and flaking may be seen at times over the whole body. The disease is easily treated with niacin or nicotinamide at 300 to 500 mg/day along with a balanced diet.

**Pantothenic acid** is an essential component of Coenzyme A which is important in linking the glycolytic cycle with the Krebs cycle and many other metabolic reactions. We need about 5 to 10 mg/day of pantothenic acid. Deficiencies are hard to determine since this vitamin is linked to all the other B vitamins and overall nutrition.

**Pyridoxine** (vitamin $B_6$) is a complicated vitamin, not fully understood, for when we say $B_6$ we are really talking about three different substances. These are pyridoxine, pyridoxal phosphate, and pyridoxamine phosphate. It is absorbed as the unphosphated form and then phosphate is added, since only the phosphated form can attach to the enzymes.

The function of $B_6$ is also complex for it is a cofactor in more than 60 different enzyme reactions. These reactions involve mainly amino acid metabolism, but fat metabolism also requires $B_6$. Since a great many amino acid reactions occur in the liver, a large concentration of $B_6$ is found in the liver of animals (making liver a good source of the vitamin). We require about 2 to 3 mg/day of $B_6$. Pregnancy and the use of certain drugs will increase the need for $B_6$. The best sources of $B_6$ are whole grains, legumes, nuts, avocados, and bananas. Liver is the only good source from meats though steak, fish, and chicken contain some $B_6$, about half the amount found in liver.

Deficiency of $B_6$ is not infrequent in chronic alcoholics, who frequently develop a skin disorder manifested by a seborrheic dermatitis, weakness, irritability, nervousness, and insomnia. There is frequently an associated anemia in which the red cells are small and pale (called microcytic hypochromic anemia).

**Vitamin $B_{12}$** and **folic acid** are usually discussed together due to the fact that they are intimately entangled in metabolism. $B_{12}$ is also known as cobalamin and is associated most frequently with a disease known as **pernicious anemia**. One of the causes of pernicious ane-

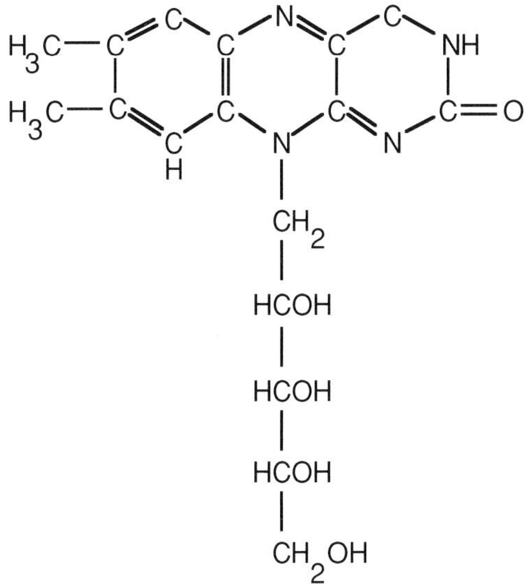

**FIGURE 10-6** Structure of riboflavin. Riboflavin is water soluble. Note the number of OH groups present in the molecule. This is avitamin B family member.

mia is the inability of the vitamin to be absorbed in the stomach. In order to be utilized, the vitamin must be cleaved from a protein in the stomach and then bound to glycoprotein, called **intrinsic factor**, which is secreted by the gastric mucosa (the cell lining of the stomach). After binding to the intrinsic factor, the $B_{12}$ is absorbed by the stomach lining and then is passed into the blood stream.

$B_{12}$ is used in two enzymatic reactions, one of which relates to acetyl CoA. The other relates to folic acid metabolism.

Good sources of $B_{12}$ are liver, kidney, eggs, and cheese. A deficiency of $B_{12}$ results in a very complex set of signs and symptoms but anemia is one of them. Peripheral neuropathy and mental disturbance also occur in the disease, which is not always easy to diagnose. Treatment is, however, very effective with administration of $B_{12}$ and proper diet. Vegetarians and alcoholics are frequent sufferers of this disease.

**Folic acid** functions in amino acid, purine and nucleic acid metabolism. The reactions are many and complex but generally folic acid is involved in one-carbon donor reactions and is intimately involved in reactions with $B_{12}$. Deficiencies of folic acid result in defects of DNA synthesis which produces abnormal chromatin and impaired DNA polymerization with arrested cell maturation. The cells of the bone marrow are affected, which results in an anemia called **megaloblastic anemia.**

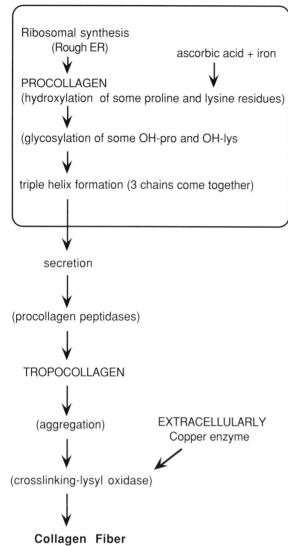

**Fibroblasts**

Ribosomal synthesis
(Rough ER)

↓                    ascorbic acid + iron

PROCOLLAGEN                    ↓

(hydroxylation of some proline and lysine residues)

↓

(glycosylation of some OH-pro and OH-lys

↓

triple helix formation (3 chains come together)

↓

secretion

↓

(procollagen peptidases)

↓

TROPOCOLLAGEN

↓

(aggregation)          EXTRACELLULARLY
                       Copper enzyme

↓                      ↙

(crosslinking-lysyl oxidase)

↓

**Collagen  Fiber**

**FIGURE 10-7** Procollagen. Collagen synthesis starts in the fibroblast and the procollagen is secreted from the cell. The collagen fiber is then formed by  cross - linking outside the cell. Adapted from Nutritional Biochemistry and Metabolism by Maria C. Linder, Ph. D., Elsevier Science Publishing, Co., 1985.

Good sources of folate are yeast, liver, green leafy vegetables, and fruit. Skin manifestations of deficiency are glycogenglossitis, cheilosis, pharyngitis, and perirectal ulcerations.

The discovery of **ascorbic acid** (vitamin C) as a vitamin is an extremely interesting story, but of more importance is the finding that by eating citrus fruits sailors could avoid the disease scurvy. **Scurvy** is a disorder that affects many tissues, but connective tissue is the most severely affected. Easy bruising, hemorrhages, swollen joints, loose teeth, and rotting gums are prime findings in scurvy. The cure for scurvy was discovered in 1753 by a Scottish physician named James Lind. It was not until 40 years later that his treatment was adopted by the British Navy.

There is a great deal written about ascorbic acid as a health food. No doubt much of it is valid, but on the other hand much is unproven. Megadoses of vitamin C do not appear to be harmful but it is important to remember if you are taking doses over 1000 mg a day, reduce your dose gradually to discontinue the high level intake. Rapid decrease in ascorbic acid levels in the serum can lead to scurvy-like symptoms.

Man, all other primates, fish, and the guinea pig, must have vitamin C in their diet, as they have lost the ability to make it from glucose.

The function of ascorbic acid is not fully known, though it has a role as a reducing agent much like vitamin E. One of the major functions of ascorbic acid is in hydroxylation reactions, particularly the hydroxylation of proline to hydroxyproline. This is the essential reaction step needed in the formation of procollagen. Lack of ascorbic acid will prevent normal collagen from forming in the tissues. Another area of hydroxylation is in the synthesis of **biogenic amines** in the central nervous system. Iron metabolism is another function of ascorbic acid, especially in the enhancement and absorption of iron from the intestine. Individuals who smoke and drink alcohol have a greater need for vitamin C. We need to look more closely at this reaction as formation of collagen is one of the prime factors involved in aging skin.

When we discussed collagen formation there was a step in which the procollagen was linked to form collagen fibers. This step requires hydroxyproline and hydroxylysine, two amino acids which require ascorbic acid to carry out the reaction from proline and lysine. The steps are outlined in **Figure 10-7**. The need for vitamin C in the skin is not fully understood but we know that it is needed for collagen formation and perhaps for precursors of elastin formation.

Ascorbic acid is also used in other reactions, such as the degradation of steroid hormones (except estrogen) and in the metabolism of drugs. There is an increased need for ascorbic acid in times of stress.

**The Fat Soluble Vitamins**

There are four major fat soluble vitamins:

**vitamin A, vitamin E, vitamin D, and vitamin K.**

### Vitamin A (retinol)

Vitamin A is one of the most useful of all vitamins to the skin care specialist, and it is certainly one of the most interesting. In plants, vitamin A exists as **beta carotene**, a yellow pigment. In the body of animals it is converted to **retinol**, the alcohol form of the vitamin. This conversion is by the action of enzymes in the intestinal wall and the liver with some help from vitamin E and the thyroid hormone. Because of the importance of **vitamin A acid, or retinoic acid** (trade name Retin A), it is necessary for the skin care specialist to understand the various forms of vitamin A and what action they have in the body. We shall use the chemical names for the various forms of vitamin A.

**Retinol** is the alcohol form of the vitamin A and is the first compound formed from beta carotene. This is a very active form of the vitamin and is necessary for reproductive function in both males and females, for differentiation of epithelial cells, and for bone growth.

**Retinal** is the aldehyde form of vitamin A and is an oxidized form of the alcohol. Retinal is chiefly used in the body chemistry of vision. Night blindness is corrected with retinal. Both retinal and retinol can be interconverted in the body (see **Figure 10-8**).

**Retinoic acid** is the next oxidized form of vitamin A. It cannot be converted to an alcohol or an aldehyde and is therefore not usable for all of the functions of vitamin A. Also, it is not stored in the body as is retinol and it does not accumulate in the body. Retinoic acid functions in cell differentiation and in bone growth.

Again, remember that all forms exist simul-

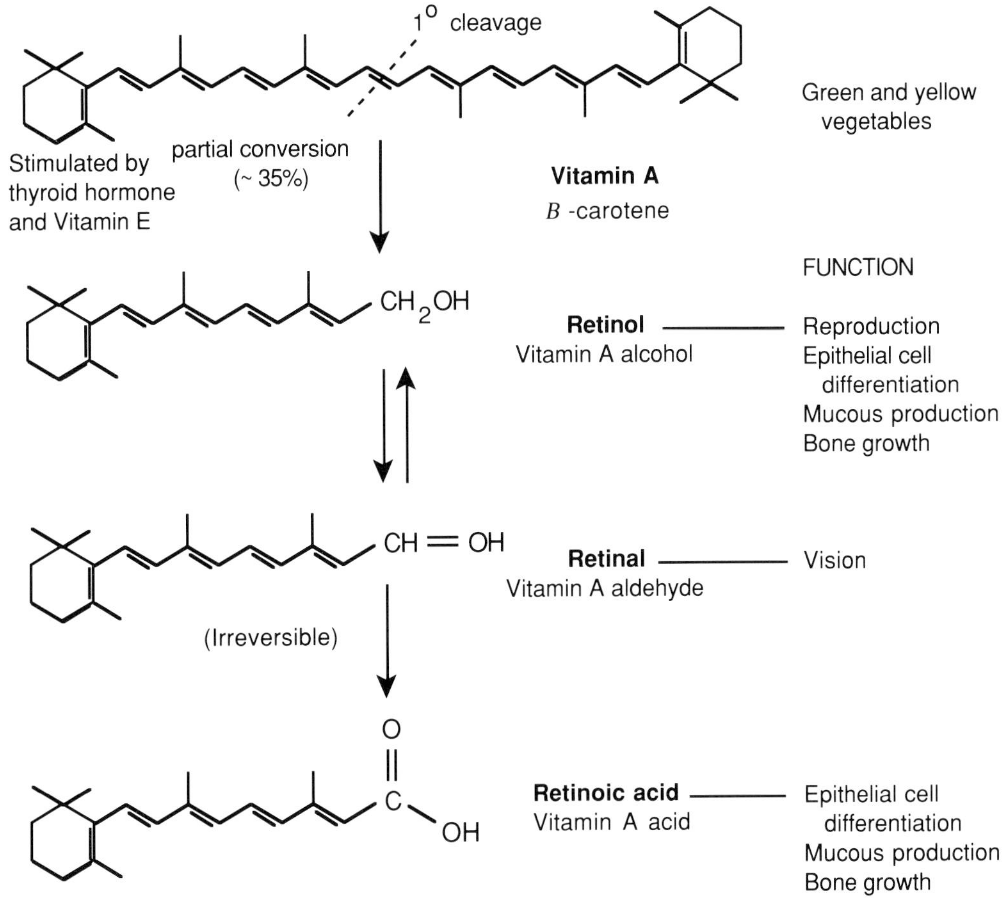

**FIGURE 10-8** Retinol and retinal interconversion. Note that the pathway from retinal (aldehyde) to retinoic acid is not reversible. This means that retinoic acid must be excreted and can not be used again by the body.

taneously in the body and that vitamin A as the alcohol form is converted into the aldehyde and acid forms.

Vitamin A is important to maintain vision. The aldehyde form of vitamin A (retinal) combines with a protein called opsin, in the eye, producing **rhodopsin** or **visual purple**. Both night vision and color vision share in this reaction. It is not important that you know the biochemistry of these reactions but you should be aware of this function. Cell differentiation is the important function of vitamin A.

**Cell differentiation** functions of vitamin A involve the maintenance of many types of epithelial cells. These include cells of the cornea of the eye, the lung, the skin, and the intestinal mucosa. We are mainly concerned with the cells of the skin. **Rough dry scaly skin is the major cutaneous sign of vitamin A deficiency**. The action of vitamin A appears to center on converting the information in the nucleus of the cell (on the DNA molecule) into an action or function. This action is called genomic expression, and it involves many biomolecular steps. Without adequate vitamin A many of the body functions would be impaired. Some of these functions include infection-defense mechanisms of the immune system, control of epidermal cell proliferative mechanisms, skin tone, and formation of glycosoaminoglycans.

When vitamin A is added to skin care products in adequate levels, it will produce an increase in cell proliferation in the epidermis, cause a stimulation of fibroblasts to produce both elastin and collagen, and induce new blood vessels to grow. All of these effects will result in a healthier and younger looking skin. You will see more and more preparations containing vitamin A as time goes on. Some of these forms of vitamin A will be new compounds. We shall discuss the various preparations of vitamin A in Chapter 14.

A major source of vitamin A (beta carotene) can be found in carrots. Collard greens, beet greens, broccoli, pumpkins, and butternut squash are other good sources. Animal sources of retinoids are milk, liver, egg yolk, and fish oils. It is well popularized that polar bear liver is toxic because of the very high vitmain A content. Cod liver oil was a major source of vitamin A many years ago and still continues to have some popularity.

**Caution!** Vitamin A and vitamin D are two fat soluble vitamins that have a toxic potential. Since they are stored in the body they can accumulate to high levels. The symptoms and signs of intoxication with these vitamins suggest a brain disorder. The **dose of vitamin A should not exceed 4000 to 5000 units a day without medical supervision**.

Vitamin E (tocopherol)

A great deal of literature has been written about vitamin E over the last 20 years. It has been reported to be good for just about every ailment known to mankind, though little proof is available. Much is known about vitamin E, however, that makes this vitamin quite important to the skin care specialist. We shall look first at the chemistry and the functions of vitamin E and then discuss the use of this vitamin in skin care.

Vitamin E has at least eight forms in nature as produced by plants. We call these various forms by the Greek letters alpha, beta, gamma, delta, epsilon, etc. For our purpose you need to remember only the alpha form. Next you need to know about the D and L forms. These designations refer to the property of chemical compounds that rotate light when examined with certain types of instruments. This in itself is not important except that the D form of tocopherol is more active biologically than the L form. The L form is about 3.5 times less active than the D form. Most commercial forms of vitamin E are sold containing the DL form (**dl alpha tocopheryl acetate**). It is this form that is used as the international standard for vitamin E. One milligram of vitamin E acetate equals one international unit. This is written as 1 mg = 1 IU.

Vitamin E has many functions in the body but the major one is believed to be its role as an **antioxidant** and as an **anti-free radical agent**. There is a hydroxyl group on the vitamin E molecule (see **Figure 10-9**) that donates a hydrogen ion to the free radical so that it becomes stable and does not enter a chain reaction. This is extremely important to remember for it forms the basis for the use of vitamin E in skin care.

Vitamin E is helpful in preventing scar formation and in reducing scars that have already formed. This is still not generally accepted by all scientists. Taking about 400 units of vitamin

E internally will help to reduce age spots on the hands and the face. Rubbing vitamin E acetate on scars will help to soften them and at times reduce them. I do not recommend the use of vitamin E capsules for this purpose. Use a commercial source of vitamin E acetate. You can buy small quantities from your pharmacist or from other specialty supply sources. Vitamin E should be used in every sunscreen product as it will help prevent the damage to the epidermis caused by ultraviolet light exposure.

Sources of vitamin E are safflower oil, sunflower oil, almonds, peanuts, whole wheat grains, and muskmelon.

### Vitamin D (D$_3$ Calciferol)

Vitamin D in nature exists as **ergocalciferol**. When irradiated with ultraviolet light the ergocalciferol forms in plants while in human skin cholecalciferol forms. Vitamin D is considered a **prohormone** because it is formed into a hormone in the body. The active form of the hormone is called calcitriol and it is formed in the liver and the kidneys. The vitamin is heat stable and is not harmed by cooking, storage, or processing; this is why it can so conveniently be added to milk (400 U per quart).

The major function of vitamin D is to promote calcium and phosphorus absorption in the body. It raises the concentration of these elements in the blood and helps to maintain normal healthy teeth and bones. The vitamin is easily absorbed from the intestine and stored in the liver and the fatty tissue.

Sources of vitamin D are limited, the best source being the sun. The amount of sun exposure and the amount of pigment in the skin will determine the amount of vitamin D produced.

Food sources are eggs, cream, butter, and liver. The recommended daily intake is 200 to 400 units for adults and 400 units for children. You will also see vitamin D listed as micrograms or mg. (One mg = 40 IU).

Hypervitaminosis D causes calcium to be deposited in tissues and yields signs of weakness, anorexia, and abnormal liver function.

Deficiency states inhibit absorption of calcium and phosphorous which results in poor bone and teeth formation. In children, **rickets** develop while in adults softening of the bones called **osteomalacia** develops. (Rickets from *wrickken* Old English for to twist. Osteo from the Greek *osteon* = bone and *malakia* = softness).

Older individuals may need more calcium and vitamin D to prevent a condition of brittle and porous bones called **osteoporosis**. This occurs usually over age 50 but it may appear in the forties.

One last word on vitamin D and the sun. As you are aware, I do not advocate sunbathing. You may see a conflict then, in my stating that the sun is necessary for vitamin D conversion. Excessive sun exposure will increase the amount of vitamin D in the skin to 5 or 6 times normal. This would suggest that sun exposure produces potentially toxic levels of vitamin D. However, as the process proceeds, the precursor of vitamin D decreases so that there is less vitamin D produced in the skin. This is nature's way of protecting sunbathers from poisoning themselves with vitamin D.

### Vitamin K (Phylloquinone)

Vitamin K is necessary for normal blood clotting. It is found in plants as phylloquinone

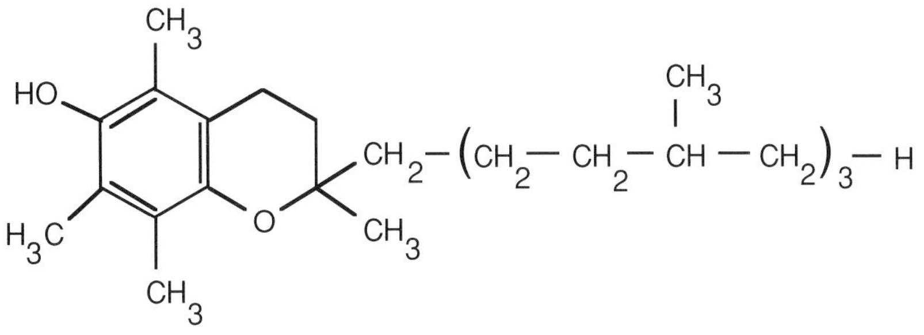

**FIGURE 10-9** Structure of vitamin E. The OH group on the left side of this molecule is the active part. The long chain carbon part on the right side functions to enter the cell membrane where it is anchored between the lipid layers. In this position the OH group is able to react with free radicals.

and is formed in the intestine by bacteria. This form is known as menaquinone. The best sources of vitamin K are spinach, cabbage, and kale. Fruits and cereals are also good sources, while animal sources are poor.

Deficiencies of vitamin K will cause bleeding disorders since it affects the clotting time of blood. An excess of vitamin K can be very dangerous since it will cause liver and kidney damage. You need only 70 to 140 micrograms a day as an adult, while children need only 15 to 40 micrograms of vitamin K daily.

## THE MINERALS AND TRACE ELEMENTS

**Minerals** are inorganic elements which are essential for normal body functions. Oxygen, carbon, hydrogen, and nitrogen make up 96% of the body chemistry, minerals make up only 4%. We find minerals in all parts of the body serving as regulators (or catalysts), electron donors, electron acceptors, and as essential components of many important proteins and other vital compounds. We obtain most of our minerals from plants, water, and from animal products. Processed foods are usually low in natural minerals. These preparations require the minerals to be added back to the finished product. Such products are called enriched, such as enriched flour. In this section we shall discuss the role of the minerals and their dietary sources.

For convenience we divide minerals into two major groups depending on our need for them. **Macrominerals** are those that we need a lot of and **microminerals** are those which we need only in trace amounts.

### The Macrominerals

**Calcium** is the most abundant mineral in the body with most of it being in the bones and the teeth. Only one percent is found in the tissues, but this is a very important one percent. Calcium gives strength to bones and teeth. Both of these organs serve as storage areas for calcium as well. In the soft tissue, calcium is required to transmit nerve impulses, to contract and relax muscles, to clot blood, and for normal heart function. One other major function of calcium is its role in enzyme function, as an enzyme activator. The best sources of calcium are milk, cheese, and dark green vegetables. High fiber diets tend to reduce calcium absorption from the intestine. Spinach contains oxalic acid which will bind calcium so that it is not available.

Calcium deficiency causes rickets, and muscle contraction called **tetany**. In adults both osteomalacia and osteoporosis may occur. Vitamin D is essential for the absorption of calcium.

**Phosphorus** is the second most abundant mineral in the body and it is the constant companion of calcium. It is needed for strong bones and teeth as well as being important in the metabolism of fats, carbohydrates, and proteins. You will recall that ATP contains phosphate as the energy carrier of the body. The sources of phosphorus are similar to calcium-dairy products, though cereal, legumes and nuts are also fairly good sources. Drinking large quantities of carbonated soft drinks may cause a shift in the calcium-phosphate ratio to the point that the amount of calcium available is reduced. A condition like rickets could result.

**Magnesium** is also an essential mineral for bones and teeth but is important for many metabolic pathways. Life as we know it would not exist without magnesium. Unfortunately, magnesium is lost with cooking and processing since it is water soluble. The sources of magnesium are primarily in plant foods. Green leafy vegetables, whole grains, nuts, and fruits such as avocados and bananas are good. We need about 350 mg of magnesium a day. In pregnancy the need increases by 50%. Magnesium deficiency is rare and is associated with general malnutrition.

**Sodium** is usually discussed with potassium and chloride which make up the body-water controlling minerals called **electrolytes**. Electrolytes are responsible for many of the body functions including pH, nerve conduction, tissue tone, water balance, kidney function, and many more. The complexity of this system is beyond our scope. Sodium is outside of the cell and controls the **extracellular fluid.**

Our major source of sodium is from table salt. One teaspoon of table salt contains as much as 2300 mgs of sodium. You will find extra sodium in many foods including most processed foods and soft drinks. Another source is "soft water". Clients with swollen legs will often have an excessive intake of sodium. This is also as-

## SIGNS AND SYMPTOMS OF MICROMINERAL DEFICIENCY

| MINERAL | SIGNS AND SYMPTOMS |
| --- | --- |
| 1. Iron | Anemia |
| 2. Copper | Anemia, depigmentation of hair, brain damage, vascular defects, kinky hair |
| 3. Zinc | Skin lesions, diarrhea, hair loss |
| 4. Selenium | Rare, but muscle and heart disease, growth retardation and tumors |
| 5. Chromium | Hypercholesterolemia, diabetes |
| 6. Iodine | Goiter, hypethyroidism |
| 7. Cobalt | Anemia |
| 8. Tin | Not seen in man, but needed for growth enhancement in animals. |

**TABLE 10-2**

sociated with heart disease and high blood pressure. A lack of sodium occurs with profuse sweating or diarrhea and is manifested by weakness and muscle cramps. A safe intake of sodium for healthy adults is between 1100 and 3000 mg daily.

**Potassium** is an **intracellular electrolyte** and is responsible for water balance and osmosis. It is potassium that keeps the water in the cell and salt that holds the water outside of the cell. If the sodium content of the cell increases, water will flow into the cell and cause **edema** or swelling of the cell. Potassium is also needed to keep the pH of the body normal and to maintain normal muscle contraction and tone. Particularly good sources are melons, bananas, oranges, and peaches. Vegetables such as brussel sprouts, potatoes, lima beans, and carrots are good sources as well. A safe intake of potassium is about 5500 mg daily.

**Chloride** is an important electrolyte for maintaining pH and for control of fluid levels in the body. In the stomach it forms part of the hydrochloric acid digestive juices. Our needs for chloride are about 1700 to 5000 mgs a day.

**Sulfur** is a component of many body proteins, including keratins of the skin and hair. The main source of sulfur in the diet is from protein rich foods of both plant and animal origin.

### The Microminerals

The microminerals include the following elements: **iron, copper, iodine, manganese, zinc, fluorine, cobalt, chromium, molybdenum**, and **selenium**. In addition, there are ref-

erences at the end of the book for those who are interested in doing further reading on these elements. **Table 10-2** shows the signs and symptoms associated with a deficiency of these elements.

### STRESS - THE WHY, WHEREFORE AND WHAT TO DO

**Stress** is a physiological condition characterized by psychological origin. Stress is a response to a stimulus either internal or external, that evokes a total body response. The physiological events of stress involve the cardiovascular system, the central and peripheral nervous system, the endocrine system, the digestive system, and the immune system. **No part of the body escapes the effect of stress.**

First, let's look at the genesis of stress and the events that occur when a stress reaction is triggered.

**Definitions** of stress vary depending on what authority one reads, but I prefer the definition given by Hans Selye who has studied stress for many years. He states that: "Biological stress is the nonspecific response of the body to any demand made upon it." This includes both positive demands, such as an extra effort in sports, and negative demands such as a dangerous external threat. Most stress is associated with conscious mental involvement (psychological stress). This appears to derive from conditions which we feel are beyond our control. The key is "beyond our control", in other words, a serious threat to our well being. The steps that follow mental stress are outlined in **Figure 10-10**.

1. The brain decides it is under stress.
2. A signal is sent to the hypothalamus.
3. A neurohormone called **corticotropin-releasing factor** is produced.
4. The **pituitary gland** secretes **pro-opio-cortin and ACTH**
5. ACTH, or adrenocorticotrophic hormone, triggers the adrenal glands
6. The **adrenal glands** release hormones from the **cortex**.
7. The **adrenal medulla** is stimulated and releases **adrenalin**.
8. The **immune system** is stimulated by unknown mechanisms.
9. These factors combine to produce a **state of readiness or alertness to danger**.

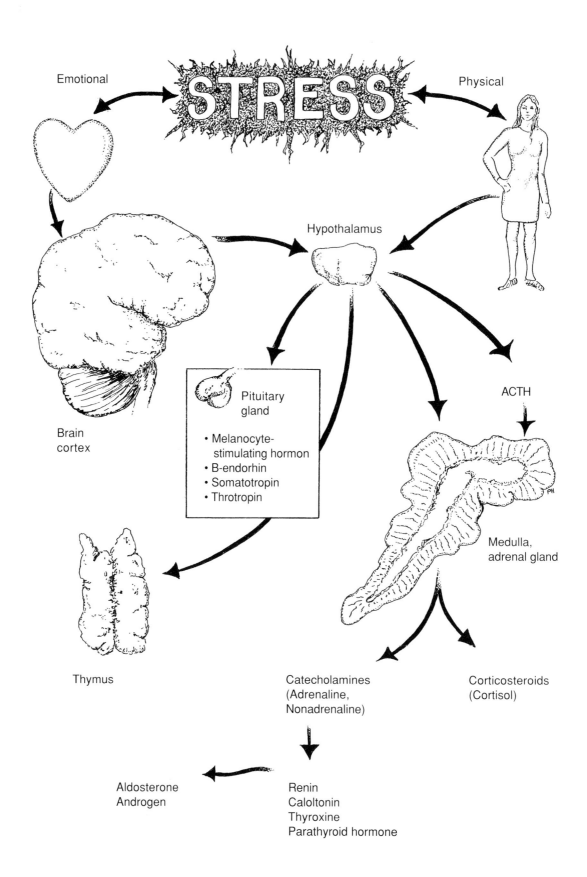

Emotional

# STRESS

Physical

Hypothalamus

Brain
cortex

Pituitary
gland

- Melanocyte-
  stimulating hormon
- B-endorhin
- Somatotropin
- Throtropin

ACTH

Medulla,
adrenal gland

Thymus

Catecholamines
(Adrenaline,
Nonadrenaline)

Corticosteroids
(Cortisol)

Aldosterone
Androgen

Renin
Caloltonin
Thyroxine
Parathyroid hormone

**FIGURE 10-10** Pathway of mental stress. All stress is not bad. We need some stress to survive and be ready for danger, to heal the body and to build bones. Excess stress or non-functional stress creates an excess of active metabolic agents in the body that can do harm to the organs.

Again, I must emphasize that in psychological stress the feeling of not being in control is the single greatest inducer of stress. The study of stress is quite difficult because of the many variable factors in the stress picture. Here are a few factors that are important to the skin care specialist and the care of the client.

Stress of short duration is different from long term stress. It is difficult for the body to adjust to short term stress so the effects may be quite deleterious.

Stress will decrease immune function initially but could increase immune function in the long term. Not all stress is negative.

Stress can produce a delay in wound healing and can accentuate a reaction to drugs or other allergens. It can aggravate arthritis and asthma.

Stress that produces a negative attitude is dangerous to the body's welfare. Efforts to reduce stress must be directed to either remove the cause of the stress or help adjust the individual to the situation.

**Stress treatment** involves a holistic approach. Dietary management as well as exercise are extremely helpful. Here are some suggestions:

**Brain food** has often been considered a joke but there are certain foods that do affect the chemistry of the brain. Tyrosine is an amino acid that is known to be a precursor of adrenalin (actually the compound norepinephrine). High protein diets contain high amounts of tyrosine.

Another compound is prostaglandin $E_1$ which is essential for normal immune functioning. A healthy immune system will fight stress. We find prostaglandins in vegetable oils and primrose oil. Along with this oil one should have 20-25 mg of vitamin $B_6$, 5-15 mg of zinc, and 250-500 mg of vitamin C a day.

General foods such as fruits and vegetables provide vitamin and fiber. Keep sugars and fats low in your diet.

**Exercise** at least 20 minutes, three to four times a week. Start with easy measures and build up. There are many good books on this subject. I do not advocate jogging. It does not make sense to me. No animal runs 2 to 4 miles every day. Exercise should be fun or productive. Few indi-

viduals stick to a diet or exercise program when it is burdensome.

Stress, in most cases, can be reduced. Remember that most of us are as happy or as miserable as we want to be. Control of our life is in our own mind. Granted, there are times we lose control of a given situation and that is stressful. These times are the exception rather than the rule. Think about it. Reduce your wants, your need for material things, love your neighbor, be considerate and be forgiving. In other words, following the golden rule is still the best advice for a stress-free life.

### Stress and The Skin

Stressed individuals have a rather characteristic appearance. They have tight or lined faces. The eyes are smaller and pulled inward with a knitted brow and the gaze of the eyes is often distant and out of contact. The mouth is a straight thin line, often blue rather than red. The whole color of the skin may be pale, or dusky red. There is no joy in the face and no spring in the walk. Movements are jerky.

Inside the body, nausea and diarrhea may be present. The cardiovascular system often shows high blood pressure and the pulse is elevated. Such a person is not a very good client for skin care. Just about anything you do for this client will be attenuated by the stress; however, if you work to relieve the stress you may help.

### Stress Treatment

The key is to **calm and relax the client**. Think of the way you would calm a fearful child or animal. Soft words, encouragement, stroking, and warming. Here is a prime example where a soothing, comforting massage may be used. The use of essential oils such as lavender, rose, borage, and camomile in a massage oil will be of great benefit.

Warm baths followed by massage are helpful. Neck massage and foot massage are of great benefit for a quick or brief treatment where time is limited.

Work to obtain the confidence of the client. Have frequent visits planned to maintain contact and continue the therapy. A sincere skin care specialist with healing hands and a warm smile is an unbeatable therapeutic combination.

## CALORIES

Much is made of calories and calorie counting. A calorie relates to our energy needs. Energy goes with heat so that the calorie is a term associated with heat. A kilocalorie is the amount of heat required to raise the temperature of a kilogram of water one degree Celsius. (A kilogram of water is 2.2 pounds of water, or roughly, a quart.)

### How Many Calories Does a Person Need a Day?

To determine caloric need simply divide the person's weight by **2.2** to convert pounds to kilograms, then multiply the kilograms by **24 hours.** Take that answer and multiply by .9 if the person is a women or 1.0 if a man. Here is an example for a 150 pound woman.

150 lbs/2.2 = 68.1 kg x 24 hrs = 1636.4 x .9 = 1472.7 kcal.

Here are some numbers for calories used during various activities:

| Activity | Kcal/min |
|---|---|
| Sleeping | 1.0 - 1.2 |
| Seated or standing | 2.0 - 2.5 |
| Walking, shopping, carpentry | 2.5 - 4.9 |
| Walking moderately, cycling | 5.0 - 7.4 |
| Walking uphill, climbing | 7.0 - 12.5 |

The values listed above are for men. Women have a slower metabolic rate.

Tables for body weight are given in **Table 10-3**.

## NUTRITIONAL ASSESSMENT

All this knowledge would be of no use if it could not be applied. First, we must have a method of assessing the nutritional status of the client. In the Western world there is not a great deal of malnutrition but subtle signs of malnutrition do exist. Here is one suggested way of assessing nutritional status that is adequate for most clients.

1. Check body weight against weight/height tables. If overweight or underweight by 20% the cause should be investigated.
2. Check the skin for dryness, flaking, hy-

## BODY WEIGHT

| HEIGHT WITHOUT SHOES | WEIGHT WITHOUT CLOTHES | |
|---|---|---|
| | 19-34 YEARS | 35 YEARS AND OVER |
| 5' | 97-128 | 108-138 |
| 5'1" | 101-132 | 111-143 |
| 5'2" | 104-137 | 115-148 |
| 5'3" | 107-141 | 119-152 |
| 5'4" | 111-146 | 122-157 |
| 5'5" | 114-150 | 126-162 |
| 5'6" | 118-155 | 130-167 |
| 5'7" | 121-160 | 134-172 |
| 5'8" | 125-164 | 138-178 |
| 5'9" | 129-169 | 142-183 |
| 5'10" | 132-174 | 146-188 |
| 5'11" | 136-179 | 151-194 |
| 6' | 140-184 | 155-199 |
| 6'1" | 144-189 | 159-205 |
| 6'2" | 148-195 | 164-210 |
| 6'3" | 152-200 | 168-216 |
| 6'4" | 156-205 | 173-222 |
| 6'5" | 160-211 | 177-228 |
| 6'6" | 164-216 | 182-234 |

SOURCE: Agriculture Department
Health and Human Services Department

**TABLE 10-3** We tend to get a little heavier with age. This is not a bad thing but we must not go overboard.

perpigmentation, and ulcerations. Look for general paleness.
3. Check the face for dark skin, scaling, and palor (paleness).
4. Check the eyes for cloudy, pale color, for dryness, and redness.
5. Check the lips for swelling, redness, and cracks at the sides.
6. Check the gums for bleeding, abnormal redness, and sores.
7. Check the tongue for swelling, redness, fissures, and magenta color.
8. Check the nails for spoon-shape, brittleness, and ridges.
9. Check the lower extremities for edema and muscle wasting.
10. Check the hair for dryness, dullness, shedding, and sparseness.

Taking a history of the food intake is required if any of these signs are found.

If you have any doubt about the client's nutritional status refer the client to a physician for an evaluation.

## SOME THERAPEUTIC FOOD SUGGESTIONS FOR A BETTER LIFE

The following list of foods is taken from Jean Carpenter's book The Food Pharmacy published by Bantan Books, New York, 1989. If you have not read this book I highly recommend it to you. Here are a few suggestions taken from that book.

**For rheumatoid arthritis** try fish food high in omega-3 fatty acids such as salmon, sardines, lake trout, and mackerel.

**For asthma** use coffee, two strong cups. Coffee contains xanthines which are used to treat asthma by doctors. Spicy foods such as chili peppers, garlic, and onions are also recommended.

**Anti-cancer** foods include carrots, beets, milk, yogurt, kale, apricots, broccoli, turnips, pumpkins, and cauliflower.

**Anti-heart disease foods** include fatty fish, garlic, onions, ginger, melon, olive oil, and kelp. Lean meats and vegetables are important in everyday diets as well. To raise **high density lipoproteins and lower the low density lipoproteins** use oat bran, soybeans, grapefruit segments, oranges, apples, and skim milk. Vegetables such as carrots, eggplant, and artichokes along with shitake mushrooms, and bananas are helpful. Alcohol at a level of two drinks a day is reported to raise the high density lipo-proteins.

**Stimulating foods** are coffee, tea, colas, and chocolate, due to their caffeine content. High protein foods and low fat foods are also helpful. (Avoid high carbohydrate foods if you are attending lectures; they will really zap you after an hour).

**Chronic lung disorders** such as emphysema and bronchitis (which all smokers will eventually get in various degrees) are helped by chili peppers, garlic, onion, mustard, and an adequate water intake.

**Psoriasis** is helped by omega-3 foods as described above.

**Urinary tract infections** benefit greatly from cranberries. It does not matter if it is the cocktail, juice, or the sauce of the cranberry, all are helpful. It was believed that the action of the cranberry was to make the urine acidic, but this is not true. The only known action is the prevention of bacteria from adhering to the bladder wall. This stops the bacteria from multiplying and thus stops the infection. Cranberries also act as deodorizers of the urine.

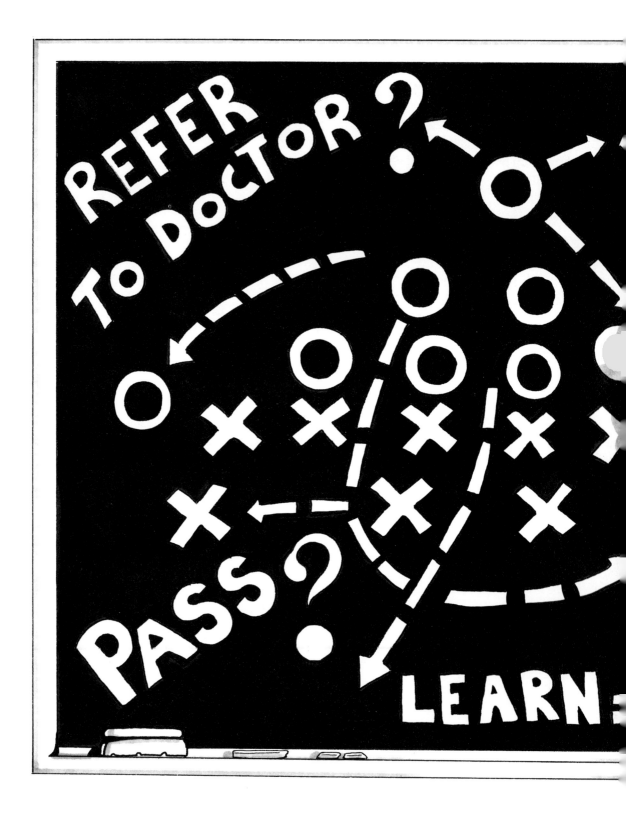

You've come this far, kid, and we're proud of you. It hasn't been an easy journey through these mean streets. If you've been paying attention, you're well equipped to recognize and handle some pretty serious bumps in the road. Now we're going to give you a break and tell you this: To be seen as an expert doesn't

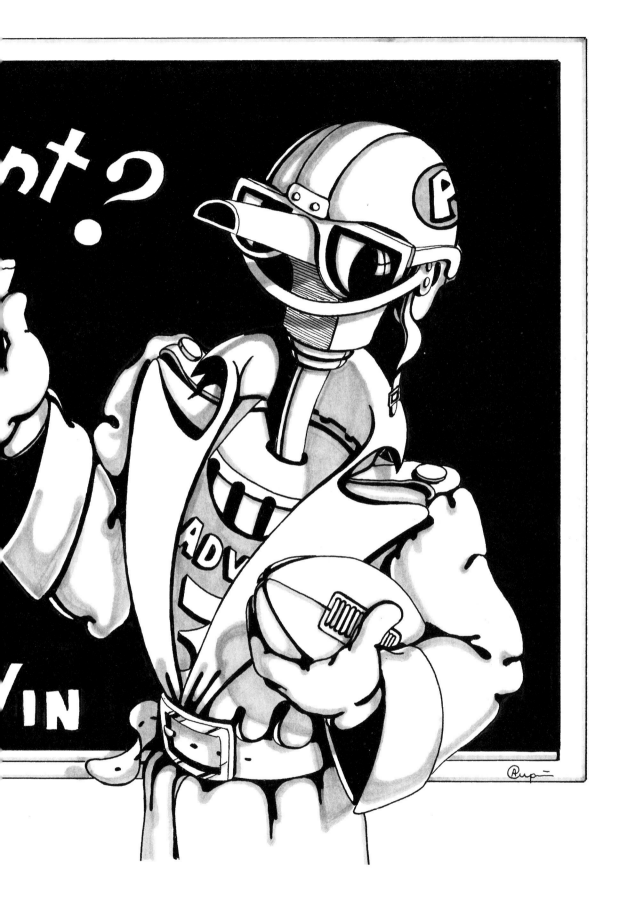

mean **you** have to know **everything**.......but rather that you know **who** knows. You've earned some friends, let's find out how and when to call them in.

# Referral Options - When and How to Punt

**REFERRAL MAKES LIFE EASIER. IT BUILDS YOUR REPUTATION AND PROVIDES BETTER CARE FOR YOUR CLIENT.**

We define a profession as an occupation that requires extensive education in a science or the liberal arts. Skin care is currently a subspecialty of the cosmetic profession. One way to enhance our professional image is to associate with members of other professions who are allied to skin care. Attend their meetings and seek their help. This chapter is all about how and when to refer clients to other professionals.

## PROFESSIONS RELATED OR ALLIED TO SKIN CARE

**Medicine and podiatry** are allied professions. Medicine has many specialties such as general medicine, dermatology, plastic and reconstructive surgery, and cosmetic surgery.

## METHOD OF REFERRING CLIENTS

Most clients will have a family or personal physician that they use most of the time. Know who this physician is by name and telephone number. This physician is called the primary care physician.

**Rule number one: never cut out the primary care physician.**

Let us take a hypothetical case. Jane Doone comes in for a facial. You recognize that she has severe pustular acne and you feel she should first be seen by a physician. In your history taking you should have marked down the name of her family doctor. Discuss with Jane that you believe she should first see her family doctor for treatment of her acute phase acne. Ask Jane if it is OK for you to call her doctor. If she says yes, then call the doctor.

Contact the doctor's office, introduce yourself to the receptionist as Ms. So and So's skin care specialist, or esthetician. If she asks you what that means, explain it to her. Next, tell her why you are calling and ask for a convenient time that you could speak with the doctor. Again, introduce yourself and your profession. Then explain that Jane is in your office and that you have found her to have acute pustular acne and you feel that she should see him for initial treatment. He normally will welcome the referral, thank you, and make an appointment for Jane. Let us say he is receptive and discusses Jane's condition with you and suggests that the two of you cooperate in her treatment. You then follow these steps:

1. Send a letter to him with your findings.
2. Thank him, or her, for cooperation.
3. State that you will be happy to follow up his treatment with your treatment and care.
4. Ask for a follow-up letter when Jane returns to you.
5. Send a periodic follow-up letter to the physician.

That's all there is to it!

## A FEW NOTES ON PROFESSIONAL LETTER WRITING AND RECORDS

It is only when you are in a court room and involved in some litigation that you really appreciate the importance of good records.

Here are a few suggestions that I have:

**Never** mention the client as **my client**, always use the client's name. Everything that you put into writing reflects your professionalism. Remember that anything you put into writing could be used for or against you in a legal sense.

Always address the letter as **Dear Doctor** So and So. Being on a first name basis with the doctor tends to reduce professional status.

Make a copy of all correspondence and keep it in the client's file.

Keep clear and legible notes, typewritten if possible. Avoid cross-outs and write-overs.

**Date everything.**

**Always note the treatment and the reasons for the treatment on the record.** Having referred a client to a physician indicates that you are acting in the best interest of the client. It also gets the physician on your side.

## WHEN TO REFER AND TO WHOM

**Cardinal Rule for Referral: Refer any client who has a condition which you do not feel absolutely confident in treating.**

If you follow this rule you will rarely, if

ever, have a serious problem with a client.

## Referral to a Dermatologist

For many years dermatology was limited to the medical management of skin problems and did not include surgical treatment except for small lesions and biopsies. The use of mechanical and electrical devices was fairly widespread, and limited to minor problems. Today we have dermatologists doing full-scale cosmetic surgery and many other surgical procedures such as dermabrasions, chemical peels, and face lifts.

The dermatologist is best trained for abnormal skin conditions. The three year training course is spent studying the diagnosis and treatment of diseases of the skin. Both primary diseases of the skin (those that arise in the skin as the first site) and skin manifestation of systemic disorders are topics for study by the dermatologist. Many dermatologists are now venturing into surgical procedures that once were the realm of plastic surgeons. While no general rule can be made, I prefer to send clients to a dermatologist for evaluation and medical treatment of primary skin disorders. Here is a list of conditions that I suggest you refer for evaluation and treatment to a dermatologist.

### Lesions of the Face

1. Cystic acne, any number of cysts, even one
2. Any pigmented lesion you do not recognize
3. Rhinophyma
4. Diffuse seborrheic dermatitis
5. Any lump or bump
6. Vascular lesions such as telangiectasia
7. Severe contact dermatitis
8. Neurodermatitis

### Lesions of the Chest, Back, and Arms

These are essentially the same as the face except, of course, for rhinophyma, but here are some more common conditions:
1. Psoriasis
2. Impetigo
3. Tinea versicolor
4. Herpes zoster (shingles)
5. Seborrheic keratosis

6. Any rash that you do not recognize. Remember that secondary syphilis often occurs on the trunk, palms of the hands, and soles of the feet.

### Nail Conditions of Hands and Feet

Any fungal infection of the nails is important enough to be referred since a fungal infection is either chronic or associated with a systemic disease. Look for monilia (yeast) infections.

There are some unique nail conditions that were covered in the Chapter 10 that should be referred. Any nail condition that requires surgical correction should obviously be referred. Nail conditions of the feet can be referred to a podiatrist or chiropodist (the same).

**Plantar warts** that are large and painful, multiple or mosaic should be referred.

A dermatologist is interested primarily in diseases of the skin, and less interested in skin beauty. A working relationship with a dermatolgist could be very beneficial for both parties. Every referral should be treated as an opportunity for learning. The day is near when the dermatologist and the skin care specialist will view each other with respect as colleagues.

## Referral to a Plastic Surgeon

The term **plastic and reconstructive surgeon** refers to a physician-surgeon who has had special training in reconstructive procedures for both congenital and traumatic defects.

The **cosmetic surgeon** has limited training in a fixed number of procedures that are called **elective** procedures. This means that the surgery is not an emergency or a life and death matter, and that the patient will choose to have it done because they will have a better or more attractive appearance afterward. Breast augmentation and rhinoplasty are elective procedures.

### Selecting a Plastic Surgeon for Client Referral

In my experience there is no way to select a physician anymore than there is for selecting a lawyer or a hair stylist. As a skin care specialist, however, you will be expected to know who is the best plastic surgeon in your area. I would suggest that you keep in mind during your search that not every surgeon is the best in every procedure. Also, while **professional credentials** are a good guide, they are in no way a guarantee. Here are my suggestions:

First, the surgeon **must have the welfare of the patient as his major interest**.

Second, the surgeon must be considerate, kind, and understanding. He must be principled, ethical, and of good moral standing.

The surgeon should be respected by his colleagues and be a member of the local hospital and local medical societies.

Make an appointment to visit the surgeon. Explain the reason for your visit, select a time that is convenient for the surgeon, and plan no more than a 30 minute stay. Introduce yourself and state your reason for coming to the office. Don't discuss his credentials at this time.

Ask to see photographs of his work. The initial visit is very important for your client so know how the surgeon handles his patients on the first visit. If the surgeon recommends multiple procedures on the first visit and your client came in for only one procedure I would view this as a caution sign.

While multiple procedures may eventually be desired by the client they often have the effect of reducing the clients self-esteem. As an example, if a person seeks help for sagging breasts and the surgeon recommends a face lift, liposuction, tummy tuck, and a brow lift at the first visit that person may feel like a physical wreck. In my experience, the best plastic and cosmetic surgeons do one or two procedures first and then suggest any additional procedures after the patient has recovered and developed a rapport with the physician.

Caution number two - **beware the surgeon who rushes the patient into surgery**.

Everyone must take time to think about a procedure that will affect the rest of his or her life.

Now, let's talk about the **credentials** of the surgeon. The word *credo* in Latin means "I believe". Credentials provide a measure of validity to a professional. Here are the major professional societies in plastic and cosmetic surgery.

1. **American Board of Otolaryngology**. Members of this group are trained mainly in head and neck surgery, and perform facial cosmetic surgery such as face lifts, rhinoplasty, brow lifts, etc.

2. **The American Board of Plastic Surgery** certifies general plastic surgeons. They are qualified to do all types of plastic surgery.

3. **The American Academy of Facial Plastic and Reconstructive Surgery**. Highly qualified in all phases of plastic, cosmetic and reconstructive surgeons.

4. **The American Board of Cosmetic Surgery** members are trained in cosmetic surgery but not reconstructive surgery.

Your best bet is to check with the local County Medical Society for the names of the various plastic surgeons trained in cosmetic surgery. From the information you receive you will be then able to determine the training qualifications of each physician.

## THE PROBLEM CLIENT AND PATIENT

Problem customers become problem clients and patients. This type of client is identified by certain characteristics and is usually avoided by most professionals. Here are some points to look for:

1. Anyone with unrealistic expectations
2. Obsessive-compulsive types
3. Rude types
4. People with imagined problems or very minor problems
5. Uncooperative types
6. The physician-shopper type
7. People who haggle over price
8. Anyone involved in a litigation
9. Depressed people
10. Anyone who considers him/herself to be a VIP.

There are many more characteristics of these individuals. These are taken from Tardy and Klemsensmith in a book chapter titled Face-lift surgery: Principles and variations, found in Dermatologic Surgery edited by Roenigk and Roenigk and published in 1988 by Marcel Dekker of New York.

Next, look at **what conditions should be referred**. I am assuming that you would have made contact with a cosmetic surgeon and have already established a working relationship.

## ESTIMATED NUMBER OF COMMON RECONSTRUCTIVE PROCEDURES PERFORMED BY ASPRS MEMBERS

| PROCEDURE | | 1988 | 1981 | PERCENT INCREASE |
|---|---|---|---|---|
| Birth defects | | 31,620 | N/A | N/A |
| Cleft lip/palate - - | 59% | | | |
| Down syndrome - - | <1% | | | |
| Other - - | 40% | | | |
| Breast reconstruction | | 34,210 | 20,000 | 71% |
| Immediate - - | 25% | | | |
| Delayed - - | 75% | | | |
| Burn care | | 46,300 | 44,600 | 4% |
| Dog bites | | 21,600 | 22,300 | -3% |
| Hand surgery | | 229,550 | 150,000 | 53% |
| Trauma - - | 65% | | | |
| Carpal tunnel - - | 17% | | | |
| Arthritis - - | 4% | | | |
| Other - - | 15% | | | |
| Lacerations | | 220,790 | 143,000 | 54% |
| Face - - | 75% | | | |
| Upper extremities - - | 16% | | | |
| Lower extremities - - | 5% | | | |
| Torso - - | 4% | | | |
| Maxillofacial surgery | | 30,740 | N/A | N/A |
| Trauma - - | 87% | | | |
| Birth defect - - | 9% | | | |
| Disease - - | 2% | | | |
| Other - - | 1% | | | |
| Scar revision | | 52,590 | N/A | N/A |
| Tumor removal | | 271,060 | 63,050 | 429% |
| Head/neck - - | 73% | | | |
| Torso - - | 13% | | | |
| Upper extremities - - | 9% | | | |
| Lower extremities - - | 5% | | | |
| Estimated totals | | 1,100,000 | 736,200 | 50% |

(Not all reconstructive operations are individually listed.)

**TABLE 11-1** A reference table for your use. Note the increase in breast reconstruction, eyelid surgery, and liposuction. Reprinted with permission of the American Society of Plastic and Reconstructive Surgeons, Inc. See appendix for additional tables on this subject.

Look only at the most common conditions which can be treated by cosmetic surgery. These are:
1. Face lifts for aging, facial skin
2. Rhinoplasty for reshaping the nose
3. Breast surgery for augmentation or reduction of breasts
4. Eyelid surgery for sagging, drooping, or baggy eyes
5. Suction lipectomy and dermabrasion for aging and blemished skin.

Limited space in this text permits me to only cover these topics with a broad, light stroke. I have listed some popular and technical references for those readers who wish to pursue the topic further. Remember, this information is for **your** use. The plastic surgeon will discuss all of this in more detail with the patient on the first visit. **Table 11-1** lists the most common cosmetic surgical procedures as compiled by the

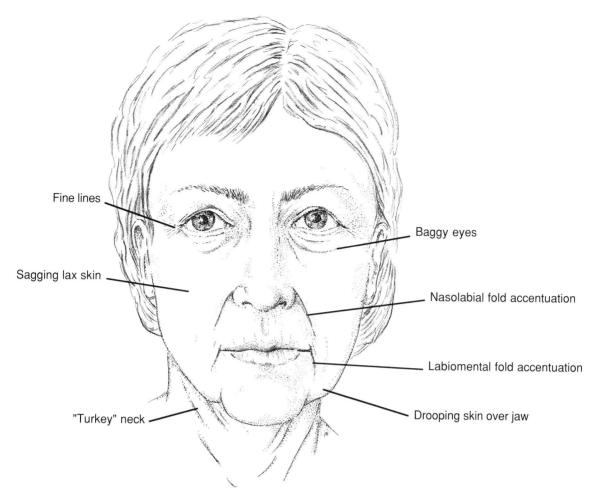

**FIGURE 11-1** Characteristics that may benefit from a face lift. All these facial aging characteristics can be changed by surgical corrections.

Labels on figure:
- Fine lines
- Sagging lax skin
- "Turkey" neck
- Baggy eyes
- Nasolabial fold accentuation
- Labiomental fold accentuation
- Drooping skin over jaw

American Society of Plastic and Reconstructive Surgeons.

## 1. THE FACE LIFT (RHYTIDEC-TOMY FROM LATIN FOR *RHYTI* = WRINKLE)

Candidates for facial surgery may be as young as 30 or as old as 85 years. There is no real upper limit of age of which face lifts are not done. The face starts its surface changes as young as 25 to 30 years so we need to think of prevention for young clients. The average age client for a face lift is between 48 and 55 years old. She will have changes in her eyes, cheeks, jawline, and neck. Many complain of jowls and baggy eyes as well as an unattractive neck, frequently described as "turkey" neck. If you see lax skin that is sagging with some fine lines about the eyes, skin drooping over the lower jaw, and a marked accentuation of the nasolabial and

the labiomental folds, you have a client that could benefit from a face lift. See **Figure 11-1** which points out these characteristics.

At this point, suggest to the client that they could benefit from plastic surgery. If the client seems amenable to corrective surgery ask if they know of a good plastic surgeon, or have heard of one. This is your opening to recommend a surgeon if they don't have one in mind. At this point, **do not discuss procedures or costs with the client**, this is the responsibility of the surgeon. Follow the steps above and make your referral. The rest is in the hands of the client and the surgeon. **Never push the client into surgery.** It is one of the worst mistakes you can make. Your job is to suggest and refer.

## 2. RHINOPLASTY (FROM *RHINO* = NOSE)

Few areas of the body are more visible or

sacred to an individual than his or her nose. While you may think a person needs a new nose they may bitterly resent you even suggesting that their nose is less than perfect. I know of no diplomatic method of recommending rhinoplasty unless there is a sound medical reason or if the client indicates to you an interest in this procedure.

The lower limit for this elective procedure is 15 years of age; there is no upper age limit. Beware of the teenager forced into considering plastic surgery either by parents or for a desire to have the appearance of some movie idol of the moment.

Consider that the nose is paramount to facial appearance and, unlike pantyhose, one size and shape does not fit everyone. There are many aspects to consider and only a skilled cosmetic surgeon can be aware of all these fine points. The skin care specialist needs to remember only a few aspects of nasal surgery. One is that **the ideal nose does not exist**. The turned-up nose of yesterday is no longer in fashion. The straight nose with slight tilt is seen most frequently as a feminine nose, however, a male with a tilted nose does not "look right". The second is that after surgery the client will have black and blue eyes and perhaps a bloody nose.

It takes from one to a few days for the bleeding or oozing to stop altogether and about three weeks for the discoloration to disappear. Complications of rhinoplasty will be covered in the next chapter on pre- and post-operative care.

### 3. BREAST SURGERY (MAMMAPLASTY)

There are three types of breast surgery.

### A. Reduction Mammaplasty

Large breasts present many problems. Large breasts are not only inconvenient in dressing but often are a source of embarassment and viewed as external handicaps. Shoulder pain, neck pain, and upper back pain are frequent complaints. Irritation of the skin under the breast, called **intertrigo**, and chronic mastitis are frequent problems. Oddly enough, even spinal curvature can result from large breasts.

Breast reduction will leave scars. See **Figure 11-2**. This will be explained to the client by

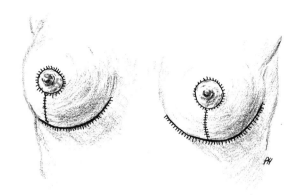

FIGURE 11-2 Breast reduction scar. Breast reduction results in a larger scar.

the surgeon, but again, be aware of it. The age of the client will be a consideration and her bra size should have been stable for at least 6 months. Pregnancy swells the breasts due to the hormonal response, so pregnancy should not be contemplated for several years after surgery.

Mature women who plan breast reduction should be of normal weight. Most overweight women who have breast reductions, then return to normal weight will appear out of proportion after surgery. The decision to have this type of surgery is profound and requires an understanding family. The skin care specialist should be supportive regardless of the decision of the pre- and post-operative care of the client and in a position to offer emotional support and physical care.

### B. Augmentation Mammaplasty

This is the most common cosmetic surgery performed in the United States. Half of the female population is considered to be small breasted based on bra size alone. The only real reason for a women to choose this operation is that **she** is unhappy with her breasts. I have never spoken with a cosmetic surgeon who will operate on a woman to augment her breast if she is happy with her current size. Pressure from her husband or boyfriend is never a valid reason to do this type of surgery. It is traumatic to the woman and almost always results in an unhappy patient and an unhappy surgeon.

Feel free to refer those adult clients who ask your opinion or seek your advice in the selection of a surgeon.

In **Figure 11-3** the two major types of breast implants are shown. The implant can be placed

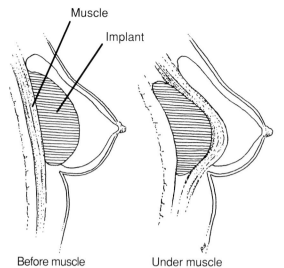

Muscle

Implant

Before muscle          Under muscle

**FIGURE 11-3** Types of breast implants. Placing the implant before the muscle is more frequent than under the muscle. This is a surgical decision.

under the chest muscle or directly over the muscle. There are four types of implants, three are of silicone and one is of polyurethane. The silicone types are the most popular. The incision is made under the breast or under the nipple and the implant inserted into the breast. Another approach to the breast is through the axilla (armpit), though I do not know many surgeons who use this method.

Post-operative care is minimal and recovery is usually complete in three to six weeks. A bra is worn night and day during that period. It is best to avoid strenuous exercise, including sexual intercourse, for the same period.

## C. Mastopexy (Breast lift for fallen or ptosis of the breast).

Sagging or drooping breasts may occur after pregnancy or weight reduction, or they may be natural. The major problem is loss of elasticity, decreased volume, or poor connective tissue in the breast. There are varying degrees of ptosis. First degree ptosis occurs when the nipple is in line with the inframammary fold as depicted in **Figure 11-4**.

Second degree ptosis occurs when the nipple is below the inframammary fold but still above the contour of the breast.

Third degree ptosis occurs when the nipple is below the inframammary fold and below the breast contour.

The breast is lifted by removing excess skin from the lower part of the breast and moving up the nipple, areola, and the underlying or supportive breast tissue. It is possible to do both a mastopexy and a breast augmentation at the same time. Recovery is similar to other breast surgical procedures.

## D. Breast Reconstruction

This procedure is also cosmetic surgery. Breast removal for cancer is a common surgical procedure and many women elect to have a new breast built on their chest wall. This is known as reconstructive breast surgery. The results of this type of surgery are of great psychological

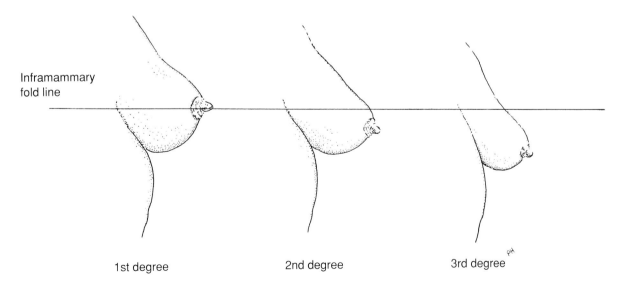

Inframammary fold line

1st degree          2nd degree          3rd degree

**FIGURE 11-4** Note that the breast folds more as it sags and the nipple points downward rather than out or up. Upturned nipples are rare.

benefit for a woman who has undergone radical mastectomy (complete removal of the breast). Techniques vary, but the aim is to match the remaining breast in size, shape, and color. Nipples may be tattooed or built up from other tissue, such as the thigh skin or vaginal tissue. These nipples look fairly natural and are acceptable to the patient.

One out of every eleven women will develop breast cancer, the most common cancer in women. Urge clients to have periodic breast examinations, including mammograms for women over 35.

## TREATMENT OF FACIAL SCARS BY FILLING AGENTS

Filling agents for scars and wrinkles have been around for some time. The early history of the use of various substances for filling has been marked with disasters. Paraffin and olive oil were injected subcutaneously resulting in pain and disfigurement. The use of silicone marked a new era in filling technology once the quantity to be injected was worked out.

I cover only a small part of the field of filling agents in this section, but an introduction to this topic will help you. Below are the current agents used in filling.

### Microdroplet Silicone

The use of silicone in microdroplets is a special procedure and technique and is not to be confused with the older form of silicone injections. The current product used is a polydimethylsiloxane of a 350 centistokes. The material is purified and sterilized and is known as "injectable grade silicone". This must not be confused with the "medical grade silicone" that is used for lubrication and topical cosmetics.

The product, used by both dermatologists and plastic surgeons in this field, is called MDX 4-4011, supplied by Dow Corning. Any other silicone product is not acceptable for this function.

Used in very small quantities (0.005 to 0.01 ml per injection location with a maximum amount of 1 ml per visit) this material works very well. There is no migration, as the small amounts of silicone injected are encapsulated by the body tissue and stay in place.

### Indications and Complications

Silicone microdroplets are used for acne scars, creases, furrows, depression lesions, post-surgical refinements, and podiatric conditions. The major complications include a transient erythema and occasional hyperpigmentation. With proper technique there is few, if any, complications.

### Zyderm Collagen Implant (ZCI)

**Zyderm (ZCI)** is collagen obtained from the dermis of cattle that has been digested by pepsin enzymes and then purified. It is 95% type I collagen with the other 5% being type III. **Zyplast (ZP)** is another form of Zyderm which has been crosslinked with gluteraldehyde.

Both of these products are injected into the dermis. The underlying theory was that the injected collagen would induce the fibroblasts to form new native collagen. The ZP appears to do this to some degree but not the ZCI. These injections last about 3 to 9 months and then are either absorbed or migrate to lower tissues.

### Indications and Complications

The indications for ZCI and ZP are the same as in the silicone microdroplets injections. Acne scars, furrows, facial lines, crow's feet, lip lines, and post-surgical corrections are all indications for this product. The three major complications are allergic reactions, intermittent swelling, and mechanical problems.

**Allergic reactions** are the most frequent complication. Since bovine collagen is a foreign material, it will be antigenic. About 8.4% of the patients tested for collagen antibodies show a positive response. More than likely, this is a food-induced antibody reaction. Tests made with Zyderm before treatment show a 3 to 3.5% reaction rate. The overall rate with treatment is about 2%. **Anyone who is planning to have a Zyderm treatment must be skin tested for an allergic reaction to the collagen.**

**The skin test** will normally be positive within 3 days. Reaction occurs as red, swollen, and hard areas at the injection site. If the test is negative, however, it is best **to wait for a month and check the site again. Some individuals do not react early**. Anyone with a positive skin test should not be treated with Zyderm.

Some of these reactions may last 4-48 months.

**Intermittent** swelling occurs in about 1% of patients. These are not allergic reactions as they occur late and are intermittent. They are not a contraindication to treatment with Zyderm but the patient should be skin tested again before treatment.

**Mechanical problems** include:

Simple over-corrections which will disappear with time.

Tissue necrosis which is serious and often due to too much material being injected too fast.

Vascular occlusion which is serious since it can produce tissue loss.

Bruising is common and often upsets the patients. Smaller amounts of material tend to reduce bruising, but there is no sure way of total prevention.

## Fibril

Fibril is a relatively new injection material which uses the patient's serum mixed with gelatin and aminocaproic acid. The product is approved by the FDA and is currently marketed by The Mentor Corporation in Santa Barbara, Calif. Gelatin is an animal derived protein. In this case it is porcine. The skin test must be done 4 weeks prior to the use of the product. 1 to 2% of patients will have a positive skin test. Fibril is unique in that the greater the wounding the better the tissue response. A 20 gauge needle is used with this type of injection compared to a small 30 gauge needle for Zyderm or silicone injections.

The positive aspect of this product is that its effect lasts for one to two years.

### Indications and Complications

The indications are similar to Zyderm or the microdroplet silicone, but its best use is for depressed scars. Lines, furrows, and other defects respond fairly well. The major complications are allergic reaction and nodules. The nodules are red and swollen and are not acceptable to the patient. These nodules can persist for a month or more. The other side effects are necrosis and hyperpigmentation. This agent still needs fur-

ther evaluation before it is widely used.

## Microlipoinjection

This technique has been used experimentally. It uses the patient's own fat cells as the transplant material. The technique depends on using live fats cells or adipocytes to make the transplant and is not firmly established because there are many unknowns. There are few if any reactions.

## PROFESSIONALISM

The expression that one is a professional is always a compliment. It denotes a high level of training and competence.

As a skin care professional you are moving from trade status to professional status. You do this by increasing your training, your skills, and your knowledge of your field. You associate with other professional fields. In this chapter I have given you only a few pointers in the right direction, the rest you learn with experience. A long time ago I was taught that you do not become a chemist by reading a book or just working in a laboratory but by working with chemists. So it is with being a skin care specialist, you learn by doing and being with other skin care specialists.

### Some Suggestions for Professionalism

**Speech**. Always conduct yourself in a manner that is above reproach. Never criticize a colleague or complain about a colleague to a client. Never say the treatment by a colleague was wrong or worthless. It is best to say only positive things about your clients and about your colleagues. Never use vulgarity. Do not show anger or depression. Keep calm and cool in times of trial.

**Dress code** is associated with all professions. The first rule is **clean** and the second rule is **neat. Uniforms** are associated with the profession of skin care, usually a white lab coat. Pay particular attention to the sleeves and hems as they often become soiled and frayed. Be careful that the items you place in the pockets do not drop out as you treat or examine a client.

**Office and treatment areas** should reflect your interest and your taste. There are no real standards for office decor. Avoid gaudy or ostentatious displays.

On a personal note, never discuss husband or wife, boyfriend or girlfriend, children or parents, unless you are specifically asked about them by the client. Do not discuss your home, possessions, or your income. None of these items are of benefit to the client. They only distract from your professional behavior and give evidence of anxiety and insecurity.

Become active in the community. Spend time teaching your colleagues and sharing your knowledge. This pratice not only raises the level of skin care practiced in your community but it also may bring you referrals from your colleagues.

Professions need active support by their members to grow. This means active participation in your local, state, and national societies.

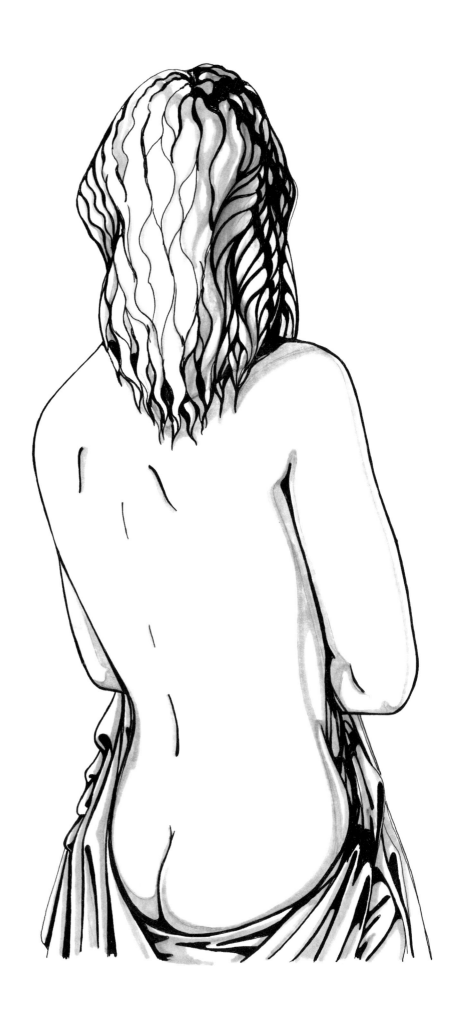

Suppose you've done all you can, and your skills and my finesse still can't completely restore the scene of too many crimes to a strong, healthy condition. Well, that's what our friends are for. Call in the Sawbones for the major work: he trusts you now and you know what he needs, too. You do the prep work, let him do the sculpting, and then follow up with the finishing touches that only you can provide. Together, you can create a masterpiece.

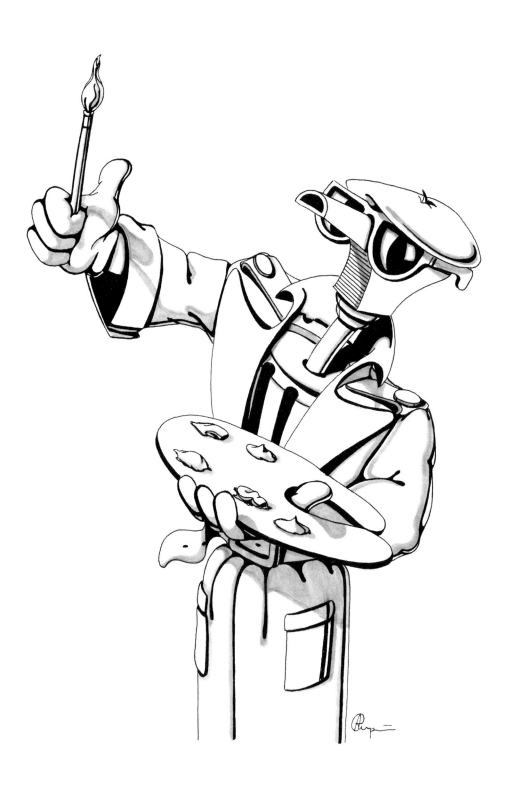

# Pre- and Post-Operative Care of the Surgical Patient

This chapter introduces you to wounds and wound care. The fundamentals of wound healing are essential to your understanding this field of treatment. You must learn this field if you plan to work with physicians. We shall start with the basics of wound healing and dressings. Next we will cover sterile technique, introduce you to the microbiology of the skin, and the complications of cosmetic surgery.

## THE FUNDAMENTALS OF WOUND HEALING

The healing of any wound is a natural process. After a wound is made in the skin, either by design (surgical) or by accident, a process of repair and restoration of the skin occurs. This is both a **cellular** and a **biochemical process**. The end result is that there is a restoration of the surface of the skin and a reconstitution of the dermis. Depending on what you read, there are four to five stages of wound healing. I prefer to combine the concepts of several research papers. My experience with wound healing agrees with the description given in **Figure 12-1**.

## The Stages in Normal Wound Healing

### Stage 1. Inflammation (Also Called the Vascular Stage)

Immediately after a wound is made the repair process begins. The blood vessels, which have been cut or torn, undergo changes to stop the bleeding. Coagulation occurs as the injured vessels thrombose. The biochemical changes are profound.

Fibrin forms to stop the bleeding and other biochemicals are secreted to allow the capillaries to dilate and bring cells to the wounded area. Platelets are small cells responsible for much of the clotting mechanism. They secrete substances that call other cells to the wounded area. These substances are called **chemotactic** and **growth factors. Platelet derived growth factor** (PDGF) is an important cell factor. These early events set into motion a very complex series of pathways necessary to heal the wound. The injured cells, including **mast cells**, will secrete **histamine** causing edema and redness as the surrounding vessels dilate. This is benefical to the wound healing process. During this stage the cellular process is initiated to control infection and clean up the cellular debris.

Two important types of cells arrive:

The **polymorphonuclear cells (PMN)** are the white cells which combat bacteria, engulf foreign matter, and remove clotted blood.

The **macrophages** also appear and serve to assist the PMN cells in bacterial control and removal of cellular debris. They have an even more important function in the total process of wound healing. At the time of injury these macrophages are biologically activated to secrete many active substances that cause further wound healing. These substances include chemotactic factors, fibroblasts, endothelial cell-stimulating factors, and a special **macrophage-derived growth factor (MDGF)** that is essential to the total wound healing process.

Stage 2. The Re-epithelization Phase

After the wound is cleaned by these cells, structural repair begins as new blood vessels and wound edge cells start to move in. The critical step is the migration of undamaged epidermal cells from the wound edges. This event may occur hours after the wound is made and does not require increased cellular proliferation. An interesting observation is that at the time of this migration a change must occur in the basal cells. They lose their attachment to other cells by retracting the tonofilaments and dissolving the intercellular desmosomes. They next develop pseudopodia or "migrating feet" that allow them to move around and over other cells. Once migration has started, a proliferation phase occurs and the cell rate increases by seventeen fold. These cells move over a specialized surface consisting of fibronectin and collagen.

**Fibronectin** is a glycoprotein of 440 kd. It is present in plasma and believed to be produced by keratinocytes, fibroblasts, and endothelial cells. This remarkable protein has many functions in wound healing that promote cell migration, phagocytosis, cell adhesion, and the binding of collagen to form a matrix for glycosoaminoglycans (the "ground substance" we spoke of earlier). The movement of keratinocytes over this matrix is determined by a "water table", that is, the migration of cells favors a route that is moist. This has importance since it leads us to the design of proper wound dressings. As ep-

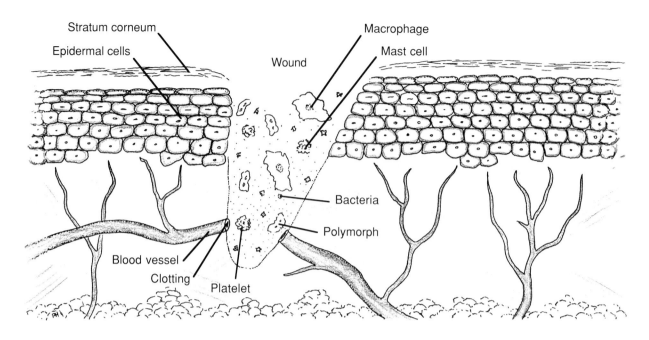

FIGURE 12-1 Wound healing. Stage 1. The blood vessels are damaged as cells are moving to defend the cut surfaces. Serum will form in the wound to impede bacteria.

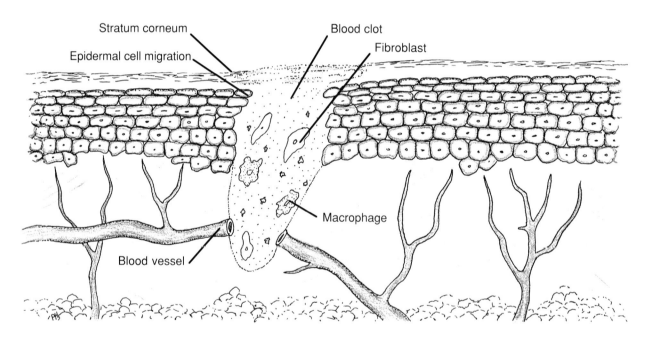

FIGURE 12-1 (cont.) Wound healing. Stage 2. A clot is formed and fibroblasts start to function. Blood is stopped as the epidermis begins to migrate over the wound edges.

ithelization occurs there is another process occurring at the same time. This is the formation of granulation tissue.

### Stage 3. Granulation Tissue Formation - Enter the Myofibroblast

Three to five days after the wound is made,

granulation tissue appears. This tissue consists of the new vasculature, the new matrix of collagen, glycoproteins, and glycosoaminoglycans.

The star of this process is **the fibroblast cell** for it functions to produce collagen, fibronectin, elastin, and the ground substance. A new type of cell differentiated from the fibroblast appears after a few days, the **myofibroblast**. This cell is

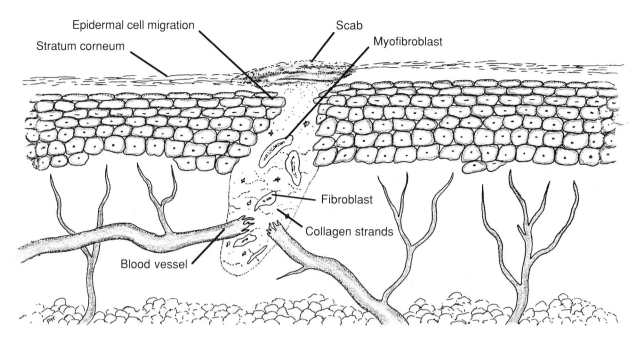

**FIGURE 12-1** (cont.) Wound healing. Stage 3. A scab forms and the myofibroblasts appear. Collagen strands form in the wound and the edges of the blood vessels start to repair the break. The basal layer of the epidermis is actively proliferating as the wound is roofed over.

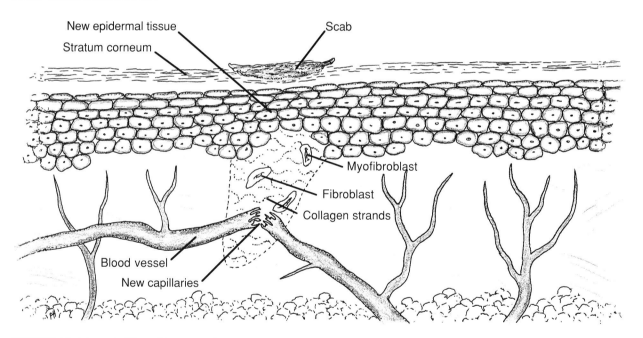

**FIGURE 12-1** (cont.) Wound healing. Stage 4. The wound is closed and contracting continues deep in the wound. The scab starts to fall off as it contracts. Increased fibroblasts and myofibroblasts actively strengthen the deeper layers of the wound.

unique in that it has tiny microfilaments in the cytoplasm that allow the cell to contract and migrate.

Many substances are involved in the direction of the myofibroblast's activity. Some of these you already know, such as the MDGF and the PDGF, but insulin, and certain substances called **lymphokines** also affect the action of this cell. In these early stages, hyaluronic acid has a role. Later in the process dermatan sulfate and chondroitin sulfate appear. These proteoglycans seem to have a role in collagen regulation and in providing the wound with a flexible resilient base.

The initial collagen laid down is Type III collagen (as we discussed in the biochemistry

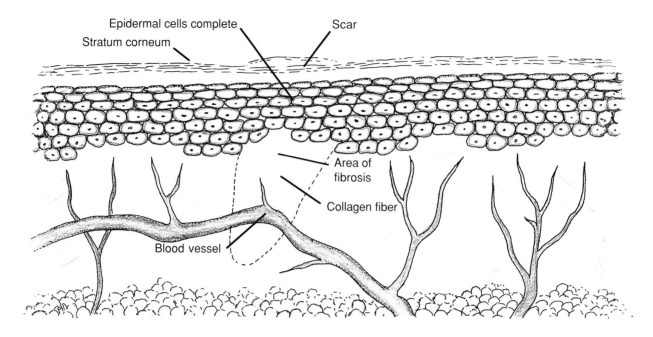

FIGURE 12-1 (cont.) Wound healing. Stage 5. The wound is healed and the blood vessels united. Now collagen and other fibrous tissue reorganize the wound area. This last process could take up to one year to complete.

of the skin), but as wound repair progresses it is replaced by Type I collagen.

At this stage the wound will begin to contract and draw the edges together. This may take place from 5 to 15 days after the wound occurs depending on the size and condition of the wound.

### Stage 4. Wound Contraction

The myofibroblast plays a central role in the contraction of the wound. It is a complex process that is believed to be controlled by a series of interconnections between the myofibroblasts and other elements of the granulation tissue. This has been termed the "fibronexus" by Singer. As the filaments in the myofibroblast contract they pull the surrounding matrix together and force the wound to contract, completely healed. It must now undergo matrix and collagen remodeling.

### Stage 5. Wound Remodeling

Even in the early stages of healing, the collagen and matrix is constantly being reformed and remodeled. This process of wound healing may take many months or years. In some cases it may never actually end. As the collagen increases, the fibronectin is replaced and the sul-

fated proteoglycans replace the hyaluronic acid as mentioned above. Water is gradually replaced in the scar while the collagen bundles and wound grow stronger. Most wounds reach a maximum strength at 3 to 4 months. They never reach full normal skin strength, attaining only 75-80% of the normal skin strength.

How the collagen is laid down and the problems attending scar formation are of interest to the plastic surgeon and the skin care specialist. There are general systemic and local factors that influence both the rate of wound healing and the quality of the final wound. Certain complications attend surgical wounds, including scars, of which the skin care specialist must be aware.

### Systematic and Local Factors that Influence Wound Healing

#### Nutritional Factors

As we noticed in the last chapter the state of nutrition can have very profound effects on wound healing. Deficiencies of vitamin A will slow down epithelization and collagen synthesis and increase infection rates. Vitamin C is needed for collagen biosynthesis. A deficiency of vitamin C will lead to delayed wound healing. Lack of certain trace elements such as zinc, copper, iron, or manganese will affect immune response, protein synthesis, and collagen synthesis. Adequate protein intake and normal glucose and fat metabolism are essential for the cellular and humoral mechanisms in wound repair.

## Aging skin

Aging skin may or may not have an effect on the repair process, although, we know that aging skin takes longer to heal. In many cases it is the attendant conditions associated with aging itself, rather than the aging skin that delays healing.

## Medications

Medications can affect wound healing, chiefly anticoagulants and glucocorticosteroids. These agents delay wound healing directly and indirectly. Anticoagulants increase the chances of bleeding into the wound. Cortisone agents directly delay wound healing.

## Local Factors

**Poor surgical technique** such as rough handling of tissues, crushed wound edges, too tight sutures, and reactive suture materials tend to produce problems in wound healing. Pulling the skin too tightly can decrease the blood supply and thus decrease oxygen.

**Infection** is the most common local condition affecting wound healing. Infection will prolong the inflammatory stage of healing and produce toxins and proteases that damage cells. Bacteria will rob nutrients, produce lactic acid in hypoxic states (low oxygen), and cause more proteolytic enzymes to be released.

**Hematoma or bleeding** into the wound can disrupt the wound and provide an optimal site for bacterial growth. **Foreign material** of any type in a wound will tend to activate the immune system and increase inflammation.

**Ischemia, or lack of oxygen and blood supply,** will delay wound healing by decreasing the cellular proliferation and the resistance to infection. Dermal healing is delayed as well, since collagen production is impaired. Causes of ischemia are tight sutures, foreign bodies, infection, and tightly stretched skin. It is axi-

omatic that poor surgical technique leads to poor healing.

## STERILE TECHNIQUE

One of the first skills that a medical professional learns is **sterile technique**. Sterile technique is the practice of producing and maintaining a sterile, or germ free, condition about a specific area. It may be required in an operating room and surgery, or it may simply be required while opening a pustule. The basic concept is to keep bacteria away from the wounded area. It may appear rather elaborate and ritualistic at first, but you will see that this is important in dealing with surgeons and surgical patients.

Let's look at the microbiology of the skin and learn the most common bacterial contaminants. Then we shall look at some available germicides, and finally, look at the steps required in providing and maintaining a sterile field.

### Basic Microbiology of the Skin Relative to Wound Infection

Microbes are often called skin **flora** by physicians. Microbes grow and flourish on the skin. You can find bacteria anywhere on the skin surface. Different types of bacteria have a liking for specific areas. We previously studied many types of bacteria in the chapter on pathology (Chapter Five). The three most common types of bacteria are Staphyloccocus, Streptococcus, and Coliform.

Bacteria can be classified by shape. Rod shaped bacteria are called bacilli. Ball-shaped are called cocci. We can also classify them by the color they stain with the Gram's stain. This is a special stain used by microbiologists to identify and classify bacteria. Gram positive bacteria stain blue and Gram negative bacteria stain red. When a physician says that we are dealing with a Gram negative infection, he is most likely speaking of a coliform infection arising from fecal contamination.

**Staphyloccus Aureus** is present in the nose in 20-30% of the population. It is responsible for many hospital infections. It is a gram positive cocci, appearing as "clumps of grapes" when viewed microscopically. When it is the causative agent of skin infection, the pus is usually golden yellow. It may be found anywhere on the skin.

**Staphylococcus epidermidis** is present on everyone's skin in large numbers. It is often the cause of minor infections and is a Gram positive coccus.

**Beta hemolytic streptoccocus** is a frequent cause of tonsillitis and may be found in about 5% of people. It may infect skin. Skin grafts appear to be particularly vulnerable to this organism. It is also a Gram positive coccus.

Bacteria that do not require oxygen are called **anaerobic bacteria**. These include a family of spore-forming organisms called **Clostridium**. Two notorious species are **Clostridium welchii** which causes gas gangerene and **Clostridium tetani** which causes tetanus. Deep, dirty wounds that are produced by trauma and have poor blood supply are the types most afflicted with these organisms. Tetanus bacilli live in the soil and easily contaminate wounds from road injuries or falls from farm or pleasure equipment.

**Bacteriodes** are anaerobic organisms that arise in the bowel and may contaminate wounds. They are relatively harmless in the bowel but they can produce sepsis when present outside.

Another group of bacteria is the coliform or gram negative rod. They are aerobic organisms that are capable of producing virulent infections in wounds. Two of these organisms are **Escherichia coli and Proteus vulgaris**. They can produce nasty, often fatal infections. **Klebsiella and Psuedomonas** are two additional organisms of the gram negative type that may produce very bad infections.

### Sources of Infections

Many infections are produced from an endogenous source, that is, from the patient's own bacteria. Remember, the skin's bacteria is usually harmless on unbroken skin but it is ever ready to take advantage of a skin break. Some wound infections occur from careless wound dressing changes or poor skin preparation prior to surgery.

Other infections are exogenous or caused by someone or something outside of the patient's body. These infections are termed **cross-infections** and are caused by transfer of organisms from the staff, by other patients, by contaminated instruments, or through the environment. The age of antibiotics ushered in a means to control infections in wounds, but alas, antibiotics also produced new strains of resistant bacteria that have been a curse to hospitals. So called "hospital staph" is a resistant strain of staphyloccus found in some hospitals. Recently it seems to be getting under control due to good Infection Control Committee measures in hospitals.

### Clinical Appearance and Onset of Some Wound Infections

The skin care specialist should be aware of the time of onset of the most common infections. Listed in **Table 12-1** are the most frequent types of post-operative infections and their clinical picture.

### Some Notes on Reducing Wound Infections in Elective Surgery

Most surgical wounds are contaminated during surgery, less commonly after surgery. Clean wounds, that is, those made under aseptic conditions have an infection rate of less than 1%. The skin is usually cleansed with an antiseptic material before surgery.

Operative sites in hairy areas should not be shaved, as the incidence of infections increases with pre-operative shaving. If hair removal is indicated, a depilatory cream should be used.

Hospitalization prior to surgery increases the incidence of wound infection; the longer the pre-operative stay, the higher the infection rate. Also, long operations increase the incidence of infection of the operative wound. The infection rate doubles with every hour of surgery.

Post-operative care requires clean hands and sterile dressings. Aseptic technique must be used at all times in the changing of wound dressings. When changing dressings of several patients, always change the patient with an already infected wound last.

**Personal hygiene is essential in all health care personnel.** Here are a few common sense rules:

1. Keep your own body clean with frequent bathing or showering.
2. Wash your hands after using the toilet.
3. Keep hands away from your nose, ears, mouth, eyes, and genitals.
4. Do not share personal items, such as ra-

## FREQUENT POST-OPERATIVE INFECTIONS

| TIME OF ONSET | ORGANISM | CLINICAL PICTURE |
|---|---|---|
| 1-3 days | *Clostridium welchii* | Brownish edema, cool intense local pain, foul exudate |
| 2-3 days | *Streptococcus* | Red, tender, warm, serous exudate, and cellulitis |
| 3-5 days | *Staphylococcus* | Abscess, erythema, tender, warm with purulent exudate |
| 5 days | Gram negative rods | Purulent exudate, erythema, tender |
| Over 5 days | Mixed infection with anaerobic and Gram negative rods | Foul purulent exudate, tissue necrosis, warm and tender |

**TABLE 12-1** This is what sterile technique is all about, preventing these infections. Adapted from Wound Care by Stephen Westaby, The C.V. Mosby Company, St. Louis, 1985.

zors or combs.
5. Always wash hands between patients or clients.

### Principles of Sterile Technique

Now that you are aware that bacteria are everywhere and your major goal is to keep them out of a new wound, you need to know how this is done. Sterile technique is best learned by practicing it with a nurse or doctor. The skills are simple, but quite rigid.

**To break sterile technique is to invite infection in the wound.** Look at the practice as a series of steps or links in a chain. One weak link and the chain is broken.

Sterile technique is best learned by observing an experienced operating room nurse in action. Study the drawing in **Figure 12-2** which lists the steps conveying the principles involved. I have outlined the basic principles for setting up a sterile field for minor surgery. These principles apply to all types of procedures. **The basic concept is to keep bacteria out of the sterile area.**

### Preparing a Sterile Field Table

Once you are gowned and gloved you must pick up only sterile objects. First place a sterile towel on a Mayo table (a common surgical table). The towel is partially opened in a sterile pack so that you can easily take the towel out without touching the sides of the pack. Place the towel on the table without touching any part of the table. Next, open an instrument pack which is handed to you in the same manner and place the instruments on the towel.

In addition to the instruments you should have 2 x 2 and 4 x 4 sterile gauze squares, sterile suture material, and sterile saline (0.85% sodium chloride) for irrigation of the wound. This procedure is illustrated in **Figure 12-3**.

### PRE-OPERATIVE CARE OF THE PATIENT FOR COSMETIC SURGERY

In researching this topic I was surprised to find how very little is written on pre-operative preparation of the skin . Most textbooks on cosmetic surgery have no mention, or at most, very brief notes on skin preparation. There have been studies on the effect of germicidal soap cleansing of the skin prior to surgery with a subsequent reduction of infections by 50% or more. The practice of shaving the hair on an operative site is usually associated with more infections. This is believed to be due to the spread of staph infections on the abraded skin.

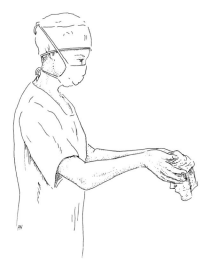

1. Cover head with cap, and mouth and nose with mask. Scrub hands with brush using germicidal soap, for at least ten minutes. Dry hands with a sterile towel as shown.

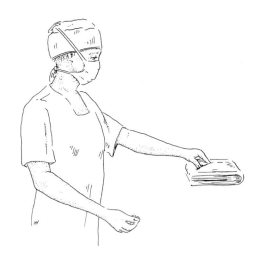

2. An unsterile person will open pack; grasp gown by inside surface.

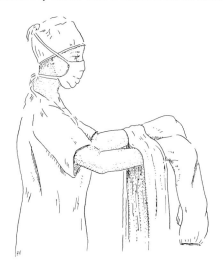

3. Place arms in sleeves.

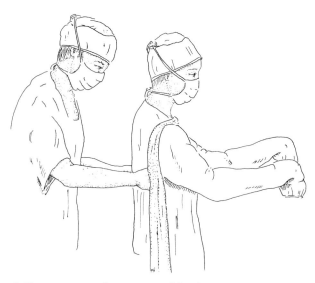

4. Have an unsterile person pull back gown.

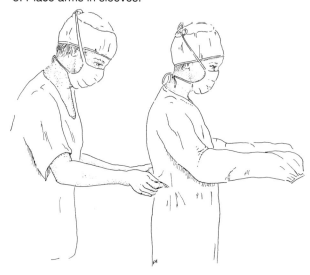

5. After adjusting the gown, the unsterile person ties strings.

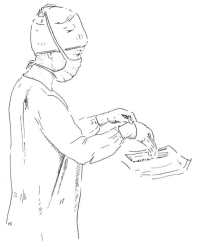

6. Unsterile person will open glove pack. Pick up one glove with thumb and two fingers of one hand. Pull glove over hand to waist. Do not touch gown.

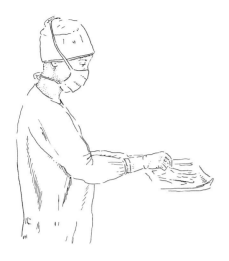

7. Slide gloved finger under folded, upper portion of second glove.

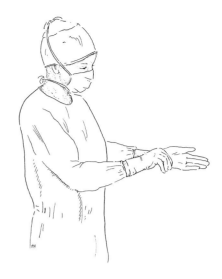

8. Point gloved fingers upward under glove fold.

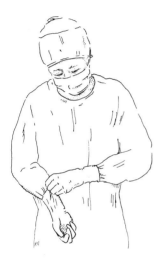

9. Pull glove onto hand, unfolding top of glove from inside, until glove covers wrist band of gown. Do not touch skin with outside of glove.

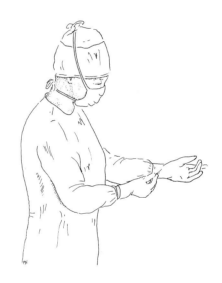

10. On other hand, cover top of wrist band of gown with glove.

**FIGURE 12-2** The sterile technique. You can only learn sterile technique by actually following the steps with a trained nurse. The diagram will help. You must keep in mind "clean" and "dirty", as "sterile" and "unsterile". No part of the sterile field must come into contact with the unsterile area, or sterility is "broken".

The type of preparation needed is determined by the type of surgery planned. I have tried in this chapter to bring together the best information available. Textbooks, journal references, interviews with cosmetic and plastic surgeons and with estheticians form the basis for the advice and suggestions given in this chapter.

Preparation and post-operative care for the following cosmetic surgical conditions, mammoplasty, face lift, rhinoplasty, dermabrasion, and chemical peels will be discussed more later in this chapter.

## MAMMOPLASTY

### Pre-operative Care

Regardless of the type of breast surgery the pre-operative care is essentially the same. I am assuming that the surgeon has discussed everything with the patient including all psychological and medical considerations. When the cli-

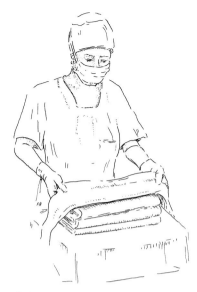

1. An (unsterile) circulating nurse opens drape pack. Nurses's hands remain on the outside of the pack, in a folded cuff, while pulling back wrapper. This will prevent contamination of the contents. The outside of the wrapper (unsterile) falls below the unsterile table level, so the inside of the wrapper remains sterile.

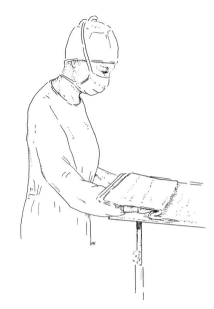

2. Draping of Mayo stand: Scrub nurse is shown with hands protected in drape cuff. Arms support folds of drape which will prevent their falling below (unsterile) waist level. A foot at the base of stand will stabilize it and prevent tipping.

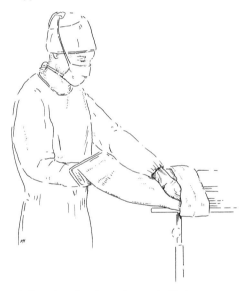

3. Completing the draping of stand. Notice hands are protected in cuff of drape.

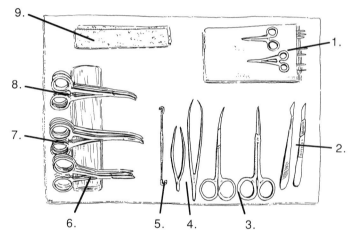

4. Contents of stand in preparation for operation: 1. suture towel and needleholders, 2. scalpels, 3. straight and curved scissors, 4. smooth and toothed tissue forceps, 5. retractors, 6. straight hemostats, 7. Kelly clamps, 8. Allis's forceps, and 9. sponges .

**FIGURE 12-3** Sterile field table preperation. The sterile field table is prepared after you are gowned and gloved. The tray of instruments is only diagrammatic for general surgical procedures.

ent is referred to you for pre-operative treatment for breast surgery you have to only make sure that the breasts are clean and that no abnormal skin conditions exists. In the case of reduction mammoplasty you must check under the breasts for intertrigo. These conditions are frequently caused by staphyloccocus or yeast and respond well to simple hygienic measures and topical antibiotics. I have found Mycostatin to be one of the best creams for this condition. It is applied twice a day after washing and cleansing the breasts. If the surgeon agrees, a total body wash the day of surgery or the day before surgery is of benefit. Washing will remove a great deal of devitalized tissue and bacteria. A moisturizing cream should not be applied, leave the skin dry.

In the case of reconstruction of the breast

after total removal for breast cancer there may be some radiation-induced tissue damage with scarring, thinning, and redness. It takes considerable experience to be able to judge these cases and I know of no hard and fast rules for estimating skin condition. Fortunately, radiation treatment for breast cancer is not as common as in the past so we see fewer of these cases. The general rule is that post-radiation tissue must be treated gently.

### Post-Operative Care

Breast surgery can be done in the office or in the hospital. In the case of the hospitalized patient, skin care is usually given by the nursing staff. Bandage technique varies widely and depends on the surgeon's preference and training. Many surgeons use an antiseptic cream, such as bacitracin or chlorhexidine, over the wound and then cover the wound with gauze. Pressure is achieved by using an elastic bandage to control bleeding and prevent a hematoma from forming. Dressings are changed in 24 to 48 hours and the bandages are reapplied. A comfortable soft brassiere can be used instead of a pressure bandage. The scar is larger in mastoplexy and reduction mammoplasty and requires more attention but the treatment principles are the same. Unless you are trained by the surgeon to remove the sutures, or you are working within a hospital setting you most likely will not see the patient until the sutures are removed. Sutures may be removed at 7 to 10 days, but usually within two weeks after surgery when the incisional lines are healing well. Some wounds have rubber drains inserted in the incision to allow serum or blood to ooze out. Special care of these drains is required and the surgeon will often give specific instructions. It is best the patient not bathe as long as the drains are in place. Sponge baths, given with care and avoiding the wounds are safe.

There is always some redness and swelling about the incision for a few days after surgery. In the absence of wound infection or a hematoma, the redness and swelling will gradually disappear over the next week or two.

Patients are advised not to work and to avoid lifting the arms above the head for about a week. Some surgeons permit hair washing a day or two after surgery but only with help. If lifting can

be limited to 2-3 lbs most patients can prepare meals within a few days to a week. Some patients have the remarkable ability to recover and heal quickly while others will take longer. Most patients can shower in about a week, after the dressings are removed. Remember to dry the area well, but gently. During this healing period of three to six weeks the client should continue to wear a soft brassiere both during the day and at night.

### Direct Wound Care

There is really little to do except to observe the wound and keep it clean. The patient will return to the surgeon once or twice within the three week period. After one week there will usually be no dressing. When you see the client, examine the incision for healing. Any complication should be referred back to the surgeon. Report any excess pain, discoloration, or bleeding to the surgeon. The major things to look for are complications which include infection and bleeding. The skin care specialist is mainly concerned with scar reduction in reduction mammoplasty or mastoplexy. Here are some general rules to help avoid scars. The most important steps in avoiding scars must be instituted by the surgeon at the time of the operation, but this is what you can do to help.

Always use an antibiotic ointment (Bacitracin[R]) on the wound. Keep the wound open after the first week. Remove the crust with 3% hydrogen peroxide. Do not use make-up on the wound unless it is a water-based material and is hypoallergenic. (Most make-up fits these criteria, but check the package insert.) Avoid any sun exposure to the scar area. Sun exposure only increases the redness and swelling. I recommend absolute sun avoidance for three months and minimal exposure up to one year.

Use a good moisturizer on the scar every day. Vitamin E has been known to reduce scar formation. It is helpful if the client takes orally 200 mg daily of vitamin E and applies vitamin E directly to the scar. Use a cream that contains at least 2% vitamin E acetate. Breast massage is often recommended by the surgeon to be done by the patient. Some patients do not like to do this so that you may be instructed on how the surgeon wants this to be done. **Massage helps to prevent capsule formation around the im-**

**plant.**

## FACE LIFT (RHYTIDECTOMY)

The care of the wound after a face lift is fairly easy. When you see the client in your office most of the difficult tasks will have been done, but if you are working with a plastic surgeon in his office you will need to know more about the immediate care. I shall present this section as if the skin care specialist is working with the surgeon in his office.

The details of the surgical procedure are not necessary for you to know, but I would advise that you obtain a good background in the expected results. This can only be obtained by working with surgeons on these cases. Observe operations, view video films, and attend training sessions.

### Dressings

The dressings for face lift surgery are bulky. A multilayered head wrap is used. Gauze is applied to the mastoid region and around the ears as padding to protect the wound. Care must be exercised to keep the hair out of the wound area. The dressing goes over the head and under the chin, then behind the ears to keep pressure in this area. Drains may be placed in the wound. The bandage is removed within 24-48 hours. Again, the wound may be cleansed with 3% hydrogen peroxide and a new dressing applied. In the office the hair can be shampooed and gently dried. Do not blow dry as this will increase swelling. Hair may be dyed at least two weeks before surgery and not until one month or more after surgery. The previous rules apply as to sunbathing, make-up, and activity. In the first few days facial expressions and talking should be limited and food should be soft or liquid to reduce chewing. Rinsing of the mouth after eating is helpful.No steaks or pizza!

Sutures are removed starting at 4-5 days after surgery and completed at about 10 days post-op. During this period have the client wear a head scarf when going outside. It is helpful not to bend or stretch the neck and to sleep with a comfortable but slightly firm pillow. Any bruising may be covered with make up, but avoid the suture line and incision area until it is well healed.

## RHINOPLASTY (NOSE JOB)

### Pre-operative Care

A good facial cleansing is about all the pre-operative care needed for a rhinoplasty. It is more important to prepare the patient for the eventual result. This is the task of the surgeon but your role should be one of support for your client. As we have discussed before, the decision to have the surgery must be made by the client for his or her own reason.

### Post-operative Care

Correction of a nasal septal defect or revision of the shape of the nose requires essentially the same post-operative care. Limit activity that involves bending, lifting, or straining. The nose is usually splinted and packed with rolled gauze. The packing is removed in 24 to 48 hours, but the splint usually stays on for one week. The function of the splint is to reduce swelling.

Invariably the patient will have two large "shiners", or ecchymotic areas around the eyes. This discoloration will last about a week and can be covered with make-up. Swelling will be pronounced even after a week. Ice packs will help to reduce swelling if used the first 24-48 hours. Blood will ooze out of the nose, at times being bright red and at other times being pink. This will gradually decrease over the first week.

It is wise to limit physical activity, including sexual intercourse, for a period of two to three weeks. Work with your client, as the post-operative swelling seems to be the major problem and concern after the first week. In some cases it will take six months to a year to achieve the final result, but most patients are content or happy with the result within a month.

## DERMABRASION

There are many indications for dermabrasions. I have listed some of the conditions that have responded to this technique. Facial scars are by far the most common reason to use dermabrasion. Acne is still the leading cause of facial scars.

**Some Conditions Treated with Dermabrasion** (adapted from Roenigk and Roenigk in Dermatological Surgery, Principles and Practice, Marcel Dekker New York 1988), are as follows:

| | |
|---|---|
| Post-acne scars | Vitiligo |
| Traumatic scars | Keloids |
| Smallpox scars | Adenoma sebaceum |
| Rhinophyma | Lichenified states |
| Tattoos | Freckles |
| Actinic Damage | Keratoacanthoma |
| Active Acne | Xanthelasma |
| Acne rosacea | Hemangioma |
| Chloasma | Stretch marks (striae) |

## Pre-Operative Care

Medication such as aspirin and nonsteroid anti-inflammatory drugs (Advil, Motrin) should be stopped. Birth control pills and estrogen may be associated with post-operative hyper-pigmentation. Doctors may also prescribe other drugs for specific conditions of the patient such as antibiotics for patients with heart disease. The current thought is that Retin A should be used in all patients prior to surgery. Besides reducing the spread of milia, Retin A also increases the healing potential of the skin. **Do not use Retin A in pregnant patients or anyone who has eczema. Caution women of child bearing age to prevent pregnancy. Do a pregnancy test before using Retin A and monthly thereafter. This is rather strict advice for a topical agent but I feel many young people do not understand the potency of Retin A.**

There are several regimens recommended, but here is the one that I advise.

### Retin A Application (Instructions for clients and patients.)

Start with a cream at 0.05% and apply a small amount (about the size of a green pea) to the forehead on one side. Rub this in an area about half of the forehead at night. Do this nightly for three to four nights. If there is no reaction such as marked redness or swelling apply Retin A to the other half of the forehead for two more days. Again if there is no reaction you may then apply the cream on both sides of the face very lightly. Keep in mind that Retin A is expensive ($25 to $30 a tube) and quite potent , so use it sparingly. After one week of use, if there is no reaction you can safely apply the product to the face and neck.

You may use a moisturizer either before or after the application of Retin A. **If you go out in the sun you must wear a sunscreen of at least 15 SPF.** Use Retin A for 3 to 6 weeks prior to surgery,applying only once a day. If you have any reaction report it to your physician. The dose may be reduced to 0.025% or application may be spread out to every other day. Only severe reactions and pregnancy are contraindications to the judicial use of Retin A. You must work closely with your physician or skin care specialist while using this agent.

There are no other general instructions for pre-operative care of the patient for dermabrasion. A clean face and few milia are forecasters of a good post-operative effect. I recommend that a facial cleansing and conditioning start at four weeks. Clean the face and remove any comedones and milia. Next, start the Retin A. Check the client each week. Apply added moisturizers if needed. Do weekly facial massage using a bland oil, such as borage oil. Massage will help to stimulate the skin by perking up enzymes, such as ornithine decarboxylase (ODC) and growth factors such as epidermal growth factor (EGF). These are natural biological agents produced by the skin that help healing.

## Post-operative Care

One can never be sure of the results of dermabrasion.

Dressings are applied immediately after surgery. The type depends on the surgeon, but Telfa[R] dressings placed over antibiotics and then covered with gauze, a roller bandage (such as Kling gauze), and a surgical net is an excellent combination. The Telfa[R] prevents adherence of the gauze and aids in healing the wound. This is left in place for 24 hours. There are several other types of dressings used, one of which is Vigilon[R]. This is a polyethylene oxide gel which is applied to the face and followed by gauze pads, usually 4 x 4's. This is a nonadherent dressing composed of 96% water and 4% polyethylene. Some other dressing classes you may find used by various surgeons:

**Films** are made of thin polyurethane which does not absorb or stick to wounds. They often allow exudate to accumulate under the dressing which is not good. Some trade names include Opsite[R], Tegaderm[R], Univlex[R], and Bioclusive[R].

**Hydrocolloid dressings** are polyurethane films with a hydrocolloid gel coating. They also allow fluid to accumulate and need to be changed often. They sometimes become bad smelling. Examples are Duoderm[R] and Comfeel[R].

**Hydrogels** are polyethylene oxide gels covered on both sides with a semipermeable polyurethane film. They are placed on the wound by removing one of the films and placing the gel next to the wound. They will absorb and do not adhere to the wound. Vigilon[R] is this type.

**Foams** are polyurethane material which is nonadherent. They absorb little fluid. An example is Synthaderm[R] and Epilock[R].

**Permeable double-layered dressings** are made of membranes that allow the fluid to permeate to the surface. Topically applied medication will penetrate the dressing to the skin surface. Omniderm[R] is the tradename for this type dressing.

All of these dressings have advantages and drawbacks. The advantages are prevention of dehydration of the skin, increase in healing rate by 50% in some cases, and rapid re-epithialization. The drawbacks are slippage, sticking, leaking, and infection.

**After the dressings are removed** most surgeons recommend showering one to three times a day. The dressing is removed 24 hours after surgery and the hair is shampooed. The water is allowed to run down over the face and the face is gently washed with soap. The face is next patted dry and and antibiotic ointment is applied over the entire abraided area. The face is then redressed or left open. After four or five days the ointment is changed to an antibiotic cream with or without cortisone. These patients should be followed by the surgeon and the skin care specialist for two to six weeks.

The client must avoid sunlight to prevent hyperpigmentation. A single extensive sun exposure within the first 3 to 6 months can produce hyperpigmentation. Make-up can be used as soon as the scabs are off. The choice of make-up technique will depend on the post-operative course.

### Complications

**Scarring** is the worst and most feared com-plication. Treatment is prolonged (several months) and requires steroid injections.

**Erythema** is less common. No treatment is usually needed as it will fade in time. Here is a good indication for make-up use.

**Hypopigmentation** may occur in 50% of patients. The area of loss of pigment will stop at the area of non-abraided skin. Blotchy areas may be seen in the abraided area. These areas are difficult to cover with make-up as it requires a great deal of skill. Some physicians advocate bleaching the skin of the pigmented areas to conform to the areas of hypopigmentation. This is an area where your skills as a make-up artist and skin care specialist will be of great benefit to the surgeon and the client.

**Hyperpigmentation** is not as common as hypopigmentation. It is seen around three months post-op and will sometimes fade without treatment. Some surgeons use hydroquinone at levels of 2% to 6% and add hydrocortisone and Retin A to the treatment. Dr. Albert Kligman has advocated the use of these three agents in equal amounts. **Infections**, while rare, do occur. They mostly occur from contamination within the scabs by bacteria. They are rarely serious as long as they are localized to small areas.

**Milia** can be controlled with the use of Retin A before surgery. Any milia present can be treated by de-roofing with a lancet and expressing the contents. They can be quite extensive.

**Acne flare-ups** occur mostly in females. Standard treatments for acne appear to work well for these conditions.

## CHEMICAL PEELS

### Introduction

Chemical peels have been around since about 1903, but it was not until the work of Dr. Thomas Baker of Miami in the 1960's that the procedure became generally accepted by the medical professions. Peels were done both in the United States and in Europe by beauty specialists for many years prior to Dr. Baker's work, but there is no documentation on the nature of these peels or the solutions used.

Baker's formula is given below as it is used by most physicians today. Note that the concentration of phenol is high at 50%, but this is important for the depth of penetration needed. The croton oil is added as an epidermal irritant to further increase the penetration of the phenol. The formula is:

| | |
|---|---|
| Phenol U.S.P | 3 milliliters |
| Distilled water | 2 milliliters |
| Croton oil | 2 drops |
| Septisol | 5 drops |

This is mixed before each use. Other formulae are published using phenol at 50% with glycerin, water and croton oil. There is much talk these days about trichloroacetic acid peels used at a concentration from 25% to 50%. This is a level used by physicians.

Cosmetic peeling formulae remove mainly the stratum corneum. The agents used are resorcinol and salicylic acid at 20%, and various plant enzymes, including papaya and pineapple enzymes. A popular formula is Jenner's formula which is:

| | |
|---|---|
| Resorcinol | 14.0% |
| Salicylic acid | 14.0% |
| Lactic acid (85%) | 14.0% |
| Ethanol 95% added to make | 100.0% |

This type of peel is used by some physicians as a "light peel" to treat fine wrinkles and irregular pigmentation. Used at intervals of four to six months peels can reduce the visibility of mild to moderate acne scars. For a skin care specialist to use these agents they must be well trained by an experienced operator. I have not gone into the technique of light peels in this text as I feel more knowledge is needed in this field and certainly more training facilities are needed. The legal matters are not fully worked out and liability is still a big question in some States. (In the companion manual for this text book I shall treat light facial peels as a complete topic, including techniques.)

Another peeling chemical is tricholoracetic acid (TCA) in 35% concentration for light peels extending through the papillary dermis. This is a physician type peel and should not be used by the skin care specialist. I know of no cardiac problems associated with TCA peels as is found with phenol peels, but there are other problems such as scarring.

## Pre-operative Care

Cleansing and degreasing of the skin are the most important pre-operative steps. It is not nec-essary to use harsh detergents or to use gritty scrubs. Most experienced surgeons do not use acetone any longer to defat the skin. It is important to protect the barrier of the stratum corneum to prevent excessive penetration of the phenol. One cleansing is usually enough. Make sure that all make-up is thoroughly removed. Work closely with the surgeon and make sure you understand his instructions for both preoperative and postoperative care. Perhaps the most important pre-operative service rendered by the skin care specialist is to describe to the patient and the family what the appearance of the face will be the day after the peel.

At this stage I do not know what the final outcome of the trials with pretreatment of the skin using Retin A will be. There is some evidence that it helps but there is too little clinical data. At present I tend to recommend its use but keep open the option for further clinical evaluation.

## Post-operative Care

The surgeon will want to see the patient in the first 24 hours when the bandages are removed. Taping is becoming controversial, so you may find that the surgeon has not used tape to cover the wound. Tape has been used in the past to increase penetration of the phenol and allow for a deeper wound. The technique of taping varies with surgeons, some being almost fanatical about the method and duration of application. In any event, after the first 24 hours when you see the patient expect to find a grayish and edematous skin. In fact, the whole face will be very edematous including the lips, with eyelids swollen shut and the face awash with a serous ooze. Here is where the skin care specialist can be of great service to the surgeon, the patient, and the family in explaining what the face will look like after a peel.

A relatively new post-operative treatment involves washing the face with soap and water as in the post-op treatment of dermabrasion. This makes sense. Follow the same procedure using antibiotic ointment for the first few days and then switch to antibiotic creams. Keep the crust soft as scabs will form during this period which will fall off in about a week to ten days.

Make-up can be applied after the scabs are removed. No special make-up has been devised for this procedure. Sunscreens and avoidance of the sun are strongly advised.

### Complications of Facial Peels

Changes in pigment are the most common complications. **Hypopigmentation** occurs with deep peels usually appearing three to six months after the peel. Some surgeon authors consider this a side effect rather than a complication. **Hyperpigmentation** occurs with some patients as early as six weeks but is not as frequent. Sun exposure may be a causative agent here.

**Itching and burning with erythema** occurs sometimes during the first three weeks but can be controlled with aspirin. In some cases it will last for six months. The use of camouflage make-up is helpful.

**Infections** occur usually within the first days but can arise later. They are often associated with patients who do not cleanse the skin properly with soap and water and/or follow with antibiotics twice daily. These infections usually respond to topical and systemic antibiotics. The most common organisms are Staphylococcus aureus and Pseudomonas. Infection with Herpes simplex virus was more common a few years ago than it is today because of an **antiviral drug called Acyclovir^R**. If a patient has a history of fever blisters (causative agent is Herpes simplex) the surgeon will give Acyclovir^R before surgery.

**Scarring** also occurs but is infrequent, appearing mostly on the angle of the jaw and on the upper lip. Treatment is complex and involves steroid injections into the scar.

**All complications must be referred back to the surgeon. Never undertake to treat a complication without contacting the surgeon.**

### CAMOUFLAGE MAKE-UP

### Introduction

The proper use of make-up as an adjunct to cosmetic surgery is an art in itself. Not only in post-operative correction but in some cases the skilled use of make-up may be all that is needed to correct certain minor conditions.

Make-up is not used simply to cover defects, but rather it is used to provide subtle enhancement of desirable features while lessening undesirable features. The techniques vary with the make-up artist but a few principles can be outlined for the beginner. I strongly advise a serious candidate for this art to obtain training from the best school available.

### Make-up Principles

The use of make-up requires a basic knowledge of the principles of art. Most high school courses in art have covered these principles. Light and dark areas are used to create a sense of dimension. The subtle shades of colors and greys will produce this effect on any surface.

### Application

In corrective make-up an opaque foundation is first applied. It does not allow skin tones to show through. Select one that matches the skin tone as much as possible. Next, a second color is added to correct the first. Mixing shades takes a lot a skill but it can be accomplished with practice. There is a great deal of discussion in some make-up books about the use of applicators in applying make-up. A tiny pored sponge which is smooth and dense seems to work best as it picks up the powder or cream quite well. Touching the sponge to the skin and rolling or dabbing gently with repetition will deposit a smooth, even, thin coat of make-up on the skin.

Aim for only 80% coverage since 100% coverage tends to look the same. This tends to prevent the caked-on appearance of heavy applications. The make-up is then set with a powder of appropriate color. The powder should be applied in the same manner as the foundation, that is, with a rolling or rocking action rather than a dusting action. An effort should be made not to have the powder "dust" about in the room, as this tends to result in an uneven application.

### A Note on Colors

There are four discolorations seen after surgery that must be covered. Red is from erythema. Blue is from early bruising. Green and yellow are from late bruising (hemoglobin degeneration) and occur during healing. Brown or white, to pink discoloration is due to pigmentation effects from melanocytes being turned off or on. A simple color scheme is as follows:

1. Use opposite colors on the primary color

wheel. Blue is the opposite of orange, red is the opposite of green, yellow is the opposite of purple.

2. For a purple bruise use a yellow color make-up.
3. For a red erythematous skin use a greenish tint make-up.
4. For a greenish skin use a pink make-up.
5. For a blue discoloration use a yellow or pink make-up.

Most skin care specialists will have a good background in make-up, far more than I can impart to you. I can give you a little direction, though, in when to use make-up after surgery. Some guidelines are:

**Face lifts** present only a problem at the neck and ears. Some bruising about the ears in the front may be covered over. It's impressive that just with hair style changes and a high collar many of these areas may be effectively masked. It's not the case for men who have face lifts. Conventional collars on shirts and coats attract make-up and rub off your good intentions. That some men are somewhat adverse to make-up application is understandable, they may prefer to ignore the discolorations.

**Blepharoplasty** sometimes presents swelling and discolorations. Many cosmetic surgeons feel it is okay to use make-up after the sutures are removed and there is no infection or disruption of the suture line. Dark colors will cause the puffiness to recede visually. Matte finishing is better than a shiny finish since shiny things look bigger. Since the lower lid may stay swollen for up to two weeks it is better to use a lighter color here, with emphasis placed on the color of the upper lid. Use eyeliner cautiously.

**Chemical peels and dermabrasion** require stages of correction. After the crusts are gone, make-up may be applied. Use a base color of green or yellow followed by an appropriate foundation. Do not apply these color cosmetics too heavily as they will be hard to remove and may look contrived. Pigmentation occurs as the next phase. You will encounter both hypopigmentation and hyperpigmentation that will challenge your skill and patience. One of the rules is to use make-up lightly and to blend the treated edges into the nontreated areas. Heavy make-up has been associated with theatrics and those unskilled in make-up application. Take advantage of your client's more youthful appearance and apply the make-up in an alluring skillfull manner.

A pretty girl...is just like a melody...let's get back to the beauty of what we're about now (which is beauty, isn't it?) You've slogged through some gruesome territory to get yourself prepared to go out there

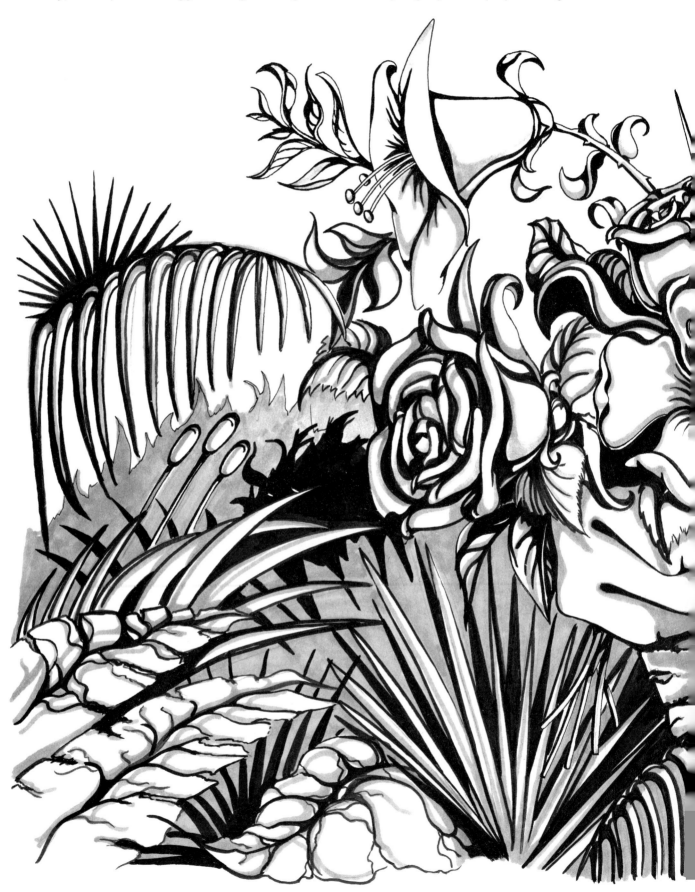

and really make a difference. It isn't always a jungle out there. Remember, to stop and smell the roses....
and some really sweet things can happen.

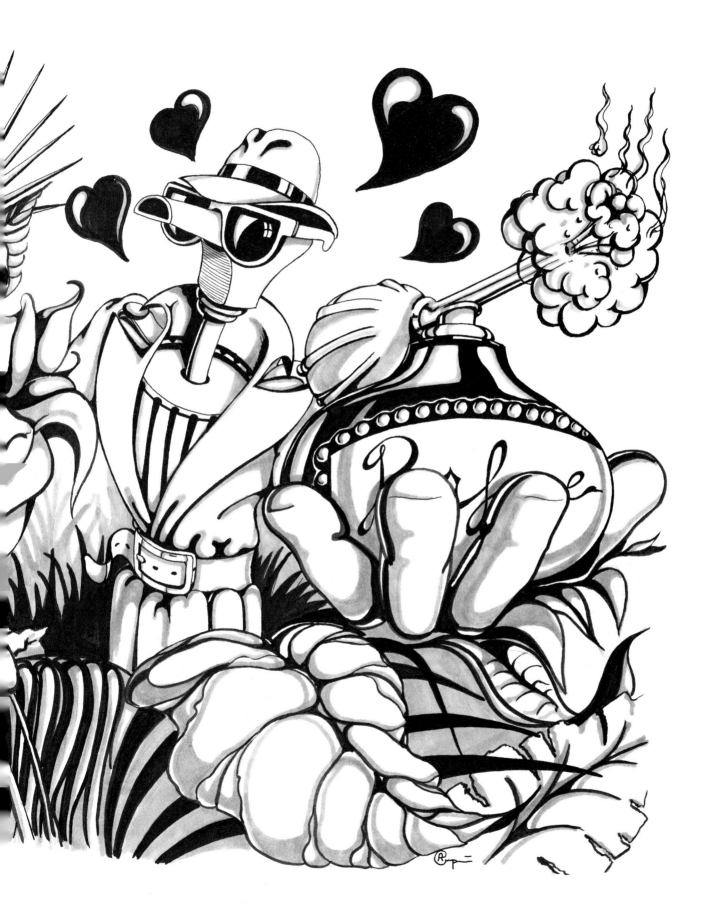

# Fragrance - The Role of Fragrance in Skin Care

Odors of one sort or another have played an important role in biological life, probably since the early days of oceanic life. We know that fish have a keen sense of smell. The salmon use their olfactory sense to guide them to their breeding grounds which are thousands of miles from the place where they spend their adult life. Considering the vast volume of the ocean, it is incredible that so sensitive a mechanism exists!

Odor is used in lower animals for food location, to find a mate, to determine willingness to breed, and as a protective mechanism. Plants use odor to attract insects for pollination and many of our fragrances come from this source. Fragrance is essentially a good, or pleasant scent as opposed to an unpleasant odor which we term a bad scent.

In man, odor is related not only to food and sexual activity but also to our social and psychological well being. In food sourcing and consumption the sense of smell and taste are bonded together for recognition of food and for excitation of appetite. Sexual activity is tied to the odor of hormones. There is a marked difference between the ability of men and women to detect sexual odor. Women, for instance, at the time of ovulation, can detect a male-like hormone called **exaltolide**, from musk and civet, with a thousand times greater sensitivity than at other times.

It is also well established that females that are living together will tend to synchronize their menstrual cycles and lengthen the cycle duration beyond twenty-eight days. The presence of males in the group will tend to break both the synchronization and the increased length of the cycle.

It is also established that males will secrete greater amounts of male hormone when in the presence of women than when isolated. A previously isolated male will maintain an increased level of male hormone for seven days after just one casual encounter with a female!

In health we know that unpleasant odor will decrease productivity on the job and increase the illness rate. Lavender, bergamot, and citrus reduce depression, elevate moods, and increase courage and resolve. Rose and vanilla tend to ease tension and tranquilize the spirit.

Perhaps the single most important aspect of odor is the inherent ability to remember odors. Fragrances can conjure up visions, paint incredible memory pictures, and piece together a beautiful panorama. Our brain can receive an odor, then search all the areas of our recent memory, reach into the depth of our past memory, and weave through the intricate pattern of information imprinted on our brain from our evolutionary development. Olfaction is one of the real wonders of biology!

## A FEW NOTES ON THE HISTORY OF FRAGRANCE

There are few subjects more exciting than the impact of fragrances on the history of mankind. The search for an easier access to the "spices" led to the travels of Marco Polo and Christopher Columbus. Our interest in this chapter is the role of fragrance in maintaining healthy skin and correcting disordered skin. It is not difficult to be carried away by an interest in the ancient uses of the fragrant extracts of plants in the health care and psychosocial areas. Many books have been written on the history of fragrances. Perhaps the pleasant olfactory experience produced by fragrance materials led the ancients to believe that these substances had to

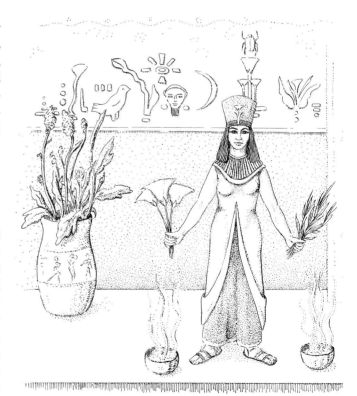

Plants played a large part in Egyptian medicine and daily life. Scented oils were placed on the head in the form of a block of fat and wax. The heat of the head melted the block and released the scented oils. A messy, but very effective use of body heat.

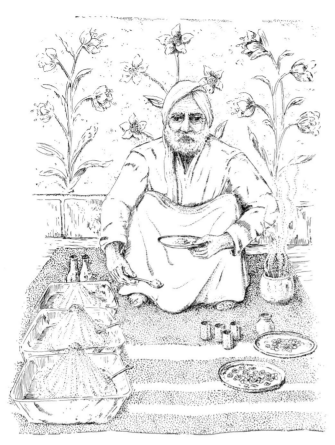

India is a prime source of exotic fragrances. Many imported ingredients for natural fragrances come from India. These fragrances are used as healing agents in sickness, and in health as promoters to maintain wellness.

analysis of the components of the natural essential oils we have been able to produce synthetic materials.

The major difference between the synthetic fragrances and essential oils is the number and type of components in each product. Essential oils contain many natural components, some in large quantities and others only in trace amounts. No one knows what effects these trace materials have on the total fragrance or its biological effects. Synthetic fragrances contain relatively few ingredients compared to natural essential oil based fragrances.

## CLASSIFICATION OF ESSENTIAL OILS BY ORIGIN (USED IN FRAGRANCES)

### ESSENTIAL OILS FROM FLOWERS

Rose, jasmine, tuberose, broom, cassie, jonquil, carnation, hyacinth, camomile, ylang ylang, boronia, champac, and lavender

### ESSENTIAL OILS FROM HERBS

Rosemary, basil, thyme, marjoram, mint, bay, laurel, coriander, caraway, cumin, and angelica

### ESSENTIAL OILS FROM THE LEAF

Lemongrass, palmarosa, citronella, patchouli, geranium, eucalyptus, oil of bay from *Pimenta acris*, spruce oil, balsam fir, cedar leaf, camphor, violet leaf oil, myrtle, labdanum, and oakmoss

### ESSENTIAL OILS FROM SPICES

Cloves, nutmeg, cinnamon, allspice, vanilla, pepper, and ginger oil.

### ESSENTIAL OILS FROM ROOTS

Valerian, vetiver, and orrisroot

### ESSENTIAL OILS FROM WOOD

Bois de rose from rosewood and sandalwood

### ESSENTIAL OILS FROM CITRUS

Bergamot, lemon, orange, tangerine, neroli (bitter orange), lime, grapefruit, and mandarin orange.

### GUMS AND RESINS

Frankincense, myrrh, benzoin, galbanum, balsum of Peru, and balsam of Tolu

**TABLE 13-1** While there are many ways to classify essential oils this method is convenient since it relates to the **parts** of the plant.

contain some "good power".

Whatever the thinking behind their use, there was no scientific rationale. Continued use over thousands of years led to an empirical body of knowledge that has been passed along through priests (or the shaman class) and healers (or physicians). Only recently have we begun to study these materials, now called **essential oils**. We shall examine the nature of essential oils, then observe how they affect the olfactory system, and finally study how the essential oils may be used to help maintain a healthy skin and mind.

Let us define some terms. **Perfume** comes from two Latin words *per* meaning through and *fume* meaning smoke. This designation most likely arose because many ancient fragrant substances were burned to create the odor. The term **incense** literally means to ignite. The word **fragrance** derives from the Latin word *fragare* meaning to smell sweet.

When we speak of essential oils as fragrances we mean only naturally derived materials and not their synthetic derivatives. By the

Some sources of the common essential oils found in many fragrances and skin care products are outlined in **Table 13-1**. This outline will also serve as one classification for essential oils.

## A LITTLE CHEMISTRY OF THE ESSENTIAL OILS

I shall not discuss how the oils are obtained from plants and trees since, again, there are excellent texts on this subject.

All essential oils are obtained from vegetable sources, either a plant, shrub, or tree. These oils are believed to serve the plant either as a defensive or reproductive material. They may attract insects, repel animals, kill bacteria or fungi, and help heal wounds in the trees. Much remains to be learned of how and why they are formed.

Essential oils are also known as volatile oils because they pass so easily from a liquid to a gaseous state. This is the reason they make excellent fragrances. This volatile property is a function of the chemical structure.

The basic unit of many volatile oils is the **isoprene unit.** This is a five carbon structure with eight hydrogens attached. The structure also includes two unsaturated bonds (see **Figure 13-1**). When two or more of these isoprene units combine we have a molecule called a **terpene**. The isoprene units in a terpene are linked head to tail. Variation in the number and type of linkage leads to a variety of essential oils. It is not important that you remember all these names, but rather, that you appreciate the relation of the structure to the molecule's function in nature. The basic groups and related essential oils are:

> **Monoterpenes (two isoprene units) -** Examples are geraniol and limonene. Pinene is a dicyclic monoterpene and is found in many essential oils such as lemon, anise, fennel, and orange flower.
>
> **Sesquiterpenes (three isoprene units) -** Examples are caryophyllene (found in peppermint), cinnamon oil, clove oil, and cadinene (found in cubeb and juniper tar).

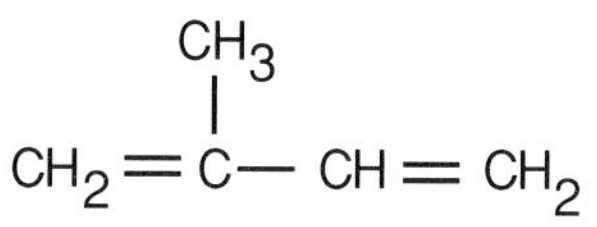

FIGURE 13-1 Structure of isoprene. The isoprene molecule is the basic unit for all terpene essential oils.

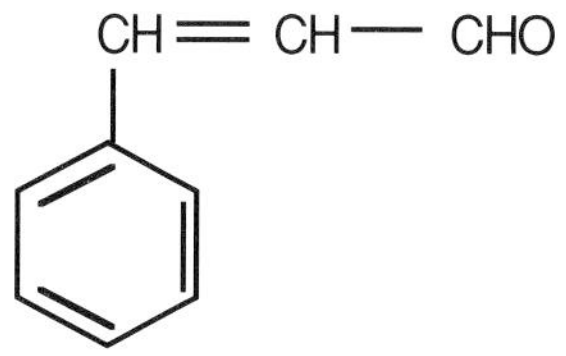

Cinnamaldehyde

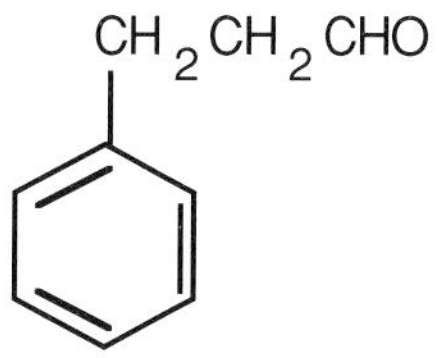

Phenylethyl alcohol

FIGURE 13-2 Structure of phenylpropanoids. Phenylpropanoids are the second group of essential oils. Note the ring structure. They are biologically very active.

> **Diterpenes (four isoprene units) -** An example is abietic acid or rosin.
>
> **Triterpene (five isoprene units) -** An example is lanosterol.

The terpenes in essential oils are mostly monoterpenes. They may be found in a single cyclic form such as limonene or in multiple cyclic configuration such as lanosterol. Oxygen can be added to them to form alcohols, aldehydes, ketones, phenols, oxides, and esters. For example, geraniol is an alcohol and geranial is an aldehyde of the same monoterpene. Listed among the more common terpene aldehydes are orange oil, lemon oil, citronella oil, and hamamelis water.

Another family of essential oils is called the **phenylpropanoids.** These compounds consist of a phenyl ring of 6 carbons and a 3-carbon side chain as shown in **Figure 13-2.** Some of the nicest fragrances and most potent germicides are in this family.

A few phenylpropanoids are **cinnamaldehyde, anethole, eugenol, methyl salicylate, and vanillin.**

These compounds all have good germicidal effects and are pleasant to the nose. Remember, **the function of the essential oil is related to the structure of the molecule.**

## BASIC OLFACTORY PHYSIOLOGY

Science has made considerable progress in the understanding of the sense of smell. Let's

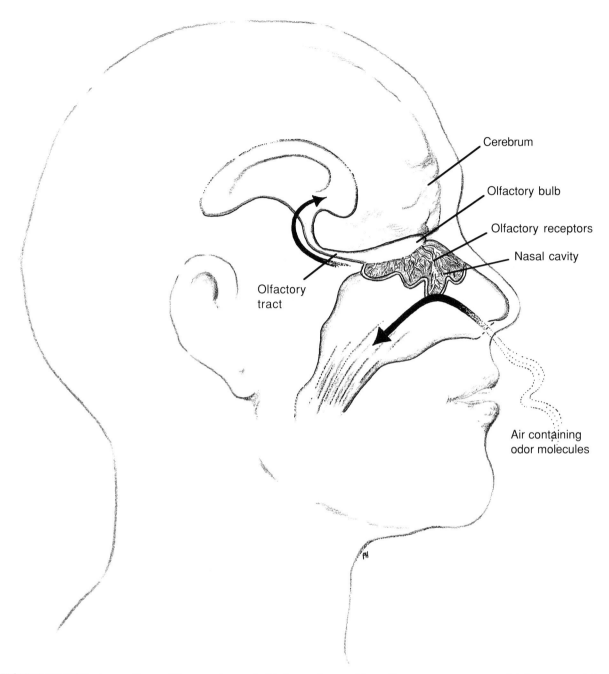

Cerebrum

Olfactory bulb

Olfactory receptors

Nasal cavity

Olfactory tract

Air containing odor molecules

**FIGURE 13-3** Olfactory pathway. The nose is needed to trap odors and keep the sensory organs moist. Long nosed dogs are better at tracing scents than short nosed dogs.

review the basic steps leading to odor perception and recognition. How does a simple chemical, landing in the nose, produce such a profound effect on the entire body?

The nose, located on the front of the face, is first, a mechanical receptor, and secondly, a chemical receptor. The odor enters the nose, dissolves in the mucous lining of the nose, and comes into contact with the olfactory receptor. **Figure 13-3** shows this pathway.

There are three parts to the nose. The outer nose is the part that we normally see. The middle

nose is the nasal cavity which receives the air. The inner nose is the actual olfactory sense organ.

In **Figure 13-4** see numerous fine hair-like projections (known as **cilia**) on the olfactory epithelium at the top of the nasal cavity. These are tiny nerve endings and are part of the olfactory receptor cell. They are connected to the olfactory nerve which in turn is connected to the brain. The cilia constantly move in the mucous covering (cells called supporting cells secrete the mucous). They are very thin, only 0.1 to 0.2

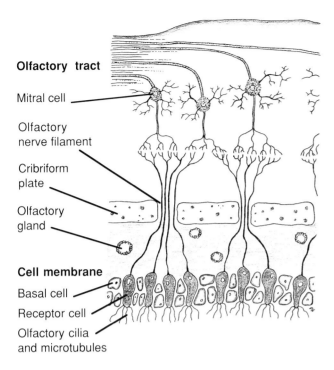

**Olfactory tract**

Mitral cell

Olfactory
nerve filament

Cribriform
plate

Olfactory
gland

**Cell membrane**

Basal cell

Receptor cell

Olfactory cilia
and microtubules

**FIGURE 13-4** Olfactory cell fiber. Note here that there are many connections. The receptor cell receives the impulse from the olfactory cilia and transfers it to the olfactory nerve. From here it goes to the olfactory tract to the brain where identification of the odor occurs.

microns thick. Their length is up to 200 microns long. Within these tiny cilia are microtubules which are arranged in a specific pattern.

When a chemical stimulus lands on the cilia, it is bound to the membrane and the signal is conducted down the dendrite portion of the cell to the cell body (**see Figure 13-4**). Within the cell body there is a **depolarization** which triggers **action potentials** that are carried to the **olfactory bulb**. Different odors produce different responses in the nerve endings. These responses vary from weak to strong. It is believed that one cell may be sensitive to 10 to 12 odors of varying degrees. The effect of "repeated exposure to an odor causing a decreased sensitivity to that odor" is thought to occur further along the nervous system pathway and not at the level of the olfactory cell.

### From the Olfactory Bulb to the Brain

When the impulse reaches the olfactory bulb, the olfactory nerve ending makes a connection, called a **synapse**, with output neurons called **mitral** and **tuft cells**. The importance of the olfactory bulb is the great variety of response patterns that occur here. Three basic patterns have

been identified: **1. an excitation response, 2. a supression response, or 3. no response**. To achieve this variety of responses requires many connections within the bulb. There appears to be a threshold function in the bulb as well. This requires the signal to be strong enough to elicit a response.

The olfactory bulb is a processing and screening center for odors. We know that odor recognition is quite complex and that it involves several areas of the brain. Scientists have observed that various regions of the bulb are sensitive to specific odors according to the chemical composition of the odor. Yet, the actual perception and relay of these odors will depend on the general state of the nervous system. For example, food odors are received differently when an animal is hungry than when it is satiated.

A most interesting aspect of the olfactory system is the relationship of the perception of an odor to its molecular structure. The identification of molecular structure is a major part of the sense of smell. This is believed to be accomplished by a process called **spatial encoding**. This means that various regions of the olfactory bulb will be specific for a particular odor. For example, camphor has a specific area in the olfactory bulb that responds to the shape of the camphor molecule allowing the brain to identify the odor as camphor.

### The Olfactory Bulb, the Brain, and Neurotransmitters

Since the olfactory bulb can yield various responses to stimulation we need to explain this phenomenon. One reason may be that the intense neuroactivity of the olfactory bulb is mediated by a series of chemicals called peptide hormones and single amino acids. Thyroid hormone, which we met in the chapter on biochemistry, is one of these. Two new ones are taurine and carnosine. We know that these neurotransmitters are complex and tend to interact with one another but we do not know exactly how this is accomplished.

Neurotransmitters like epinephrine and acetylcholine are not the same as the neurotransmitters we just described above. In fact, this is an unknown area of neurochemistry. We do not know how all these peptides and nonpeptide transmitters work together.

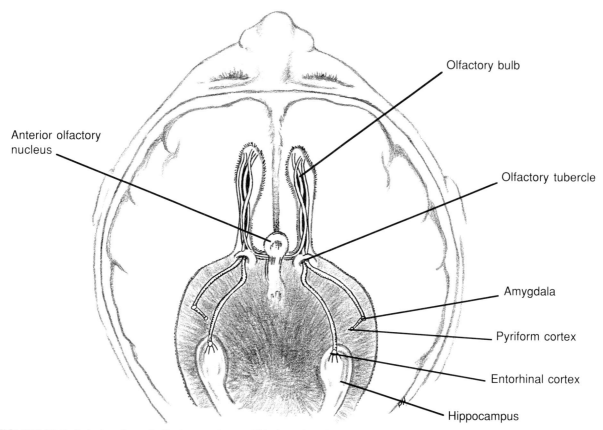

**FIGURE 13-5** Anterior view of olfactory pathway. This is a view from the top of the head. Note the olfactory connections with many parts of the brain. Each area contributes recognition and action. Terribly complex actions and associations with most parts of the brain are required to identify and to respond, or react to an odor.

As we look at these chemical transmitters we must also consider the other connections between the rest of the brain and the olfactory bulb. Keep in mind that the brain is a vast computer-like organ. It needs to have a lot of associated data to be able to interpret what it receives. All of these associated areas must, therefore, be interconnected. If you do not feel well, if you are angry, if you are disappointed, or in pain, these conditions will modify how you interpret a particular event. So it is with a simple odor. The five major connections are shown in **Figure 13-5**. Looking from the top of the head at a cutaway view of the brain you see the olfactory bulb starting at the front and running back to the midbrain where it is connected by the **anterior olfactory nucleus**. Next, you see a long nerve bundle that connects the olfactory bulb to the **pyriform cortex** on each side of the brain. This is the most important area for odor discrimination. Now look at the end of the olfactory bulb and find the **olfactory tubercle**. Fibers from the midbrain coming from the limbic system connect here. Deeper into the brain there are fibers that connect to the **corticomedial amyg-**

**dala**. Finally, there are fibers that connect to the **entorhinal cortex** in the posterior part of the brain. The entorhinal cortex projects fibers into the hippocampus.

In summary, there are three basic concepts about fragrance which you must keep in mind to understand their action on the body:

1. The action of the natural essential oils is a function of the chemical structure of the components of the oils.
2. The perception of odor is the composite of the olfactory system and the associated peptides.
3. The interpretation of the odor is a function of many associated areas in the brain.

## SOME ASPECTS OF THE SCIENCE OF PLANT AND FLOWER ESSENCES

No one knows how long natural plants have been used to treat man's disorders. My guess is that it extends far back into pre-history. We do know that the use of many plants and extracts of trees goes back five to six thousand years into

Egyptian history. While some of the names of these plants are known to us, many remain unknown. The obscure language of written Egyptian employed no vowels, so it is difficult to determine the names of plants known to them. Some which have been identified by scholars are balsam, hellebore, cypress, juniper, turpentine, myrtle, daisy tops, date-palm, lemon, apple, and a plant called Pistacia terebinthus, a turpentine plant from the Near East. We know also that frankincense and myrrh were widely used in ancient times and well known to the Egyptians. Animal fats, including lanolin and greases of all types, honey and milk, and many other agents, both holy and profane, were used to treat illnesses. Today we have literally thousands of natural products at our disposal. They come in many forms and have many uses.

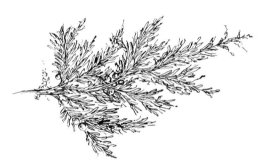

**A System of Classification**

As we have noted, every body of knowledge must be organized into a system. In the case of botanical sciences, we use a system of classification based on the physical structure of the plant. In chemistry we also use structures. We could also use the function of the chemical, for example, oxidizing or reducing agents. For our purpose, the function of the essential oil is the best method of classification. We can't classify all 4000 essential oils in this way since the function of many are not known, however, we can classify the more common ones in use today.

We shall employ the scheme of classification of the essential oils into a practical use related system and then discuss the use. There are four broad groups of essential oils based on physiological effect:
  1. **Calming**
  2. **Energizing**
  3. **Fortifying**
  4. **Correcting**

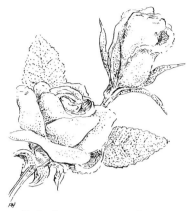

Some oils belong to more than one group as they have multiple properties. This classification is based on the action of essential oils on the skin and may not be applicable to other uses. I have included in this section some plant components and extracts that are not essential oils but are nevertheless useful as skin care products.

The Calming Group

All of the calming essential oils have the characteristic of decreasing redness or inflammation in the skin. They are also termed anti-inflammatory agents because of this property. The major ones are rose, camomile, borage, lavender, glycyrrhiza, hyssop, sarsaparilla, gotu kola, geranium, rosemary, pasiflora, melissa, and neroli.

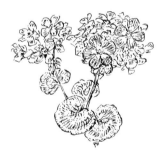

How do these natural chemical agents work? You will recall the process of inflammation and how a series of reactions are needed to produce the signs of inflammation. The calming essential oils are believed to block one or more of the steps in the inflammatory process.

The Energizing Group

This group of essential oils and plants are capable of increasing blood flow to the skin by dilating the capillaries. They may or may not

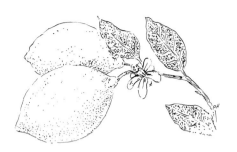

make the skin visibly red, a condition called subclinical erythema. There is a feeling of warmth and vigor with these agents. The major essential oils of this group are fennel, arnica, cinnamon bark, peppermint, pennyroyal, gotu kola, eucalyptus, echinacea, nutmeg, cloves, lemon oil, ginger, and sage.

Some of the same basic ingredients of this group may be found in the calmative group. There are terpenes in this group along with compounds known as tannins, flavanoids, and phenolic acids. These compounds have multiple biological activities, including germicidal activity. An important aspect of using the natural essential oils is that you are able to obtain multiple benefits. Let us look at peppermint as an example. This widely used essential oil has many components which include the following; menthol, menthone, menthylethoxyacetate, cineole, phytol, azulene, tocopherols, and tannins to name a few. Each of these compounds has a special function, yet when taken as a whole the effect on the biological system is pronounced. To further illustrate this complexity, a review of one of these compounds, **tannin,** is given below.

Tannin is composed of polyphenols, that is phenols that have undergone polymerization. These tannin polymers are tough to break down into smaller components. We know that tannins react with proteins to form contracted masses that precipitate from a water solution. Tannins are used in witchazel as an astringent just for this purpose.

## The Fortifying Group

I call this the fortifying group because, while it does not actively change things, it does act to strengthen the body. These are nice essential oils and plants. A few examples are: camomile, hi-biscus (as a tea), valerian root and linden flowers (also as teas), melissa, bergamot, astragalus (also known as huang qi), licorice, evening primrose, echinacea, angelica, fennel, and cardamon.

These materials are not single action chemicals, but like all other natural materials they have more than one biological action.

## The Correcting Group

This group of oils and plants are designated as correctives because they have a specific action on a particular condition as well as a general biological action as seen with most natural products. In this section I shall only list those essential oils and plants that are useful in skin care. Savory in healing, sage as an astringent and antiseptic, peppermint as a local analgesic, thuja for warts, onion for insect bites and infections, lemon for infections, lavender for inflammations of all types, hyssop for eczema, marigold for irritated skin, melissa for both fungal infections and irritations of all types, and camomile which is useful for skin irritations.

## Some Notes on the Use of Essential Oils

In classical philosophy there is an old adage *"in medio stat veritas"* which translates, in the middle stands the truth. It is impossible to have too much knowledge about essential oils, but on the other hand, a limited knowledge can be dangerous. So learn all that you can about how essential oils work and how to use them. Your best source of instruction is from someone who has a long experience with the use of essential oils. Some pharmacological points that will help you to understand some of the ways essential oils work are given below.

Before any active ingredient can have an effect on the body as a whole, it must first have a **cellular effect**. The essential oil is applied on the skin by massage, a large area is covered, and the oil penetrates the skin to the lower layers, eventually reaching the blood stream. Once in the blood stream, it circulates around the body and reaches all the cells. The effect on the cell will be related to the amount of essential oil that reaches the cell. The amount that penetrates the skin is related to the amount applied, in what vehicle it is applied, and the condition of the skin.

**Cellular effect = amount of essential oil reaching the cell = amount applied to the skin + vehicle + skin condition.**

Essential oil applied on inflammed or broken skin has a greater potential for an adverse effect than essential oil applied on normal, intact skin.

## HOW TO MAKE A DOSE RESPONSE CURVE

A basic technique of pharmacology that will help you to understand the actions and uses of essential oils is the dose response relationship. This relationship is represented in the form of a graph. A graph is nothing more than a visual display relating two parameters such as time and distance, speed and distance, or blood pressure and the dose of a drug. The vertical line on the graph is the y-axis and the horizontal line is the x-axis. You see this in **Figure 13-6**. If you wish to plot the blood pressure of an individual on the y-axis (the conventional term, for blood pressure is millimeters of mercury or mm Hg). Write at the bottom of the vertical line 0 and at regular intervals along the line write 10, 20, 30, 40, and so on up to 250 mm Hg. These numbers will be the actual values you will record on the graph after you take the person's blood pressure.

A drug, which we shall call K5R-2, is given to the individual in a dosage form based on the

weight of the subject. The subject is male and weighs 72.2 Kg. The amount that you give will be in milligrams (mg) of drug for every kilogram (kg) of body weight of the subject. Let us start with 1 mg for every kg; write this as 1 mg/kg. This means that if you have a 70 kg subject you will use 1 mg x 70 kg = 70 mg of K5R-2 drug. See what effect this drug will have on the blood pressure if you keep doubling the dose. Put the data first into the column.

| Blood Pressure (mm Hg) | Dose of K5R-2 mg | Note |
|---|---|---|
| 120 | 0 | Baseline |
| 120 | 72.2 | No effect |
| 130 | 144.4 | Slight effect |
| 140 | 288.8 | Slight effect |
| 160 | 577.6 | Marked effect |
| 200 | 1152.0 | Marked effect |
| 200 | 2300.0 | No effect |
| 200 | 5000.0 | No effect |

Notice three things: 1. only the systolic blood pressure was measured, 2. the dose was rounded off as you got higher, and 3. after a certain dose you no longer had an effect. Now plot the graph. There is a flat line at 200 mg Hg regardless of how much of the drug was given. It would be useless with this drug to keep raising the dose to get a greater effect, since the body does not respond with a blood pressure increase after about 1000 mg or (1 gram).

This does not mean that there will be no effect on other body functions. For instance, we did not record side effects like nausea, dizziness, vomiting, headache, and so forth. Only systolic blood pressure was measured.

**Figure 13-7** shows a **linear response curve.** As you increase the dose the effect increases in the same way. If you double the dose you double the effect.

**Figure 13-8** shows a **sigmoidal curve.** It tells us that there is only a narrow range of efficacy with this drug. As you increase the dose you only creep up on the maximum effect and suddenly you are there! These are very difficult drugs to work with as the dose is tricky and potentially dangerous.

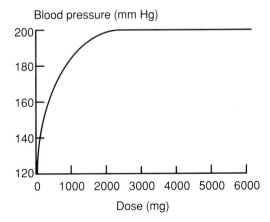

**DOSE RESPONSE
K5R-2**

Blood pressure (mm Hg)

Dose (mg)

**FIGURE 13-6** K5R-2 dose reponse curve. Here we have an increase in blood pressure with increasing doses of K5R-2 depicted by the graph. At 2000 mg there is no futher increase in blood pressure. At this level you would expect toxic effects to increase without any beneficial effects.

## DOSE RESPONSE LINEAR

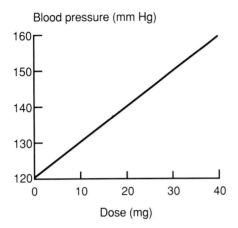

**FIGURE 13-7** Linear dose response curve. In this dose response curve there is a constant increase in effect (blood pressure rise) with an increase in dosage of the drug. This is a very rare effect in a biological system because of the homeostatic mechanism in the body.

Each time you use an essential oil automatically ask yourself: 1. do I have the right essential oil?, 2. do I have the proper dose?, 3. am I seeing the response I expect?, and 4. are there any side effects?

If you use the oils premixed in proper dosage with instructions showing how to use them, it is unlikely that you will experience difficulties. Remember, to mix your own you need to know a great deal about what you are doing and how the oils work on the cells.

## SPECIFIC CONDITIONS AND USES OF PLANT AND PLANT EXTRACTS

### Introduction

Possibly 70% or more of our medical treatments are derived from plant materials. Some of the most potent of these are digitalis from foxglove, opium from poppies, vincristine sulfate from periwinkle (an anti-cancer drug), quinine from cindona bark for malaria, colchicine from colchicum for gout, belladona from nightshade, and many others. The major difference between natural product use and the use of plant material in medical science is that medical science prefers to use the isolated active principle rather than a whole plant extract. There are many active agents in the plant extract while the isolated agent will have only one activity. In the latter case, the active principle is identified and may thus be characterized and quantified which makes dosing easier to control. Digitalis, for example, was used as the powdered leaf for many years to treat heart failure, or dropsy. It was given in water or as a compressed tablet; the patient was instructed to take enough leaf over one day to become nauseated and vomit.

This product was far more difficult to prescribe for patients than pure digitoxin when it became available. We must use common sense when we select products for client treatment. The most important consideration must be safety followed by efficacy.

### Acne Treatment

This is the most common skin condition seen by the skin care specialist. It will be the reason for more visits than any other skin condition. We must distinguish active, maculo-pustular acne from comedo-laden acne.

### Maculo-pustular Acne

The first step is to quiet down the inflammatory acne with calming agents. A few drops of lavender and rose essential oils should be placed into a steam apparatus and allowed to run for 10 to 15 minutes. The pustules should

## DOSE RESPONSE SIGMOID

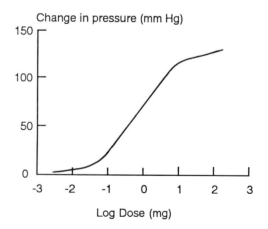

**FIGURE 13-8** Sigmoidal dose response curve. The sigmoidal curve tells us there is a fairly narrow range between the effective dose and the maximum dose. The steepness or slope of this curve is important to pharmacologists. Note the x-axis is labeled "Log Dose". This means the dose in mgs has been converted to logarithmic form for convenience in graphing the result.

next be opened with a lancet and the contents drained with a gauze pad or a cotton tipped applicator. Only the most gentle pressure should be applied to these lesions. Next, soak with two 4 x 4 gauze pads previously prepared by immersing 4 x 4's in a camomile and cajuput infusion with 50% witch hazel (10 drops of chamomile oil plus 5 drops of cajuput oil in one ounce of hot water , then add one ounce of warm witch hazel). Have the client repeat this treatment of witch hazel and camomile compresses at home twice daily for the next 4 days. See the client on the fifth day. Most of the pustules and macules should be gone or greatly decreased. Do not do extractions at this time. If the face is free of pustules and only a few macules are seen you should do a facial cleansing, opening milia, but do not do extractions. Extractions should be done only when the face is quiet, that is, no macules or pustules.

Each time the client comes in for treatment, steam the face again and apply the witch hazel-camomile-cajuput infusion. Do extractions as needed. The client can be maintained on a cream or lotion that contains an extract of echinacea and camomile along with vitamin A and vitamin E. I prefer the use of vitamin A acetate rather than vitamin A palmitate. Remember that acne is a lifelong treatment problem and will frequently flare-up and then subside.

## Treatment of Aging Skin with Natural Products

Natural products can benefit aging skin both in prevention and in treatment. The condition of the skin is very important. If you are faced with a deeply lined, sun damaged client with a leathery-looking skin you are best advised to refer that client to a plastic surgeon. You will have much better results after the surgery in maintaining the new youthful appearance of the client's skin. The key is to avoid the sun and to continue to use proper skin care. Here is my suggested treatment for a moderately aged skin, or a post-surgical skin.

### Professional Treatment

Make a comprehensive evaluation of the client's skin including all lesions and the degree of elasticity. If you are unable to measure the elasticity with an instrument, use a visual method such as observing the lines on the client's face in both the lying and sitting positions. The lines in the sitting position will generally run in a vertical direction (see **Figure 13-9**) with some curvature. With poor elasticity in the supine position the lines will appear to fade or change directions. The only lines that will be apparent in skin with good elasticity will be the creases known as the nasolabial folds at the angle of the mouth running to the nose. Sometimes, even in a young person, there may be a fold at the corner of the mouth running to the chin. This fold will fade when the client is on her or his back (supine). It is easily seen even in the skin of the young adult, but is far more noticeable in the lax skin of the older client.

### Natural Product Program for Aging Skin

Document all lesions on the client's face. Then do a thorough cleansing and moisturization program. Next, use a steam treatment with lavender oil for about 5 minutes. Follow this treatment with a facial massage that will provide lymphatic drainage, taking care not to use excessive pressure, and follow the direction of lymph flow. This operation should not take more than 5-6 minutes.

The next massage is a stimulating action to the skin in which the skin is alternately pulled and tapped to create a pumping action. This is done rather vigorously to affect a flush or erythematous reaction in the skin, but obviously without trauma. It is a learned technique familiar to all trained massage therapists.

Having completed the massage, the skin is ready for a fresh mask. I prefer a fresh parsley mask with a high level of echinacea root, or echinacea extract. There are several reasons for the use of these agents: 1. fresh parsley contains high levels of vitamin C and carotene as well as minute amount of essential oils, and 2. echinacea contains certain glucosides and dipentenes that are beneficial to the immune system. I suggest the following formula to prepare the mask; you will need a high speed food blender to make this mask.

## Parsley-Echinacea Mask Formula

Place into a blender a half bunch of parsley

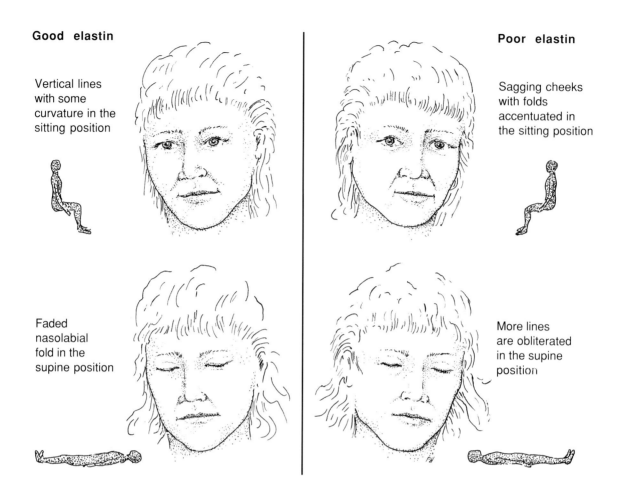

Vertical lines
with some
curvature in the
sitting position

Sagging cheeks
with folds
accentuated in
the sitting position

Faded
nasolabial
fold in the
supine position

More lines
are obliterated
in the supine
position

**FIGURE 13-9** Good and poor elastin comparison in sitting and supine positions. When the body is in a sitting position the force of gravity tends to increase the facial lines. In the supine position the lines are effaced, or diminished. Only the nasolabial fold is visible in individuals with good elastic tissue below age 30.

well washed and with the stems removed as much as possible, leaving only the leaves. Then add the echinacea aqueous extract (about one ounce), along with whole wheat flour (about one tablespoon).

To this mixture add three to four drops of energizing oils. Blend at high speed until smooth and apply to the face. Let the mask dry about 10-15 minutes and then remove with a gauze sponge. Finish cleansing the face with a rose water-echinacea toner and apply a day moisturizing cream that contains vitamin C, vitamin E, and beta 1,3 glucan.

I recommend this treatment be done professionally at least every two weeks for the first two months and monthly thereafter. The home treatment routine should consist of a gentle cleanser, a day and night product, and a toner. The routine use of these products is described in Chapter 9 where we covered the treatment of aging skin.

You need to be well trained in the techniques of lymphatic drainage and stimulating massage to make this treatment effective.

**Fragrances, Stress, and the Skin**

We discussed some aspects of stress when we wrote about nutrition and the skin. It is time again to look at some other aspects of stress and how stress affects our skin, particularly in regard to aging. In the aging process the effect of stress on the blood circulation to the skin is profound and is capable of producing an ischemic condition (ischemia is decreased blood and oxygen to tissue). What is most remarkable is that a state of calm is able to increase this blood flow.

We have a tendency to associate anxiety with increased functions of the nervous system, things like being jittery or jumpy. In fact, the newer research now indicates the opposite effect. While there may be some increased motor activity in the early stages of anxiety, what follows is a slowing down of physiological functions. These complex effects combine to make the anxious person feel very bad.

It is important to remember that we need some stress to function normally. It is not the stress that produces the damage, it is how we react and respond to the stress. This is a key observation as it forms the basis for all stress treatment.

The role of fragrance in stress reduction continues to be studied throughout the world. A great deal of information has been generated on this subject with very positive results. Fragrance in the work place has reduced illness and absenteeism while increasing overall productivity.

In the treatment of skin conditions that are associated with inflammation or aging, stress must be dealt with constantly. As we saw in the chapter on nutrition, excess or uncontrolled stress will cause a profound biological reaction that will interfere with normal physiology. The essential oils that are associated with stress reduction are lavender, rose, and camomile. These may be inhaled, used in a relaxing bath, or applied in a massage oil.

**The Anatomy of a Fragrance**

There are a few very great fragrances that have retained the public interest over many years. Some of these fragrances have been the starting point for new industrial growth. Sometimes it is difficult to determine if the ingredients or the names were more important to the success of fragrances. We do find that the success of a commercial fragrance can never be guaranteed. Some are very successful, then disappear from the market, others will last for many years, from one generation to another.

The Nose Knows

The creative perfumer is not endowed with a special nose. It is a well trained nose. Having experienced thousands of fragrance materials and how they interact has produced a very sensitive detection system for the perfumer. No two individuals will have the same response to a fragrance, any more than a fragrance will be per-

ceived as identical on two individuals. So it is not an easy matter to create a widely acceptable, commercial fragrance, let alone a very successful fragrance. To construct a fragrance, remember that creative ability requires not only skill but imagination.

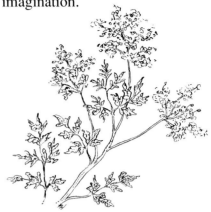

Scent Classification

1. **Floral scents** may be single or bouquet. Single notes are jasmine, hyacinth, tuberose, gardenia, lilac, lily of the valley, and rose. Bouquets are scents that have several floral singles together.
2. **Green scents** are like the odor of a crushed leaf. Here we have pine and mint, while camphor is stark green with lavender being less green.
3. **Citrus scents** are familiar to everyone and include lemon, orange, tangerine, bergomot, and neroli.
4. **Chypre** is a complex scent (from the French word for cypress). It includes a group of scents that end up having a warm, soft, and sweet fragrance.
5. **Oriental blends** are heavy perfumes that have heavy animal notes and include spices, incense resins, and woody notes such as sandalwood, cedar, and patchouli.
6. **Aldehydics** are also called modern perfumes. They have strong top notes that have a pungent but pleasant smell.
7. **Leather scents** are strong animal scents. Ambergris, musk, and civet yield these lasting scents.

Other terms used by many perfumers are **mossy, fishy, metallic, burnt, maritime, spiritous, fruity,** etc. Often terms are combined such as green-spicy, or spicy-floral, etc.

**Tone** refers to odors that are sharp, mild, or low. A low tone is a warm heavy odor. Fixatives are used to make a fragrance last longer. They are high molecular weight materials like ambergris. Low molecular weight materials will give a **lift** to the blend (**zingy** is the word used today). A well made perfume has "body" rather than being "light". Notes are of three types. The **top note** comes off first, giving the perfume an immediate acceptance, the **middle note** gives the sniffer the desire to buy the fragrance, and the **base note** is the lingering essence that complexes with our being.

Now you have the materials, that is, the essential oils; you know what types of oils have what kind of scent; and you know that a fragrance usually has three notes. Next, you must decide what you want to create. The rest is simply experimentation. The technical part of perfumery is very complex when you intend to produce a fragrance for a particular product. Many chemical aspects of the product and the fragrance need to be known before you may be able to do this. Here is a simple fragrance that consists of only six essential oils.

Top note: bergamot and lemon, middle note: neroli amd thyme, base note: vanillin and patchouli. Play around with the percentages of each until you find a good blend.

Finally, let us look at a few other aspects of fragrance and perception of odors. Perception is complicated word in the English language for it means not only to be aware of something received by our senses but also to know or to recognize the object or "thing" which we sense. In the case of odors, this is a most complex phenomenon which we shall look at briefly with the eyes of the psychophysicist.

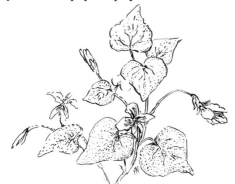

## PSYCHOPHYSICS OF OLFACTION

Psychophysics is a branch of psychology that studies the laws that relate physical stimulation to psychological response. In the realm of fragrances, psychophysics attempts to relate the intensity or the response to an odor, to some physical characteristic. For example, does the number of molecules of an odorant presented to the nose affect the response of the person detecting the odorant? Let us look at a few of the variables that have been studied by psychophysicists.

### Smoking

Does smoking affect the perception of odors? Well, when researche workers tackled this problem they found that there were many variables in the study. Actually, too many variables to draw valid conclusions. We know that the number of cigarettes smoked, the number of years of smoking, and the type of odor presented all influence the degree of perception by the subject. Most people who quit smoking experience an increase in appetite that they attribute to better tasting food, or a keener appreciation of the taste of food. We do not have the answers yet.

### Male Versus Female

Do women have a keener sense of smell? Research is this area indicates that women do have a keener sense of smell and can detect certain odors better than men. This phenomenon is related to hormones and thus may have a cyclic nature.

### Effect of Age

It is known that older individuals have a reduced sensitivity to certain odors, perhaps as much as three to eight times less than a younger person. Further research now indicates that the older nose can be trained to identify odors and reach a higher level of detection. Again, many factors influence this phenomenon, particularly, the type of odor present. The odor in cooking gas has been added to help detect a gas leak, but unfortunately this is an odor not easily detected by older persons.

### Odor Intensity

A great deal of research has centered on the intensity of odors as a function of concentration of the odorant, the chemical nature of the odorant and the magnitude of the response perceived by the subject. It appears that there is no simple law that governs this relationship since doubling the concentration does not double the perception of the odor. Certainly, the size and shape of the molecule influences the detection, but with larger molecules increasing the concentration does not produce a proportional increase in detection. This is one case in which knowing this fact will prevent you from using too high a concentration of an odorant such as an essential oil.

### Odor Fatigue

We have all experienced some obnoxious odor that other people do not seem to notice or mind. This is called an **adaptation phenomenon** and it has been measured. With continual exposure, perceived intensity will decrease to about 30% of the initial preception. This is a blessing in some ways.

### Other Factors - The Trigeminal Influence

The trigeminal nerve is a sensory nerve that conducts sensations from the nose and oral cavity. The ophthalmic branch and the maxillary branch of this nerve are responsible for the "cool" sensation of menthol and the sharp pungency of ammonia. Now, it is a curious fact, but the concentration of a material that activates the trigeminal nerve is very important to the intensity perceived by the subject. Unlike olfactory perceptions, the trigeminal nerve has the ability to sense high concentrations of potent irritants. In effect, this is a warning system that helps to protect us from these potentially dangerous substances. A small change or difference in concentration produces a large increase in perceived intensity.

Another finding in trigeminal nerve research is mixed signals that stimulate both olfactory and trigeminal nerves. In these cases one signal may totally blunt the other signal.

### Some Observations on Olfactory Cortical Output

As we have discussed in this chapter the actual body response to an odor is extremely complex. We are not sure if there is a **direct** chemical effect of the odor or if there is **only a recognition factor**. We know that various essential oils, for example, when studied for electrophysiological response will produce either "calming or excitatory responses." These are physiological responses that are measured by physical means, such as brain wave pattern, pulse, breathing rate, blood pressure, sweating, and many others. We are able to classify many agents in this manner but we do not know why they produce these various responses. The multiple connections of the olfactory cortex may provide some clues to this mystery, so let us look at a few of these connection.

### The Thalamus (pronouced thal'ah-mus) Gr *Thalamos* = inner room.

Activity from virtually the entire olfactory cortex is funneled through a small number of cells in the thalamus. This is called the transthalamic olfactory pathway. Just consider what goes on in the thalamus, for an instant and you will be impressed with the complexity. Over 20 nuclei function in the thalamus which integrate sensory information, acting as a relay center to and from the cerebral cortex. Impulses arriving from the olfactory cortex interact with or are modified by other sensory information. There is more complexity, however, since the neocortex which projects from the olfactory cortex receives the direct input from the olfactory bulb. The thalamus receives all other sensory impulses. We do not know the reason for this, but it is believed that the **neocortex** processes olfactory impulses and the thalamus in some manner modulates these impulses.

### Hypothalamus

Parts of the olfactory cortex project down to the lateral hypothalamus. The accessory olfactory system has a key role in olfactory information transfer within the hypothalamus. Without going further into the neuroanatomy of this system, there are fibers that connect with other nuclei in this area, that process and control activity in sexual reproduction and the neuroendocrine system. Even more, the hypothalamus controls many vital processes associated with the autonomic nervous system. The hypothalamus is concerned with regulating temperature, wa-

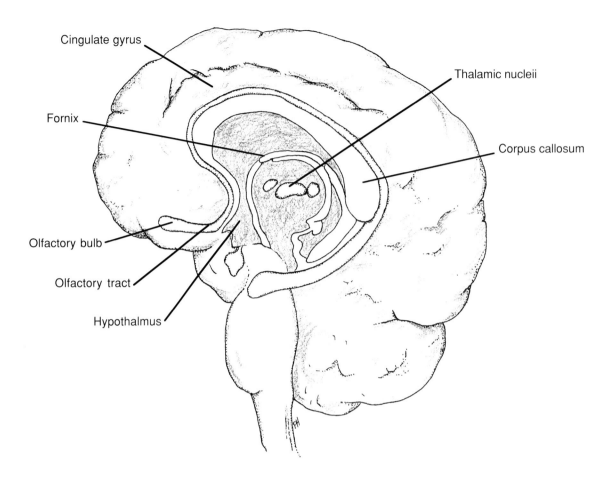

Cingulate gyrus

Thalamic nucleii

Fornix

Corpus callosum

Olfactory bulb

Olfactory tract

Hypothalmus

**FIGURE 13-10** The limbic system represents an important group of brain structures. Remember that while these individual structures have specific functions of their own, they are integrated into the limbic system which is concerned mainly with expression of emotions.

ter balance, appetite, gastrointestinal activity, and expression of emotion, particularly, fear and rage. Imagine the effect of a dysfunction in this area!

### The Limbic System (L. *limbus* - a border or hem)

The **limbic system** is often mentioned in discussions on the action of essential oils. The **limbic system** regulates emotional behavior and consists of the following structure, **the olfactory bulb, the fornix, the cingulate gyrus, basal ganglia, mammallary bodies, thalamic and hypothalamic nuclei**. See **Figure 13-10**.

**Why is all this information needed for a skin care specialist?** I believe it is very important to know what you are doing with various fragrances. The art and science of fragrance is still in its infancy. We are only now starting to take this subject seriously. You must understand that when you **activate the olfactory sensors you are having a profound effect on the entire brain, and thus on the whole body**. What I have outlined is only the very basic information needed to appreciate the complexity of the olfactory system. If you find this interesting then you need to study more of the basic physiology, neurochemistry and biochemistry. You can, of course, use essential oils and other fragrances in your practice but the more you know about them the better you will be able to use them.

You've gotten to know me, your Topical Agent, pretty well, and I know you'll never forget me and you're always going to want me around. I'll always be here for you, kid, but like Gramps and Dad, my time will soon be past. So I want you to keep an open mind about those smoothies that will come after me...give

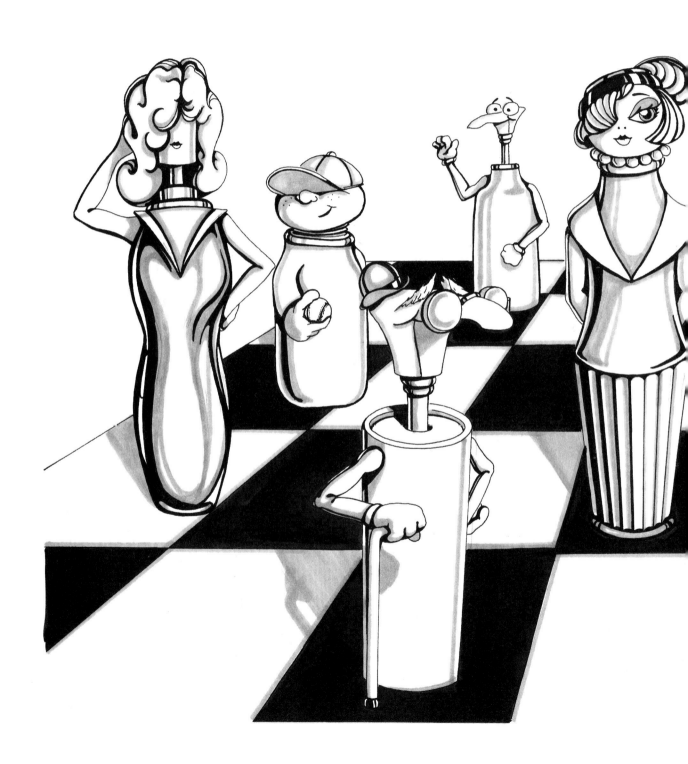

them a chance. But, just like choosing friends--look for what's inside, what they're made of...that's what really matters.

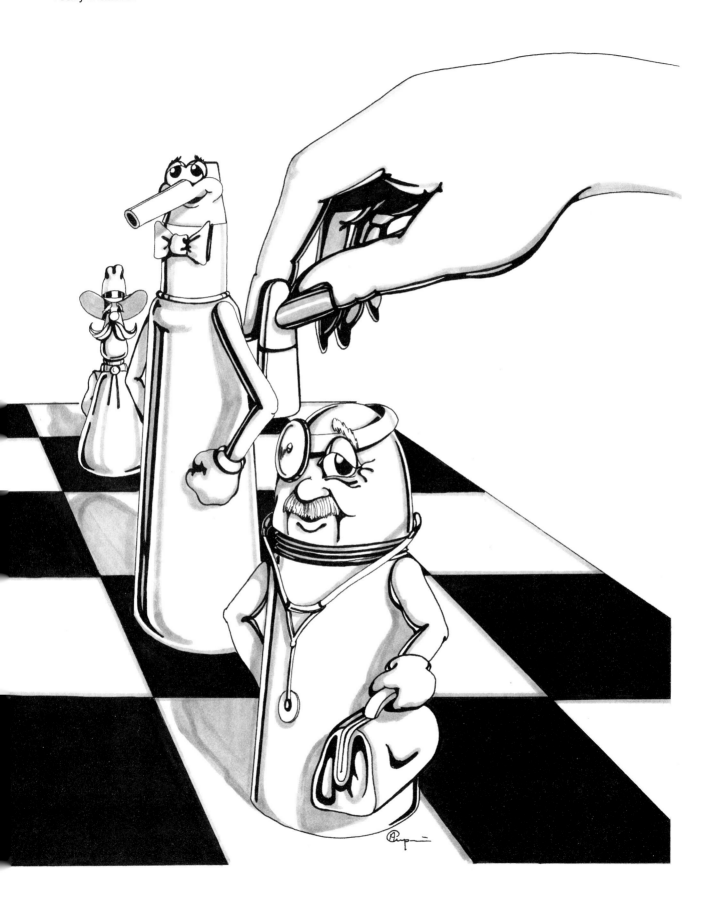

# Skin Care Products - What They Are and How to Use Them

Skin care product development is both an art and a science. It is not possible to learn, either the art or the science of formulation from one book chapter on the subject. At best, I plan to introduce the reader to the subject, provide acquaintance with the terminology and present some basic formulations. This introduction, hopefully, will help to guide the reader in the selection and appreciation of skin care products. It is a worthy habit to ask what and why of each new product you plan to use. It is my purpose in this chapter to provide for you the necessary information to ask the proper questions in order to be knowledgeable about the product.

The ideal product should be cosmetically acceptable, not stain or have an unpleasant odor, be able to hold and release active ingredients, and be safe and effective.

All skin care products may be divided into two types, **corrective, that is, treatment, or maintenance, which includes protective**. Color cosmetics will fall into either category or both. Skin care products are used to keep our skin looking good, that is, attractive, or to correct a bad or blemished skin. If you think in these terms you will have little difficulty understanding what follows. A good starting point is to look at some products on the shelf, analyze the claims, and then see if the ingredients inside the product actually fulfill this promise.

In this chapter we must look at what makes up a product, how the product is put together, and how it is tested for efficacy and safety. You will also learn in this chapter how to analyze a product for ingredients and predict with reasonable accuracy whether it will work or not. I shall touch briefly on the FDA's role in cosmetic product regulation.

## A WALK THROUGH THE PRODUCT JUNGLE

A skin care specialist with sufficient background knowledge must be able to understand the ingredients in a skin care formula, and how the formula is designed to work as a whole. First, we need to look at the basic parts of a skin care formula. Look for the **active ingredients**. Then look for the **emulsifier ingredients**, the **auxillary ingredients**, the **fragrance** and finally, the **preservatives**. **Most products will have these four basic groups of ingredients**.

Now, let us look at how each of these basic groups function in the formula.

Creams, ointments, and lotions are the most common physical forms of cosmetics. Ointments are usually formulations that do not contain water so they are called **anhydrous products**. The other two forms, the creams and lotions, present the greatest difficulty in formulation. A cosmetic formulation must be pleasing to see, smell, feel and use; in addition, it must be safe. Putting together all the ingredients to achieve a cosmetic product is the art and science of formulation. The key problem is the emulsion system. Understanding the emulsion system helps you see how the product is put together, what distinguishes a cheap product from an expensive one, how elegance is achieved, and why some systems just don't work.

## EMULSIONS AND SURFACTANTS

An **emulsion** is a combination of water and oil that is stabilized by an emulsifier. In order to keep the emulsion together, since water and oil do not mix, it is necessary to have some agent that will allow this union to take place. This is the role of the emulsifier. The oil may be dispersed in the water, or the water may be dispersed in the oil. Either system will produce a stable emulsion depending on the **surfactant**. **Surfactant** is a short form of "surface-active agent". These agents reduce the energy at the surface of a material with which they come into contact. There are five reasons for their use in cosmetics: as **detergents** for cleansing, as **wetting agents** in perms, as **foaming agents** in shampoos, as **emulsifiers** for creams and lotions, and as **solubilizers** for perfumes and flavors. We shall look at surfactants as emulsifiers. Before we get into this section, a word of comfort first. You will meet new terminology which I shall define, but it may still be somewhat confusing. Do not worry about this, it will come to you after a bit of repetition. Below, I have listed the most important group of emulsifiers, defined them, and added examples of each.

### Classification of Emulsifiers

1. **Anionic surfactants** have a surface active ion that is **negatively charged. Negative is the important word**. They are the most com-

mon emulsifiers used in cosmetics as they are cheap and stable. An example is soap. Soap, as you know, is fatty acid neutralized with lye, or sodium hydroxide (NaOH). This will produce a chemical that has a negative charge on the fatty acid and a positive charge on the sodium part. Here is the reaction.

Oleic acid + NaOH (sodium hydroxide) = sodium oleate (a soap) and water.

When you place soap in water with some fatty material, such as grease, the sodium oleate will dissolve (ionized). The sodium part seeks water and the oleate part seeks fatty material. Since they are charged molecules they hold the water, fat, and emulsifier together forming an **emulsification**. That is all there is to it! Now, let's look at another type of emulsifier.

**Cationic emulsifiers have a positive charged surfactant**. Many cationic emulsifiers are also called "quat" emulsifiers because their chemical nature involves a nitrogen with a valence of five, that is, 5 positive charges. Usually three of these charges are taken up by methyl groups, one charge is taken up by the long chain surfactant group, and the other charge is left positive to react with the anionic or negative molecule. This we saw in the soap emulsifier. Quat cationic emulsifiers are often germicidal as well. Cationic emulsifiers bind to the skin and leave a smooth, conditioned feeling. You may be familiar with chlorahexidine which is a cationic material used as a germicide.

**Nonionic surfactants are essentially uncharged surfactants.** They have, as a rule, either hydroxyl groups (OH) or ethylene oxide groups that aid in the emulsification. They can be used with either cationic or anionic emulsifiers as an auxillary emulsifier. The chief disadvantage to this group of compounds is that they tend to react with the germicidal agents and make them less active. An example is the Tween product line, which is also called polysorbs, and glyceryl monostearate.

**Ampholytic surfactants have the ability to form both a positive and negative surface-active ion**. They can be made to be very gentle and find frequent use in low irritation shampoos, such as baby shampoo.

The properties of emulsifiers differ according to the charge and the fatty acid they make

up, the active-surface agent. Below are some effects on the skin.

<u>Effects of Surfactants on Skin</u>

The two major effects are skin wetting and degreasing. Excellent cleansing properties derive from these actions. Excess cleansing can defat the skin, breaking down the lipid barrier and causing irritation and chapping. As a rule, surfactants with long chains and the addition of many ethylene oxide groups will reduce irritation potential. Cationic surfactants should not be used near the eye as they bind to protein and may cause damage. On the other hand, this is why they make such excellent conditioners for hair.

Toxic properties of surfactants also vary by types. Cationics are more irritating then anionics and anionics are more irritating than nonionics. Most surfactants are of such low irritation that they are safe for cosmetic use.

## THE ACTIVE INGREDIENTS

Now that you are familiar with emulsification we are ready to look into active ingredients. These agents actually do the job of making the cosmetic product effective. It is why the customer buys the product. Since there are so many active ingredients we shall limit our discussion to those used in **antiaging products**. First, we will need a rationale basis for selecting these ingredients. To do that we need to know what is aging? What are the physiological causes of aging? What physiological systems can we try to correct? How do these systems relate to the changes in the skin? There are many more questions to be asked but these are starting questions for the formulator.

Assuming that we accept the theory that aging skin is due to environmentally induced damage, we have a starting point. This theory states that free radical damage is one of the major causes of reduced skin functioning. **Aging can be defined as physical and biochemical changes in our body characterized by reduced physiological functions**. Our job is to find agents that will prevent further damage and try to correct the damage that is present. The physiological changes in aging of the skin are mostly known. They are 1. a decrease in epidermal proliferative activity, 2. a decrease in normal elastin production, 3. a decrease in collagen production, 4. a change in the secretion of ground substances, 5. a decrease in capillary circulation, 6. decreased enzyme activity, and 7. decreased immune function. We have agents that will help many of these negative conditions.

## A List of Known Active Antiaging Ingredients

### Vitamin A and Vitamin A Derivatives.

This group includes Retin A, a prescription drug; retinyl palmitate, retinyl acetate, and other newer forms of retinol esters. This group is a very essential part of the current agents effective against aging.

### Vitamin E and Vitamin E Derivatives

Vitamin E is alpha tocopherol. We use tocopheryl acetate, tocopheryl linoleate and tocopheryl nicotinate. This is an important antiaging vitamin. More than just an antioxidant, vitamin E is finding use in many areas of modern medicine. It has a wide margin of safety, both orally and topically. As much as 3000 mg may be taken daily without serious side effects, though 1000 mg daily is considered a high dose.

### Vitamin C and Derivatives

Vitamin C is needed for connective tissue building and maintenance. It is difficult to stabilize in an emulsion. The natural form is ascorbic acid and is not stable in cosmetics. Ascorbyl palmitate is used but it also has some problems. Recently, ascorbyl phosphate has appeared and it seems to be stable.

### Panthenol and Panthenol Derivatives

Pantothenic acid is essential for normal body function. It is used in products as the alcohol, panthenol. It has many uses in the body and is essential in all phases of metabolism.

### Immune Active Agents

This is a relatively new group of compounds that you will hear more about over the next few years. Some of these are proprietary while others are well known. Beta 1,3 glucan is a natural immune stimulant that is effective on the skin. Echinacea augustifolia contains immune ingredients that may be used as isolated extracts or whole extracts. Certain mushrooms are effective as general immune stimulants. A few of these are zhi ling, shiitake, and enokidake.

### Antioxidants

Many new antioxidants have come into use in cosmetics in recent years. Some of these are vitamin E, wheat germ oil, ascorbic acid, dihydroguaretic acid and certain tannins.

## Auxillary Ingredients

### Moisturizers

Many vegetable oils act as effective moisturizers. Some of the better ones are jojoba oil, avocado oil and almond oil. Natural waxes, such as beeswax, perform as moisturizers in emulsions. The lanolin series of compounds also serve well as moisturizers. Remember, **moisturization must occur from the bottom of the skin and not from the top**. Moisturizers afford some partial occlusion of skin thereby retaining skin water, and thus, providing moisture to the upper layer.

### Emollients

**Emollients** are products that soften the skin. This covers many oils and other materials, such as mucin and other polysaccharides from plants. Many synthetic materials are available for this purpose. The general rule is the smaller the chain length (number of carbon atoms in molecule that makes up the material) the quicker it will penetrate and the more fleeting will be the effect. Silicone is an excellent emollient as well as an excellent moisturizer. It is available in many forms.

### Essential Oils

The essential oils serve as both fragrance materials and as product preservatives. It may be necessary in some cases to add an auxillary preservative depending on the type of formulation and the use of the formulation.

## Humectants

**Humectants** are agents that hold water. They usually contain a lot of OH groups. The most widely used humectants are glycerine and propylene glycol. Glycerine is also known as glycerol and is a natural product.

There are over 4000 ingredients a cosmetic chemist can choose from to make a single formula. A great deal of study and experience can lead to skill in making a superb formula. As mentioned before, even with great skill, trial and error are often needed to polish a formula into being a great or superior product. It is now time to look at a few formulae and see how they are put together.

Let us put together a simple formula for skin moisturization. We shall look at both **oil-in-water and water-in-oil emulsions**. At the same time we shall explore the different types of emulsifiers we discussed above.

## HOW TO PUT TOGETHER AN EMULSION FORMULA

When baking a cake you need the ingredient list and the directions for mixing and baking the cake. This is called a recipe, in cosmetic chemistry we call it a **formula**. The general directions are part of the formula. The few simple rules are easy to learn. You will have an oil phase and a water phase, just as in cake baking you have dry and wet ingredients. You must weigh out the ingredients in grams or pounds; for a small amount of product we shall use grams. After weighing out all the ingredients in the oil phase put them into a glass beaker, then weigh out the water phase ingredients and place them in another glass beaker. Next, heat both beakers to 60-70 degrees C while stirring. This can be done conveniently on a hot plate equipped with a magnetic stirrer. You will need two thermometers. After you reach a temperature of 70 degrees carefully pour the water phase into the oil phase while constantly stirring. The mixture usually turns color (white) and will thicken as it cools. It is best to keep stirring until the product reaches 35 degrees, or even to room temperature. Fragrance should be added when the temperature reaches 40-45 degrees C. Do not add fragrance to the product at a hotter temperature.

That is it. Keep in mind that anything as hot as 70 degree C will burn if it spills on you.

## Oil-In-Water Emulsions

Most of the creams and lotions used in the cosmetic industry are based on oils that are emulsified in water. These formulae will evaporate if exposed to air. (The top is left off the jar.)

They are also called "vanishing creams" because they disappear when rubbed into the skin, unlike cold cream which is a water-in-oil emulsion. Soap is the most frequently used emulsifier for oil-in-water emulsions. By adding stearic acid fat to the formula in the oil phase and triethanolamine (TEA) to the water phase, heating both to 60 to 70 degrees C, then pouring the two together, an emulsion will form. The combination of stearic acid and TEA will make TEA-stearate (a soap). These emulsions are stable and cheap, but they are most often alkaline. They tend to break down in the acid states. Here are some examples of oil-in-water formulae.

### Two Hand Lotions (Cheap, Easy, and Stable Formulae)

| Oil Phase | % by Volume | | Function |
|---|---|---|---|
| Cocoa butter | 2.0 | 5.0 | emollient |
| Spermaceti | 3.0 | 2.0 | moisturizer |
| Stearic acid | 4.0 | 4.0 | emulsifier |
| Propyl paraben | 0.15 | 0.15 | preservative |

| Water Phase | | | |
|---|---|---|---|
| Methyl paraben | 0.15 | 0.1 | preservative |
| Potassium | | | |
| Hydroxide | 0.40 | - | base for soap |
| Triethanolamine | - | 1.50 | base for soap |
| Glycerol | 7.00 | 3.0 | humectant |
| Water | 83.00 | 83.9 | |
| Fragrance | 0.30 | 0.30 | |

Here is a nonionic/anionic cream that may be used for hand or body. This is an old timer that uses mineral oil and lanolin with glycerol monostearate as the nonionic emulsifier. Note again the formation of the TEA-stearate soap.

| Oil Phase | % by Volume |
|---|---|
| Mineral oil | 2.0 |
| Modulan$^R$ (lanolin) | 2.0 |

| Amerchol l-101[R] | 4.0 |
|---|---|
| Stearic acid | 6.0 |
| Glycerol monostearate | 12.0 |
| Propyl paraben | 0.15 |

| Water Phase | |
|---|---|
| Methyl paraben | 0.15 |
| Triethanolamine | 1.00 |
| Water | 72.40 |

Finally, a nonionic cream for general use on the face, hands, or body. This cream uses polyethylene glycol which functions as a co-emulsifier as well as adding "feel" to the cream.

| Oil Phase | % by Volume | Function |
|---|---|---|
| Anhydrous lanolin | 2.0 | moisturizer |
| Isopropyl palmitate | 4.0 | emollient |
| Polyethylene glycol -1000 monostearate | 5.5 | co-emulsifier |
| Silicone oil 550 | 10.0 | emollient |
| Stearic acid | 6.0 | base for body |
| Glycerol monostearate | 4.0 | emulsifier |
| Propyl paraben | 0.15 | preservative |

| Water Phase | | |
|---|---|---|
| Methyl Paraben | 0.15 | preservative |
| Propylene glycol | 2.50 | humectant |
| Water | 65.68 | |
| Fragrance | 0.20 | |

Notice that this formula uses some petroleum derived ingredients. These are examples of old formulae which used most of that type of ingredient. Current formulae do not necessarily avoid the use of petroleum products altogether. It is unfortunate that we are not at a state of expertise in cosmetic formulation where all petroleum derived ingredients may be eliminated. One can be a purest in this but, I think as long as we heat our homes with oil, and drive cars, and fly in airplanes powered with oil-derived fuel we can accept that we have a way to go to eliminate oil derived ingredients entirely from all skin care products.

Petrolatum

A note here must be said about petrolatum. This material is widely used in medicine, particularly in dermatology. It is a good moistur-

izer in that it occludes the skin, preventing escape of skin water. It is greasy, messy, cheap, and not very esthetic. While much is written about petrolatum as being safe if not harmless, I am less enthralled about this product. There are many ways to produce petrolatum and thus there are many different products out there on the market. Basically, it is a hydrocarbon that is yellow until it is purified.

**Water-in-Oil Emulsion**

One of the first water-in-oil formulas must be the ancient olive oil and beeswax with water formula of Galen, a physician who lived in 150 A.D. This was a difficult and tedious formula to make since there was no emulsifier added. As the years went by rose water was used, almond oil was substituted for olive oil, and borax was added as an emulsifier. This final formula was called Rose Water Ointment and was the orginal "cold cream". Here is the formula as listed in the United States Pharmacopeia XV.

| Ingredient | % of Volume |
|---|---|
| Spermaceti | 12.5 |
| Beeswax | 12.0 |
| Almond oil | 56.0 |
| Borax | 0.50 |
| Rose water | 5.00 |
| Distilled water | 14.0 |
| Rose oil | qs |
| (qs = quantity sufficient) | |

Today many beeswax-borax formulae are used, mainly in cleansing creams. Many old formulae were based on this combination and a few are still around. The borax serves to neutralize the fatty acids, the beeswax. In this formula, heat the water and the borax together, then add it to the other heated ingredients. Add the rose oil as the product cools.

Here is another simple water-in-oil formula that uses beeswax and borax with a nonionic emulsifier called Arlacel 83[R] and a co-emulsifier called Tween 80[R].

| Oil Phase | % by Volume |
|---|---|
| Lanolin, anhydrous | 7.00 |
| Mineral oil | 31.00 |
| Beeswax | 5.00 |
| Arlacel 83[R] | 5.00 |

| Tween 80$^R$ | 1.00 |
|---|---|
| Propyl paraben | 0.15 |
| | |
| Water Phase | |
| Methyl paraben | 0.15 |
| Borax | 0.30 |
| Water | 50.55 |
| Fragrance | 0.30 |

Note that the amount of water in this formula is much lower than in the oil-in-water formulae. You can substitute various vegetable oils for the mineral oils and with slight adjustments in the emulsifier obtain a stable emulsion.

Now, let's go on to working up an active modern formula. Keep in mind that the principles are the same. As we go along, I shall give reasons for using each ingredient. Our plan is to formulate a cosmetically elegant cream that will be effective as an antiaging product. We shall not look at the cost of ingredients, or what the selling price of the product will be, though this is important. Our major interest will be how well the product functions and how safe the product is.

## ONE DESIGN OF AN ANTIAGING PRODUCT

First, the product concept.

This product will be a soft white cream that will have the following functions: 1. immuno-stimulation to the skin, 2. anti-oxidant properties, 3. reparative properties for the dermis, 4. epidermal stimulation for new cellular growth, and 5. the ability to increase capillary blood flow.

For a second set of functions we want the product to moisturize and soften, adding a healthy glow to the skin. We want the product to rub in smoothly, leave no visible residue, and provide a dry after-feel.

Second, the product ingredients. We are limited to cosmetic ingredients since we are not producing a pharmaceutical product. We can not use any ingredient that is a known drug. If we stick to natural plant ingredients that are "generally recognized as safe" (GRAS) it will make our job easier. The cosmetic chemist starts with the ingredients he knows best and then begins to ask for help from the cosmetic raw material suppliers, specifically, are there any ingredients that have the effect that is sought.

## Choosing Active Ingedients

Immunostimulants would be my first choice. Knowing that certain plants have this property, I select from a group that have a previous history of use as immune system stimulants. The beta glucans are such a group of compounds. They are available from the yeast cell wall and from certain cereal seeds. We need a particular type, called beta 1,3, glucan. You need not know the chemistry except that it is a large molecule composed of linked sugars (glucose), and that it is not soluble in water or oil. Farnesol is another ingredient that is a natural material and has a good antiaging effect.

I shall choose vitamin A for an epidermal stimulant. It has a long history of use in topical skin products and is known to be essential for the normal functioning of the skin. There are many types of vitamin A, the most commonly used is vitamin A palmitate which is an ester of retinol, the vitamin A alcohol.

One of the best agents for repair of the dermis is vitamin C. There are few stable forms, the most common known as ascorbyl palmitate but there is an ascorbyl peptide which is now available. This ingredient is water soluble as well. Panthenol is another good addition to this formula for it will provide good support function to all metabolic pathways.

Vitamin E (as tocopheryl acetate) will make a good antioxidant as well as provide benefit to the dermis.

There are many ingredients to stimulate capillary blood flow, but the one I like best is tocopheryl nicotinate.

This is our active list of ingredients. We could have chosen others, but these are known to be safe and effective.

### The Moisturizer Emollient Group

Again, we have a large number of ingredients from which we can choose. First, we shall add silicone since it is waterproof and will add a good feel to the skin. Then, jojoba oil which is a waxy smooth oil that proves an excellent moisturizer. To provide body we shall use cetyl alcohol, this is a solid white, fatty material. Next, we'll add an ester oil that allows a dry rub in, for example, isopropyl palmitate or caprylic/capric oils.

## Emulsifier Selection

Now, we must decide if we are going to go anionic, cationic, or nonionic. We decide to go nonionic and will use self-emulsifying glycerol monostearate. You will notice that I did not use a humectant, but we shall add glycerine to the formula to give shine and more body.

## Fragrance and Preservation

Ideally, this should be the same agent, but not all essential oil systems provide adequate preservation for repeated use products. We can take advantage of other properties of the essential oils as stimulants, activators, and skin penetration aids. I would add rose oil, camomile, eugenol, and lemon oil to this formula. Not having a good nose for fragrance, I would have a perfumer make up a special essential oil combination that would be a preservative and still have a pleasant fragrance.

## The Making of the Emulsion

| Oil Phase | % of Volume |
|---|---|
| Silicone oil | 5.00 |
| Isopropyl palmitate | 5.00 |
| Cetyl alcohol | 5.00 |
| Vitamin A palmitate | 0.50 |
| Vitamin E acetate | 1.00 |
| Tocopheryl nicotinate | 0.50 |
| Glyceryl monostearate  SE | 8.00 |

| Water Phase | |
|---|---|
| Beta 1,3, glucan | 0.01 |
| Ascorbyl peptide | 1.00 |
| Panthenol | 2.00 |
| Farnestol | 2.00 |
| Essential oils | 0.20 |
| Preservative (if needed) | 0.30 |
| Water qs to 100% (in this case) | 70.50 |

## Procedure

Combine the oil phase ingredients and heat to 65 degrees C. Heat the combined water phase ingredients to 65 degrees C and add to the oil phase with constant stirring. Let the emulsion cool down to 45 degrees and add the essential oils and preservative if needed. You will only be able to tell if the preservative is needed after you have the product tested for microbiological preservative efficacy. This is done by special laboratories that are equipped to perform these tests.

## Product Testing

### Stability

When the product is completed you will need to test it for stability and safety as well as preservation. Product testing for stability involves cycling the product three times by repeated freezing and thawing. If it does not separate into layers, it is stable to freezing. Next, you must heat the finished product to 40-45 degree C for 30 days. If the product does not fall apart into layers, change color or appearance it can be considered stable. This test also provides an indication of  shelf life. Thirty days at 40-45 degrees C is equivalent to one year at room temperature.

### Safety

If the ingredients have approved human safety use, animal testing is not required. Human patch testing would be performed. The standard test is a 48 hour repeat insult patch test on 100 human volunteers. This test is done by placing a small 0.5 ml amount of product on a special patch. The patch is put onto the back of the human volunteers. After 24 hours the patch is removed and scored on a rating of 0 to 4. The higher the score, the more irritating the product. **See Table 14-1.**

After reading the test score, a new  patch with product is applied for another 24 hours. After 24 hours the test site is read again. Non-irritating products will score between 0 to 0.25. Scores over 0.50 have potential to be irritating.

### Allergy Testing and Hypoallergenic Products

A patch test does not tell you whether or not that product is allergenic. To test for allergy producing products requires a much more complicated series of tests and takes a longer time. In order to make a claim of hypoallergenicity for a product you will need a series of tests. Companies who wish to make a strong hypoallergenic claim will have these studies performed on their products. See **Table 14-1** for this recommended series.

### A Word About Allergy and Hypoallergenicity

I do not know of a single product in the cosmetic industry that has not had a reported case of allergic reaction by someone. The most common allergy producing substances in cosmetics have been identified some years ago and are listed in the order of frequency. (See **Table 14-2**.)

Now it is time for us to look at all the products out there and try to make some sense out of them. One good method would be to look at the various types of products and analyze the ingredients. The key to product knowledge is to understand how the ingredients function on the skin. Since this list is very long we shall limit our coverage to skin care products only, which includes make-up items.

## COMPOSITION AND RATIONALE OF SKIN CARE AND MAKE-UP PRODUCTS

### Moisturizers and Cleansing Creams

Most, if not all, moisturizers will use an occlusive substance to retain water in the skin. You cannot add water to the skin from the top surface so you must slow down normal moisture loss from the skin. The majority of products on the market are water-in-oil emulsions with an anionic emulsifier or a combination of anionic and nonionic emulsifiers. The most common ingredients seen in these preparations are mineral oil. petrolatum, beeswax, propylene glycol, glycerine, cetyl alcohol, stearic acid, triethanolamine, glyceryl monostearate, isopropyl myristate or palmitate, and methyl and propyl parabens.

None of these ingredients are terribly exciting.

### Cream Cleansers

Cream cleansers have gone through some changes in the past years. The original formulae were designed for convenient use, to reduce harshness of soap (drying), and to prevent lipid loss from the skin's surface. To do all this and still clean away make-up and industrial grime required some fairly stout products. Most were of the cold cream type. The most common ingredients were beeswax, borax, mineral oil, lanolin, paraffin wax, stearic acid and triethanolamine, cetyl alcohol, and the parabens. New cleansers use the more modern surfactants, and are usually clear solutions or gels. Gels, incidently, are not mysterious compounds. They are usually made from polymers that bind water and trap the oils within the interspaces. Some gels are oil-free and some are all oil. Gel cleansers may contain the following: sodium magnesium silicate, sodium lauryl sarcosinate, hydroxyethylcellulose, propylene glycol, lanolin, and water, plus fragrance and preservatives.

### Toner, Astringents and Skin Freshners

Whoever came up with the word "toner" produced a great word! I do not believe toners physiologically "tone" the skin, but they can be formulated to do a number of things: smooth, exfoliate, reduce oiliness, etc. Astringents are chemicals that react with the protein in the skin and actually modify the skin's surface keratin. They are made from three basic materials and they all react in a similar manner. Metals, such as zinc, aluminum, and zirconium in various forms, such as acetates, chlorides, tartrate and citrates, make very good astringents. Citric and lactic acids are also effective astringents. Alcoholics probably the most common astringent and toner used today. Witch hazel is alcohol plus tannin and tannic acid from the Hamemelis virginiana plant.

There are many forms of astringent products, such as sticks for bleeding after shaving, emulsions for colognes, aftershave lotions, and face masks. The most common ingredients in these preparations are the following items: alcohol, potassium alum, zinc sulfate, glycerin, propylene glycol, and lanolin, along with fragrance and preservatives.

Toners can provide a "physical and psychological lift" if they contain appropriate herbal extracts. When combined with essential oils they offer a stimulating and healing effect.

Beware of toners that are mostly alcohol, the effect is fleeting and of limited value. Water based toners do not dry off fast enough for most

# REPEATED INSULT PATCH TEST (RIPT)

## PURPOSE

To determine the irritation and/or allergic contact sensitization potential of a test article after repetitive patch applications to the skin of human subjects.

## EXPERIMENTAL DESIGN

### Subjects

Usually 50, 100, or 200 subjects, male or female, over 18 years of age are selected. The subjects will be informed of the nature of the test, and any possible reactions that may occur. A signed Informed Consent Form will be obtained from each subject. Additionally, the subjects will be considered dependable and able to read, understand, and follow the directions.

Prior to test initiation, each subject will complete a medical history form. The subjects will not exhibit any dermatological condition that would preclude application of the test product.

### Test Article

A sufficient quantity of each test article should be submitted by the Sponsor:
    Liquids (including lotions)- approximately 250 ml (8oz.) per 50 subjects.
    Powders, semi-solids- approximately 250g (1/2 pound) per 50 subjects.
    Fabrics, fibers- approximately 600 sq. in. per 50 subjects.

### Induction Phase

Approximately 0.2ml or grams of the test article is applied to the subject's back, using occlusive patches. Semi-occlusive tape may be recommended when evaluating known irritating and/or volatile materials.

Twenty-four hour patch applications are generally made on Monday, Wednesday, Friday schedule. Twenty-four hour rest period follow Tuesday and Thursday removals and a 48 hour rest period follows Saturday removals. The site is scored by a trained examiner just prior to the next patch application. This procedure is repeated until 9 induction applications of the test article are made to the same site.

If a subject develops a 2-level reaction or greater during the induction phase, the patch is applied to an adjacent fresh site for the next application. If a 2 or greater reaction occurs at the new site, no further induction applications are made. However, any reactive subjects will be subsequently patched with the test article at a virgin site during the challenge phase of the study.

### Challenge Phase

Approximately 2 weeks after application of the last induction patch, a challenge patch is applied to a previously unpatched (virgin) site, adjacent to the original induction patch site. The challenge site is scored 24 and 48 hours later. The subjects are asked to report any delayed reactions which might occur after the final challenge patch reading.

Skin responses are scored according to the following 6-point scale:
    0 = No evidence of any effect
     - = Minimal, faint, uniform or spotty erythema
    1 = Pink, uniform erythema covering most of the contact site
    2 = Pink-red erythema, uniform in the entire contact site
    3 = Bright-red erythema with/without petechiae or papules
    4 = Deep red erythema with/without vesiculation or weeping

Accompanying edema (swelling) at any test site is recorded with an "e" and described as mild, moderate, or severe. Other possible dermal sequelae are similarly recorded.

## REPORTING

The final report will include: Purpose, Test Article Identification, Panel Selection and Dermatographics, Experimental Design, Results, and Conclusions.

Results of dermal responses will be presented in tabular form.

**TABLE 14-1** Note the number of subjects and the type of testing needed.

## MOST FREQUENT COSMETIC PRODUCTS CAUSING ADVERSE REACTIONS

1. Bath soaps and detergents
2. Deodorants and antiperspirants
3. Eye shadow
4. Hair dyes
5. Mascara
6. Moisturizers
7. Permanent waves
8. Shampoos

## MOST FREQUENT COSMETIC INGREDIENTS CAUSING DERMATITIS

1. Fragrance ingredients
2. Preservatives
3. p-phenylene diamine
4. Lanolin and derivatives
5. Glyceryl thioglycolate (used in "acid" perms)
6. Propylene glycol
7. Toluenesulfonamide/ formaldehyde resin (nail polish)
8. Sunscreens and other UV absorbers
9. Methacrylate ("sculptured nails")

## MOST FREQUENT FRAGRANCE INGREDIENTS CAUSING DERMATITIS

Fragrance, unspecified
Cinnamyl alcohol
Citronellol
Musk ambrette
Isoeugenol
Geraniol
Cinnamal (Cinnamic aldehyde)
Coumarin
Eugenol

**TABLE 14-2** These are the most frequent causes of dermatitis. Printed with permission from A. Fisher: Contact Dermatitis, 3rd ed., Philadelphia, Lea & Febiger, 1986.

users, but when formulated effectively they can evaporate fairly rapidly. Skin freshners are composed mainly of alcohol and citrus oils or citrus scents.

## Bath Products

Bath products, for many years were mainly crystal materials such as bath salts. The agents were mostly water softeners and were needed because of the hard water in most areas. The bath tub "ring" was common in the old days. It consisted of soap that had reacted with the calcium in the hard water and other suspended minerals in body dirt. Instead of remaining in suspension they fell out and collected on the skin and on the tub walls. Soft water and improved foaming action has put an end to this ugly beast.

Bath products now include bath oils, bubble baths, after bath gels or lotions, shower gels, bath salts, and therapeutic bath preparations. It is rather sad that the custom of bathing has lost ground to the shower. The shower is an effective and quick body cleanser but it has little relaxing potential. The bath as a luxury phenomenon will never pass from the scene, and as a treatment method is in a class by itself! The bath is one of the best ways to use essential oils. Many different types of oils may be used in the bath to help soothe and heal both the skin and the psyche.

The most common ingredients in bath products are foaming agents. Of these, the fatty alcohol ether sulphates are the most popular. This is due to the ability of these agents to suspend dirt and maintain foam independently of water hardness, soap, or oil content. We shall look at the composition of several of these product types. Many considerations are needed before a bath product can be put together. Baths are primarily for cleansing, but the product must not injure the skin, it must have a pleasant fragrance, and must not precipitate dirt. Also, physically the product must be appealing and easy to use.

**Liquid foam baths** are usually clear, thick products. They contain some of the following ingredients: sodium lauryl ether sulfate, coconut diethanolamide, citric acid, fragrance, preservatives, and perhaps some sodium chloride for thickening the product. You may also see the following ingredients on more expensive products: coconut imidazoline betaine, lauryl alcohol polyglycol ether sulfosuccinate, and alkyl amido betaines.

From a safety point of view, the products with disodium lauryl alcohol polyglycol ether sulfosuccinate are the better products. You will also find alpha-olefin sulphonates and paraffin sulphonates, amine oxides and ethoxylated alkanolamides. Finally, you may also find coconut imidazoline betaines listed. These are gentle agents and good foamers. Avoid any product that lists linear alkyl benzene sulfonates as they are suspected of producing vaginal irritation.

**Gel bath products** are composed of the same ingredients as the liquid products except they have a gelling agent. This may be increased surfactant, a salt or some foam stabilizer, or a cellulostic material. **Dry bath products** are composed essentially of the same ingredients as the liquids except they contain fillers to help the product flow and not cake. Also they will contain agents that soften hard water. A typical formula may contain lauryl sulfate, alpha-olefin sufphonate, lauric isopropanolamine, sodium sesquicarbonate (water softener), and calcium silicate (filler).

**Bath salts**, which were popular some years back, are still around. They are essentially water softeners and fragrance. You will see some herbal baths that contain these ingredients as well. The major ingredients are sodium sesquicarbonate, sodium carbonate and sodium bicarbonate, and many types of phosphates, such as sodium hexametaphosphate which is in Calgon[R]. Borax and rock salts are also used, as is tartaric acid and citric acid, in combination with bicarbonates to make fizzy salts.

Bath salts arose to reduce hard water and soap scum. The fragrance is pleasant and the salts are mild to the skin. I believe with the resurgence of natural products we will see new bath salts products on the market that will be very functional and attractive.

## Bath Oils

Bath oils are a separate group of products that have considerable benefit in skin care programs. Initially they were used for dry skin. They remain the easiest and most effective way of treating generalized dry skin conditions. The basic concept is that oil on the skin will retain water for a longer period and reduce the drying tendency. This is true in many respects. Bath water loosens skin scales and hydrates the skin while the person is bathing. Upon leaving the tub, the oils cling to the skin trapping the moisture beneath the oil. With good oils very little towel drying is needed and only light towel patting should be used. There are interesting reference papers if you wish to read more about the retention properties of bath oils.

There are four types of bath oils: 1. spreading or floating types which do not mix with water, 2. blooming or dispersion types that will make the water cloudy or milky on addition, 3. soluble types that form a clear solution with the water and, 4. foam types. We shall only consider the first three, because the foaming types are not effective skin lubricants.

**Spreading bath oils** float on the top of the water in a thin film. They are usually very fragrant as they sit on the surface and can yield up the aroma easily. To produce the spreading requires a surfactant that changes the surface tension and allows the oil to spread. As for oils, mineral oil is widely used, but I do not like it. There are some excellent propoxylated lanolin oils and silicone oils that make a very effective bath oil. Addition of light oil, such as isopropyl myristate, will carry the fragrance quite well.

You can easily check the spreading quality of a bath oil. Here is how. Add warm water almost to the top of a basin or bowl. Sprinkle the surface lightly with any body powder. Now, put **one drop** of the test oil in the center of the bowl. The powder should move rapidly to the sides of the bowl leaving the water clear in the center. A good spreading oil will move the powder faster than you can see it move. See **Figure 14-1**.

**Blooming bath oils** are dispersed into the water. You can use the same oils, only the dispersant must be different. Here we use a polyoxyethylene(2)oleyl ether, known as Brij 93[R]. A typical formula would contain vegetable oil 60%, isopropyl myristate 20%, silicone oil 5% , Brij 83[R] 10% and fragrance 5%. These are excellent preparation to add essential oils for therapy. Addition of rosemary, camomile and lavender will make an excellent skin healing blend.

**Soluble bath oils** are formulated to dissolve in the water, and as a result have a very high surfactant level. They are used mainly to prevent the residual bath tub ring and as a result have no skin emollient effect. I do not recommend their use. Typical formula will contain high fragrance and high surfactants such as polyoxyethylene sorbitan monolaurate (known as Tween 20[R]), and polyoxyethylene sorbitan mono-oleate (known as Tween 80[R]).

Keep in mind that bath oils allow a great

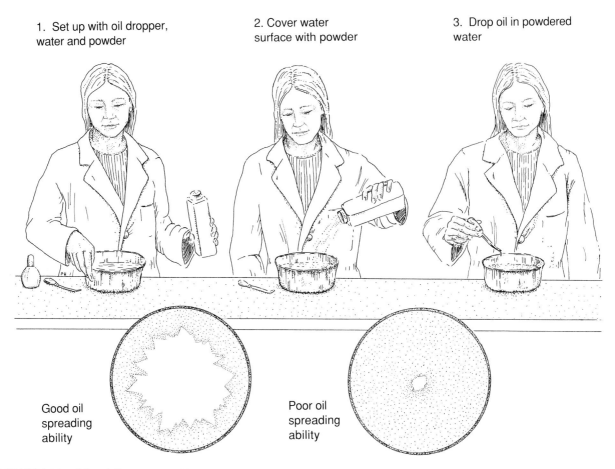

1. Set up with oil dropper, water and powder

2. Cover water surface with powder

3. Drop oil in powdered water

Good oil spreading ability

Poor oil spreading ability

**FIGURE 14-1** Oil's ability to spread in water. This is a simple method to check the spreading action of a bath oil. Baby powder or magnesium stearate may be used.

range of treatment types. Keep the water comfortably warm, let the client be the judge of the comfort level. Do not exceed 20 minutes in the bath, after that period you will begin to get keratin dissolution. Be very careful of slippery preparations, check them first by using them in your own bath.

## Depilatories

Depilatories have been used since ancient times. This is one of the oldest uses of cosmetic preparations next to eye make-up and primitive foundations, i.e. mud. The original formula was called rhusma and was made up of quicklime and arsenical powders on a ratio of 1:2. The powder was mixed with wood ash as a source of alkali. This was obviously quite toxic, though very effective.

The three types of hair removal used today, besides shaving are: 1. **epilation** which refers to pulling the hair out either with tweezers or waxing, 2. the use of electricit or **electrolysis**

which destroys the hair at the shaft, and 3. the use of chemicals that destroy or weaken the hair called **chemical depilation**.

Epilation by Waxing

This is the most common method used by the skin care specialist to remove hair. Most doctors are not enthused by the use of this method because of the incidence of infection associated with its use, however, in the hands of a skilled operator this is a safe and effective method. The formulae for most waxes are based on the use of beeswax and rosin, with the major component being rosin. Rosin hardens and holds the hair. Some preparations use paraffin and petrolatum as well. The use of camphor in the preparation reduces discomfort. An antimicrobial agent also reduces the chance of infection. I am currently working on a new form of depilatory wax.

The only caution I can give the reader is to be careful about using a wax treatment on any area that has any redness or signs of infection. Also be careful of individuals with psoriasis or chronic eczema. People who bruise or blister easily are not good candidates for this type of treatment.

## Chemical Depilation

Chemical depilatories should be non-toxic and non-irritating to the skin as well as being effective in three to six minutes. Most depilatories contain an alkaline reducing agent that will break the disulfide bridges (the cystine group), between the polypeptide chains in the keratin molecules of hair fibrils. Here are some preparations and how they work.

**Sulfides**, such as strontium sulfide, are effective in 3-5 minutes after application. While effective, they generate hydrogen sulfide, a gas with an unpleasant odor (like rotten eggs). You can cut down on the odor by removing most of the product with a wooden spatula before washing it off. It is the combination with water that makes the smelly hydrogen sulfate. However, it is imperative that the product be washed off as it will damage the skin and is toxic to lower tissues. A typical preparation may contain the following ingredients: strontium sulphide, talc, methyl cellulose, glycerol. fragrance and water. The formulations are not easy to put together.

**Stannites** are tin derived products that are relatively odor free. They have not been very popular because they are not stable. Attempts at using various stabilizers has not been very successful.

**Thioglycollates** are the current choice for depilatories. They are used in a concentration of 2.5 to 5% and are non-toxic and stable at that level. They work in 5 to 15 minutes depending on the concentration and formula. For rapid action the pH should be around 9.5 to 12.5 though more advanced research suggests that the pH can be lower. There are many formulae on the market and more will continue to appear. The use of thioglycolic acid is an effective way of producing a thio compound. You will find several of these preparations on the market. They may be combined with other agents, such as glycerol, to form a thioglycerol.

**Enzymes** that attack keratin are a new form of depilation. There is a keratinase available from the microbe called Streptomyces fradiae which will dissolve keratin. An old patent on this type of product, US Patent 2 988 485 (1961), was issued thirty years ago. New enzyme technology promises to improve this method. At present, the system is slow and costly. Unfortunately, much of the newer technology is still proprietary.

## Depilatories for Black Skin

Black males have a problem with regrowth of hair into the skin after shaving. This condition arises out of the curved nature of black facial hair. As the sharp, shaved hair enters the skin it sets up a reaction that is called **pseudofolliculitis barbae**. There is a preparation used for this condition that will remove facial hair in 3 to 7 minutes. The current formula is a powder that uses barium sulfide and calcium thioglycollate. This is an area that needs more work.

Now, let us look at another area of skin products that is gaining popularity - **sunscreens**.

## Sunscreens and Tanning

As a review we need to look at the process of tanning again and see how this process is integrated into sun-related products. Tanning is a color change produced in the skin as a response to ultraviolet light. We can divide the tanning process into three stages or types. **Immediate tanning** involves immediate darkening of the unoxidized granules in the upper epidermal layers. An energy ban of sunlight between 300 nm and 600 nm with a peak at 350 nm is the most effective energy to produce this effect. This tanning appears about an hour after exposure but fades in 2 to 3 hours after exposure.

**Delayed tanning** is produced by the oxidation of melanin granules in the basal layer and their subsequent migration to the upper layers. This tanning also begins about an hour after exposure and lasts perhaps for 4 to 8 days after exposure. The effective range of sun's energy is between 295 and 320 nm; this region is also called the erythemogenic region.

**True tanning** starts about 2 days after exposure and reaches a maximum at 2 to 3 weeks after exposure. The same mechanism is involved as in delayed tanning.

Not all sun exposure is bad. It is hard to conceive of a world with out bright sun light to bring cheer to the day to day existence. We know that the sun is beneficial to our psyche and to our bones and perhaps to our circulation and central nervous system. The danger, as in all other aspects of life, is overexposure or excess sunlight. Here are four levels of sunburn based on an article by Luckiesh. The exposure is at mid-day in June in the USA.

1. Minimal perceptive erythema - slightly red or pink skin produced by 20 minutes of exposure. This is called 1 MED or minimal erythema dose.
2. Vivid erythema - bright red skin but no pain, after 30 minutes of exposure. This is caused by 2.5 MED.
3. Painful burn - vivid erythema and mild to intense pain 100 minutes of exposure. This caused by 5.0 MED.
4. Blistering burn - extremely high level of pain with vivid erythema and blistering with some systemic symptoms after 200 minutes exposure. This is caused by 10 MED.

Severe sunburn takes 4 to 8 days to heal and will usually peel.

Now, let us look at the products that are available to protect us fromthe ravages of the sun. The sun can produce cancers and hastens aging.

## The Sunscreens

Sunscreens are chemical materials that either block the sun's ray or absorb specific energy levels of the sun's rays. We call that an **absorption band**. A band is just another way of saying a group of wavelengths. Only a tiny fraction of the sun's energy is in the visible range of the electromagnetic spectrum. We are dealing with a band in the ultraviolet range, from 290 nm to 320 nm for UVB and from 320 to 400 for UVA. Many chemicals will absorb light in these bands. For an effective sunscreen the chemical must be safe for use on the skin and non-penetrating.

I cannot go into all the details about sunscreens for the subject is both vast and complex. I shall try to lay out what I feel is essential for the skin care specialist to know. First of all, the concept of **skin protective factor or SPF must be understood**. Next, you must appreci-

ate the difference between skin types. Finally, you need to know the difference between a screen and a block and what a tanning accelorator is. Let's look at SPF first.

SPF is the number produced by dividing the MED of protected skin by the MED of unprotected skin. So, it is a ratio. Here is an example, if a type III person has an MED of 20 minutes without sunscreen and an MED of 200 minutes with a sunscreen we then divide as follows:

$$\text{Sun Protective Factor} = \frac{\text{Time in minutes for 1 MED with sunsreen 200}}{\text{Time in minutes for 1 MED no sunscreeen 20}}$$

therefore, SPF = 10

See, no real complicated calculation. Now, here are the skin types and the recommended SPF's:

| Skin Type | SPF Needed |
|---|---|
| I. Always burns; never tans | 8+ |
| II. Always burns; minimal tan | 6-7 |
| III. Burns moderately; tan gradually | 4-5 |
| IV. Burns minimally; always tans | 2-3 |
| V. Burns rarely, tans profusely | 2 |
| IV. Never burns, deeply pigmented | 0 |

Again, what the SPF tells us is that the time you may stay in the sun is a measure of your skin type MED times the SPF. If you burn in 20 minutes and you have a sunsreen with an SPF of 4 you may stay in the sun for 20 minutes times 4, or 80 minutes without burning. If you use an SPF of 15 you could stay out 15 x 20 = 300 minutes or 6 hours. This is provided the sunscreen does not wash off.

Now, the products. Most of these products will be used at the beach, will have to cover large areas, and must not penetrate the skin to be effective. Some of the factors that influence the sunscreen is the thickness of the film on the skin and the stability of the formulation. Certain media in the formula can shift the absorption peaks of the sunscreen away from the best absorption band. It is important then that the sunscreen be tested for changes in absorption after it is formulated. I shall list some sample preparations for the reader and then list all the approved ingredients for sunscreens. Ideally, a sunscreen should protect from 295 nm to 400 nm, but most only protect in the 295 to 320 range.

You will find sunscreens in lotion forms, oil forms, creams of the water-in-oil and the oil-in-water types, and spray types. The only difference in these formulations is the sunscreen. When a claim of waterproofing or water resistance is made the sunscreen must be tested for that property. **Waterproof** means that the sunscreen will not wash off with 80 minutes of exposure to normal swimming. My advice is to select a sunscreen for your client after you have determined the client skin type (Type I to Type V) and considered the use by the client.

The negative aspects of sunscreens are that they tend to sensitize certain individuals. Using a lower SPF is better and using a sunscreen product only when exposed to the sun is important. I do not recommend sunscreens in every cosmetic product any more than I recommend that a laxative be in every food.

The strange part of this mixed up society is that we have light people who wish to be dark and dark people who wish to be light. Even if we were all a homogenous shade of tan we would have some people opting for the two extremes. So we go on to the next topic, **skin lighteners**.

## Skin Lighteners

We need to look at the melanocyte before we explore the products used in lightening the skin. Three things contribute to skin color: 1. the blood circulation, 2. carotene, and 3. melanin pigment. Melanin is by far the most important of these, so we need to look again at the melanocyte and review a few basics.

The melanocyte is a dendritic cell in the epidermal basal layer which produces the pigment melanin. Briefly, the melanocyte produces the melanin and then combines it with a protein matrix called a melanosome. The melanosomes are transferred to keratinocytes that then migrate to the top of the epidermis. Melanin production is a function of direct ultraviolet stimulation and melanocyte stimulating hormone, or MSH, which is secreted by the anterior pituitary.

Caucasoids and blacks have the same number of melanocytes. The melanosomes in black skin are larger and nearer to the surface of the skin in the horny layer, and they are scattered individually. The melanosomes in white skin are usually in the basal layer. See **Figure 14-2**.

## Depigmenting the Skin

There are several ways to decrease pigment production and stop transfer of melanosomes. Here are some ways:

1. destroy melanocytes
2. inhibit melanosome production
3. stop or decrease tyrosinase production
4. inhibit melanin production
5. block the transfer of melanosomes
6. degrade the melanosomes

Most current approaches attempt to discolor the melanin and damage the melanocyte. The agent most commonly used to lighten skin is hydroquinone. This chemical is known to inhibit the oxidation of tyrosine on its way to becoming melanin and it also inhibits the enzyme tyrosinase. There is some evidence that hydroqui-

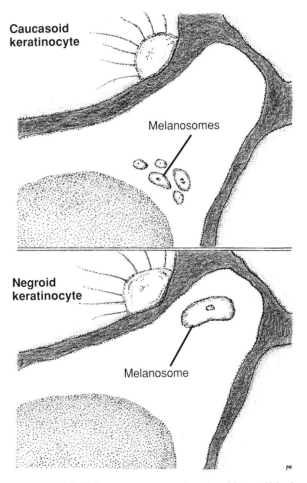

**FIGURE 14-2** Melanosome comparison in white and black skin. The white skin melanosome is small and multiple in the cell, while in black skin they are large singular bodies. Picture the difference between grapes and cucumbers. More light would pass through grapes scattered in a given area than would pass through cucumbers scattered in the same area.

none also damages the cell membrane of the melanocyte and thereby destroys it.

There are many formulae that have been published; some excellent ones are in <u>Harry's Cosmeticology</u>. Most commercial preparations have only 2% of hydroquinone, but up to 10% has been used. Only prescription drugs contain over 2% hydroquinone. One of the best is the Kligman formulation. This can be made up from two existing over-the-counter preparations. Dr. Kligman suggests a skin lightening formula made from Hydrocortisone cream 1%, Hydroquinone cream 2-4%, and Retin A 0.05% mixed in equal quantities. This is applied twice a day to the area to be treated. One point must be kept in mind, that an area to be lightened must be protected from sun exposure.

A relatively new product that is appearing in Europe and may soon be on the market in the US is azelaic acid. This is a compound that is used in 20% concentration as skin lightener. I have had some experience with this product but the general experience with dermatologists is quite mixed. I have heard reports of results from excellent to no effect, so just keep an open mind and be aware that there is something new around that may be of benefit. I do not know of any toxicity with the use of azelaic acid.

## Masks and Packs

Masks had their beginning in the use of mud packs. Today we still use mud packs, but the facial mask is a more sophisticated application and fundamentally more scientific. Animals have used mud to protect them from insects, the sun, and heat as well as to help skin hydration. One of the beneficial aspects of a mask or pack is the debridement effect on the skin after removal. There is also a temporary hydration effect on the stratum corneum providing a better condition for the delivery of any active materials in the mask.

The properties of a good mask are well known: the material should be smooth and have a pleasant scent, drying should be rapid (not over 15 minutes and preferably in 5 minutes) with a drawing or tightening effect; the material should be cleansing and effective as a debridement, and finally, active ingredients for treatment of aging or acne should be incorporated in the mask to take advantage of the delivery system.

## Mask Systems

**Wax masks** may contain paraffin wax and cetyl alcohol along with a little clay and mineral oil. These masks are solid at room temperature and must be heated before application. Generally, they are formulated to melt at 32 to 35 degrees centrigrade. They are popular since they are inexpensive.

**Latex or rubber-based masks** are popular since they are easy to apply and easy to remove. They are occlusive and therefore hydrating, also they are effective in mild debridement. A typical formula would include a 20 to 30% latex emulsion with various clays and thickeners such as methylcellulose.

**Vinyl-based masks** are usually made of polyvinyl alcohol, or vinyl acetate resin as a film former. These are nice preparations and had a high popularity a few years ago. You can add a lot of different agents to these masks as they are compatible with both water soluble and oil soluble ingredients. A typical formula will include polyvinyl alcohol 10 to 20% with clay, glycerine or propylene glcyol, water or alcohol, and perhaps a titanium dioxide. I like this type of mask for it is an excellent debriding mask as well as a superb vehicle for transporting actives into the skin.

**Hydrocolloid-based masks** formed from a variety of materials have a high molecular weight polymeric base. Examples of some of the natural materials that are used, include gum tragacanth, gelatin, casein, carrageen and guar gum. Polyvinylpyrolidine and methylcellulose may also be used. The addition of propylene glycol, glycerine, or sorbitol will allow the film to be plastisized and become not only easier to remove but will also serve as a humectant. While these masks dry rapidly they do not contain much in absorbant materials so they are not very good cleansers or oil absorbers. If the amount of clay or other solid matter is increased the film will not form. The result is an imperfect and unattractive application. The use of zinc oxide and camphor in these masks allow for germicidal and healing activity. Masks can be made from these preparations, but seem to me to be more for feel than effect.

**Clay or earth-based masks** are popular because they can be prepared dry and then mixed with water immediately before use. The most frequently used materials are: china clay, colloidal kaolin, fuller's earth, bentonite, and a variety of other materials. Most of the masks with which I am familiar are derived from bentonite clay. There are many forms of this clay since they depend on where they are mined. (The name derives from The Benton layer of volcanic ash in the earth. It is named after Fort Benton in Arizona where it was first described.) One property of Bentonite clay is its absorption of 15 times its volume in water.

A typical formula will include glyceromonosterate, oils such as lanolin and isopropyl myristate, bentonite, kaolin, and sodium lauryl sulfate. Titanium dioxide and fragrance are added as well. Fuller's earth , I believe, is the best oil absorbant, but it has an ugly color that is not easy to mask. (No pun intended!)

Hot masks and cold masks are variations on the mask theme and have a place in your treatment regimen. Masks allow a great deal of therapeutic ingenuity and I believe we are just at the technological beginning of this old beauty aid system. Now, let us take a look at color cosmetics.

## COLOR COSMETICS FORMULATIONS IN SKIN CARE

At one time the skin care specialist was advised not to use make-up items after a facial as it just undid, or negated, the results of the facial. At one time that was probably good thinking when many make-up items were heavy and occlusive. Today, with lighter make-up products and therapeutic make-up products it makes good sense to use color cosmetics as a continuation of the facial treatment.

Color cosmetics include loose powder, pressed powder, concealers, foundations, lipsticks, mascara, eyeshadows and eyeliners. Essentially, make-up tones down certain areas and emphasizes the eyes and the lips. The skillful use of color cosmetics is important in our society, which is as many societies, beauty oriented. (I really do not know of an "Ugly Oriented Society" unless it was the Hippies' Society of the 1960's.) We need to look at what goes into these formulations and what these various ingredients do to the skin. Each ingredient has a function in the formula, but it also has some effect on the skin itself.

## Facial Powders

Face powder is designed to produce a uniform smooth texture of finish to the skin, to cover minor blemishes, and to reduce shine from moisture or oil. Face powders are one of the earliest of cosmetics, ante-dating recorded history. An effective face powder must be reasonably opaque, lasting, adherent, and resistant to sweat and sebum. In addition, it should be pleasant to use, able to carry a fragrance, and be harmless to the skin. These qualities are expressed in **covering power, absorbancy, slip, adhesion, bloom, color and perfume**.

**Covering power** is achieved by titanium dioxide, zinc oxide, kaolin, and magnesium oxide. Zinc oxide has less covering power than titanium dioxide but it provides some astringency and antiseptic qualities. The smaller the particle of the covering material, the better the coverage down to a range of 0.25 microns. Once a particle reaches that small size it will begin to allow increased light transmission rather than blocking light.

**Absorbancy** is made possible with colloidal kaolin, starch, and magnesium carbonate. There is still much debate about the use of starch in powders since it breaks down and favors bacterial growth. Kaolin is a naturally occurring aluminium silicate that is partially hydrated. It is an excellent absorber of moisture, provides good coverage, and resists skin grease while providing good adhesive properties to the face powder as a whole. It is used below 30% since it reduces slip.

**Starch** in face powder is usually from rice grounded to 3 to 8 microns. It was used as a principal ingredient of face powder for many years but has now lost popularity. There are newer forms of rice starch now available that make up many of the defects of the older product. I have had no experience with these new products. My major objection to starch in a leave-on product like face powder is the tendency of starch to hydrolize and provide a medium for bacteria to multiply.

**Magnesium carbonate** is a good material to use in face powder as an absorbant. In levels of 5% it will absorb oil and water and help prevent balling up of the powder.

**Slip** means easy spreadability during application. Talc and zinc stearate are used to add slip to a face powder. Talc is chemically a hydrated magnesium silicate. To be of value talc must be ground well, be white and bright, and must be free of any amorphous material, including asbestos. The type of talc used in face powder is a **foliated** type which has flat plates that slide easily over one another, providing slip.

**Adhesion** is the property that allows the powder to stick to the face. Magnesium stearate and zinc stearate are used for this purpose. The level is usually around 3 to 10 percent. Some powders contain fatty acid derivatives to increase adhesion. Cetyl alcohol and glyceral monosterate have been used for this property.

**Bloom and color** are two important aspects of a face powder. Bloom refers to the appearance of shiny or dull qualities of the powder. Chalk, rice starch, and powdered silk have been used for this property. Powdered silk is produced by a complex process ending in a very fine powder. It has good slip, adherence, and high absorbancy. It is a good material, though, being a protein, it has a potential for allergic reactions. Color in face powders is derived mainly from inorganic pigments like iron oxides, ultramarines, chrome oxides and chrome hydrates.

Perfume is the final ingredient in the face powder which we must consider. It is frequently difficult to obtain adequate fragrance for a face powder since there are many reacting substances with the powder that may adversely affect the fragrance characteristics. It is the skill of the perfumer who can overcome these problems with the experience of many years. This is not an area for an amateur.

None of the ingredients we have mentioned are toxic and can be used without fear of trouble. In the case of open inflamed skin, ordinary face powder should not be used. Both infection and foreign body reactions are likely. As far as I am able to determine there are no other contraindications to face powder use in skin care other than a sensitivity to one of the ingredients. Here are some basic formulas.

This is a very light transparent powder: talc 80%, zinc oxide 6%, zinc stearate 6%, chalk 8%; add perfume and color.

Here is a complete formula for a face powder that will impart a shimmer to the skin (from the mica): talc 75%, mica 10%, zinc stearate 5%, zinc oxide 2%, kaolin 5%, magnesium carbonate 2%, red iron oxide 0.36%, yellow iron oxide 0.35%, black iron oxide 0.04%, and perfume 0.25%.

Mica is a form of aluminium hydrate that separates into shiny sheets.

Pressed Powders

Pressed powders and loose powders have essentially the same ingredients except that the pressed powder must have binding properties. Higher levels of kaolin, zinc oxides, and zinc stearates are used in these powders. Starch and synthetic gums are often added as binders as well.

The manufacturing of these products is complex and requires special equipment. Check the labels on these products for soap content and surfactant content since occasionally they contain as much as 8 percent soap or detergent as binders.

**Liquid Foundation**

Liquid foundations are pigments dispersed in an emulsion. To achieve the best application it is necessary to produce a uniform stable suspension of the pigments. The pigments are the same inorganic pigments we used before and the emulsifying materials are the same we used in the moisturizing formulae. To achieve the various shades we vary the levels of the four pigments: red-iron oxide, yellow-iron oxide, black-iron oxide, and titanium dioxide. The pigments are usually from 5 to 10% and the most frequently used emulsifers are stearic acid and TEA. Again, there may be as much as 5 to 7% soap in these foundations. You will also find waxes and mineral oil as well. Today many companies are using a combination of anionic and nonionic emulsifiers and many moisturizing ingredients. In addition, some products will contain sunscreens. I have some reservation to the use of sunscreens as a routine ingredient. Considering that products are used all year round there is little need for a sunscreen in the winter in many parts of the US and Europe. When they are indicated, as in the case of skiers, the amount needed will be far more than is present in a foundation product.

Many foundations also contain elastin and collagen, placental extract, and other animal derived ingredients. I see no real benefit to the consumer for these ingredients in a foundation product since they add nothing to the product except cost. The addition of vitamin A and vitamin E to these products is beneficial, however, and should be continued. I do not give a representative formula since there is nothing unique about these products.

**Stick foundations** are the same color ingredients as liquid foundation except that they are not emulsions but are anhydrous formulations. They contain waxes such as paraffin, carnuba, and beeswax, and mineral oil. Here is a formulation that is used for heavy coverage. Lanolin alcohols 3.0%, ozokerite wax 7.0%, paraffin wax 7.0%, lanolin 3.0%, mineral oil 20%, isopropyl myristate 11%, titanium dioxide 35%, kaolin 8%, black iron oxide 0.5%, yellow iron oxide 2.7%, red iron oxide 2.0%, and perfume 0.25%. This formula can be used to cover blemishes.

## Lipsticks

Lipsticks are also very old cosmetics and have had a beneficial effect on lip health as a consequence. Being made mainly of lipid materials they provide emolliency and protection from the sun. A good lipstick should be safe, provide bright color, be ultrasmooth, be stable, and easy to apply. Newer lipsticks do not run up into creases about the lips.

**Colors for lipsticks** are of two types, those that dye the lip tissue and those that cover the lips. The staining dyes are very popular with eosin dye being one of best available. Eosin as a water soluble dye and certain derivatives of fluorescein, known as bromoacids, are widely used. Dye selection for lipsticks is regulated by the FDA in the US and by the EEC in Europe. These dyes are identified by a color index number and by a common name, and there are currently 25 of these colors on the approved list.

Titanium dioxide and iron oxide are approved colors, as is certain metallic salts of certain approved colors. These metallic salts are called **lakes**. The range of added color will vary from 0.5 to 3% for the staining dyes and up to 10 % for the insoluble pigments, such as lakes. Lip color, again, is a very special skill that is acquired only after many years of experience.

**Bases** for lipsticks are selected for the ability to dissolve the dye and to hold the color well. The major ingredients: are castor oil, fatty

alcohols, various kinds of esters such as isopropyl myristate, polyethylene glycols (also known as carbowaxes), and lanolin alcohol derivatives. Since a lipstick must have stability during application, waxes are added that control the melting point and hardness of the product. Two of these materials are carnuba wax from vegetable origin and candelilla wax from the plant world. Carnuba is a hard brittle wax while candelilla while hard, is less brittle and melts at a lower temperature.

Other ingredients you will find may include lanolin, petrolatum, lecithin, silicone waxes, cocoa butter, beeswax, and microcrystalline waxes derived from petroleum.

Some lipsticks contain sunscreens as an additive and this may be a good practice, but I do not favor it. I am a firm believer in lipsticks as I feel we have not fully explored the potential of this product category. There are natural agents now available to help control viral infections on the lips and soon these will find their way into lipsticks. I have not included a formula for lipsticks as they require special equipment to manufacture and even molds for tiny lab batches.

Most of the lipstick ingredients are very safe. Only sensitization to specific ingredients presents problems.

### Eye Make-up

We shall discuss only mascara, eyeshadow, and eyeliners. Eye make-up also has a very long history. Big, dark, bright eyes have always been a sign of beauty, the power to wilt the hardest of hearts. Blessed is the women who is skilled in this art. I need not review any of the history of eye make-up here since most of the readers will have studied this in their courses; it is a most fascinating subject.

**Mascara** is a black pigmented product used to augment the eyelash color and to increase their apparent length. The signs of a good mascara are easy application, no running or smudging, no caking and non-irritating. Only a limited number of pigments are permitted in mascara, including: black iron oxide, ultramarine blue, umbers (which are brown ochres), burnt sienna, titanium dioxide and zinc oxide, carmine, alumimium lake of cochineal, chromium oxides, and soluble oil blue. Again, this is skill acquired with long practice as good mascaras are not easy to make. We shall look at a formula of a simple liquid mascara.

Using a gum, such as tragacanth, at less than 1%, lampblack at 8%, alcohol at 8%, water, and preservative makes a simple mascara. This product will smudge. A waterproof, smudge-free mascara will require an entirely different formula. Again, you could use lampblack but you will need a resin material dissolved in alcohol and little oil to plasticize the resin. This is a product that has a higher potential for irritation because of the resin and the alcohol.

Your first consideration when recommending a mascara should be safety and then efficacy.

### Eyeshadow and Eyeliner

Eyeshadows are used to accent the eyelids. They may be in the form of a cream or emulsion, stick, or pressed powder. Pressed powders seem to dominate the market at present. They are mostly talc and pigment with a binder, such as zinc stearate.

**Eyeliners** are either liquids, cakes, or pencils. An eyeliner will accentuate the position of the eyes, thereby increasing the expressiveness of the eyes. These products contain about 30 to 50% pigment and the rest is a carrier, binder, or emusifier. In the pencil form, an anhydrous preparation is used that allows easy application. Waxes and petroleum-based lipids are used in these preparations.

All eye preparations must be free of bacteria as they could be a major source of infection. Always check for a preservative, if none are present ask why.

### HOW TO READ A LABEL ON A COSMETIC PRODUCT

All products must carry a list of ingredients if they are sold to the public. These ingredients are **listed in the order of concentration (largest amount)**. You will find that most products will start off with water as the first ingredient. If an extract of a plant is used you may find the first ingredient listed as "extract of horsechestnut". This means that the first ingredient is still water. Next, you find either the humectant, glycerine or propylene glycol, or the emulsifier which is either stearic acid or glyceryl monostearate. The third item will be the moisturizers, oils, co-emulsifiers or emollients. By this time you are down to ingredient levels of less than 1%. Colors, preservatives, and fragrance are usually at the end of the list, less than 0.5%.

Active ingredients are listed separately if the product is designated an OTC (over-the-counter) product. These products are regulated by the FDA and must comply with set standards for activity and functionality. Sunscreens, antiperspirants, and skin protective products are examples of OTC products.

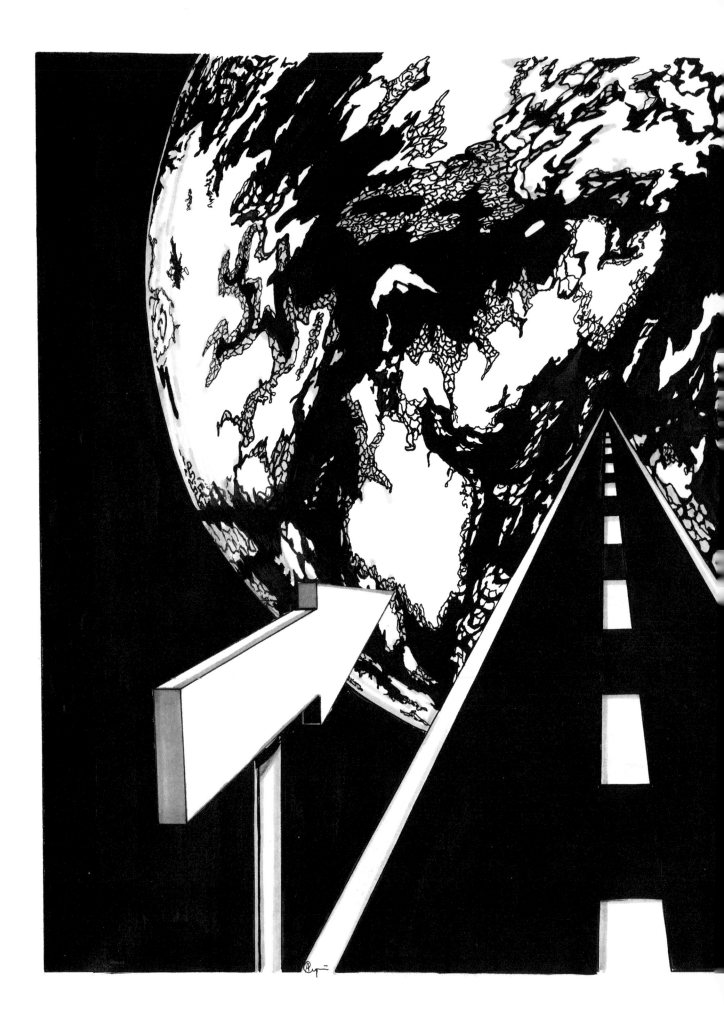

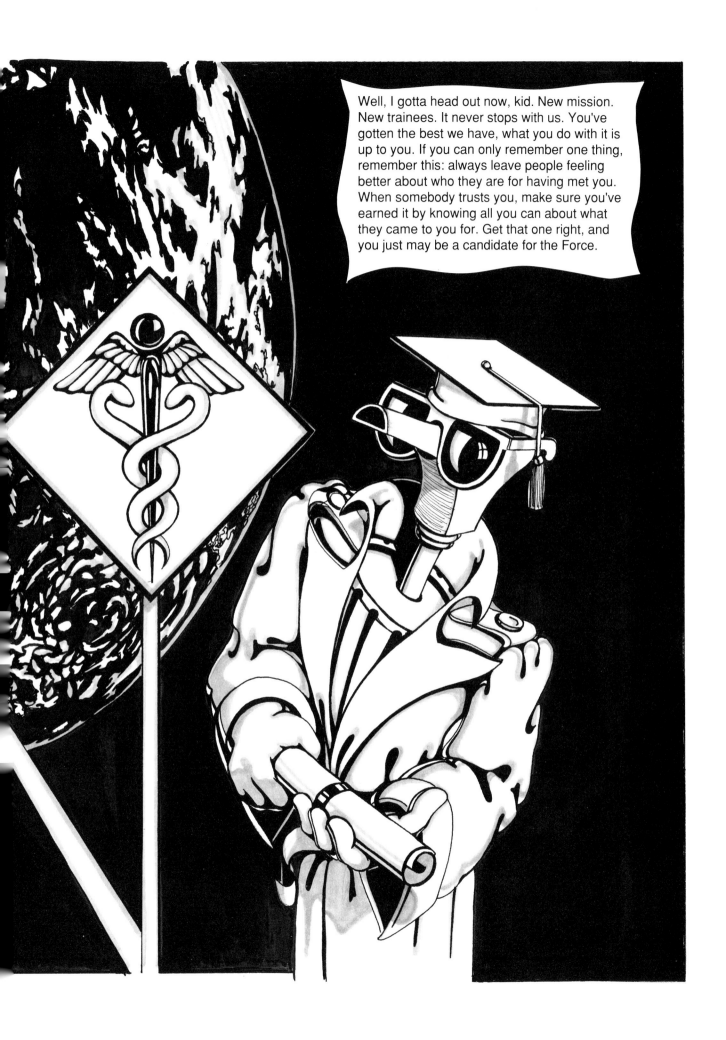

# The Future of Professional
# Skin Care

I am certain that anyone who attempts to forecast or prognosticate is extending his or her neck into a vulnerable position. Nevertheless, it is my duty to venture into this unknown area to help provide some type of guidelines for the future training and direction of the skin care specialist. The days of marketing hype in skin care are over and the day of science is at hand. This is the starting point of my discussion of the future of skin care.

## THE PROMISE AND HOPE

Selling hope in a jar was for a long time the basis of the cosmetic industry. Since very few product were effective a gimmick was needed to push the sales. Fear and hope and buzz words dominated the market theme. Somewhere in the dim past the word "moisturizer" came into being and that started a whole series of investigations into the nature of skin moisture. About the same time more interest in the physical nature of skin and the biochemistry of skin was evident. Many of the early cosmetic chemists were quite serious about the efficacy of the final product but limited raw material, cost constraints, and crude methodology hampered their efforts. It has been my privilege to know many of these fine men and women personally and to have worked with some of them. They represented the driving force of the new wave of products and are largely responsible for our present movement toward effective products. These pioneers recognized the "hope in a jar method" would last only as long as the consumer remained naive.

## THE NEW CONSUMER

Somehow many of the buying public have become aware that the something was missing in the available cosmetics and they started to ask for more- effective products. Today we are dealing with an educated consumer who has a driving need to maintain an attractive appearance.

We are also dealing with an older, more challenging population who present different needs and desires. This is a consumer who will have more disposable income but will be more discreet in how that income is spent. The shifting of the mean national age from a young to an older group presents both opportunities and challenges for the skin care specialist. This new market will be more sophisticated and more expectant of positive results with services rendered. This is one aspect of our future needs. Another aspect is the role of preventive skin care. In medical practice preventive medicine has been taken seriously by pediatricians and by gynecologists but to a large extent it has been ignored by the medical profession in general. After all, physicians are trained to treat disease so why try to prevent it? That is both a callous and stupid statement for we have many more people trying to keep healthy than we do people who are seeking treatment for illness. Here is a potentially large market for the skin care specialist, one that extends over all age groups. But there is yet another aspect to consider - the role of science and advancement in knowledge of skin and skin care.

## THE NEW SCIENCE OF SKIN PHYSIOLOGY

The last twenty to thirty years has seen a large expansion in our knowledge of skin care. Much of this work derives from the investigations of dermatologists who have a keen interest in the why's and wherefore's of skin disorders. A large portion of this work arises as a desire to understand normal skin anatomy, biochemistry, and physiology. The impact of the new information on skin im-munology and role of the pigment, melanin, on skin care will be tremendous.

Out of this research has come several new findings that are changing the treatment of skin disorders rather radically. The use of Retin A, or retinoic acid, for aging skin and the treatment of premalignant disorders has added new dimensions to the our therapeutic armamentarium. There is now new hope for the age and sun ravished faces. More interesting than the use of retinoic acid in treatments is its role as a preventive measure. This finding is leading us down the pathway to look at more serious preventive methods over the horizon. Surely a new and better world is dawning for the skin care professionals and their clients.

## THE MOVEMENT TOWARD MEDICINE

The new science and the new technology in skin care coupled with the growing trend in our population to maintain youthful skin and vigor is moving skin care specialist closer to the field of medicine. The term **cosmoceutical** coined by Dr. Albert Kligman points the way. Medicine, on the other hand, is making a slow move toward the cosmetic industry, in particular, in the direction of the skin care specialist. Surgical patients are asking their physicians for expert advise in post-operative skin care and they do not have this expertise. The rise of the skin care paramedical is here!

## A GIANT LEAP BACK INTO TIME - THE USE OF NATURAL PRODUCTS

For many thousands of years the only treatments available to mankind were magic, plant and animal substances in various porportions. All of this knowledge gathered over the years seemed to be destined for total oblivion until it was revived only a few decades ago. Granted that much of it is sheer nonsense, there is a valid core of real knowledge that we must not ignore. It is foolish to even think that we no longer use plants in our modern pharmacopeiae for about 50% of our current drugs are based on natural products or naturally-derived products. Today, we are beginning to see a reversal of this trend as new products are appearing that are of plant origin. Let us understand, however, that because it is natural does not mean that it is automatically safe and effective. The old Latin saying "caveat emptor" (let the buyer beware) is true for all ages and all things. This means that all skin care specialists must be able to evaluate the current products in terms of the data supplied with them. This is a heavy responsibility but one that we all must bear.

The current research in this field is growing. Most of it is being done in Europe, China, Japan and India. We in the USA are lagging behind a good ten years. There is hope, however, as the tiny spark of interest is being fanned into a little blaze of commercial products.

## THE ROLE OF THE FOOD AND DRUG ADMINISTRATION

How much regulation is needed in the cosmetic industry? Here is a sticky question. The FDA is here to protect all of us against the unscrupulous marketer. We need a regulatory body in government in this area. The question of how much regulation we need in the cosmetic industry and what kinds of regulation is needed is still not answered. There is no doubt that we need some regulation in some areas. It is unfortunate that we can not eliminate all the bad actors from any field of endeavor. Some natural products will eventually fall into a category that will require FDA ruling. Scientists are looking closer at the many ingredients even in a single natural product and are finding them quite active. What is most interesting is that in some cases the individual ingredients when isolated and mixed together do not have the effect that the whole plant extract has. So, this is a difficult field and one that I know will require a great deal of research before we understand the plant activity. Until then no one really knows what role the FDA will play in natural plant use for skin care. The major effort we should make is to be sure that the products we use are safe and effective.

## THE NEED FOR CONTINUING EDUCATION

If we consider the task ahead, mainly of presenting the best skin care available, we shall need to keep up with the new developments - and that means education. Many of the skin care specialists are eager for new knowledge and new techniques. It is impressive to see how many are attending the current educational programs. Many of these programs are quite good while others are simple rehashing of outmoded data. A great deal is also pure nonsense.

A national standard is needed for basic education in skin care and there is a slight movement toward this goal. The National Cosmetology Association (the NCA) is the natural choice to lead this movement. There is a skin care section within the NCA that is able to focus on this task, but at the time of this writing there is no assigned task force.

I have outlined below what I feel is needed for a mininum course in skin care science to produce an adequately trained skin care specialist. The course covers 1800 hours, or 225 days. There are four sections to the course: basic biological science, skin anatomy and physiology, basic clinical skin care, and advanced clinical skin care. Within each of these sections there are specific topics . I have used as a guide in this outline the theoretical training program as suggested by CIDESCO. While the grouping is different, the course matter is similar.

### Section One - Basic Biological Science (320 Hours)

The objective of this section is to provide the

student with an overview of the biological sciences as they pertain to skin care. Zoology, botany, genetics, basic chemistry, physics, general anatomy, scientific method and classification, terminology, general microbiology and principles of sterilization, cytology and histology, and an introduction to general physiology will form the subject matter of this section.

This course will need a laboratory with student microscopes and demonstration microscopes as well as a basic chemistry laboratory. The skills needed to put together simple skin care products will be taught in this course, but enlarged upon in the advanced course. Emphasis is placed on core knowledge and practical application of facts. The role of natural products in skin care is taught in this section. The use of plant extracts and the difference between fresh and prepared products is discussed. Essential oils are covered in all aspects from preparation to actual use including the classification of these natural products as to activity and efficacy.

### Section Two - Skin Anatomy and Physiology (240 Hours)

The objective of this section is to provide the student with a thorough understanding of the anatomy of skin and related underlying structures. In addition, emphasis on skin physiology, pathophysiology, basic skin pathology, pharmacology and biochemistry will be stressed. Slide shows and live demonstrations are a part of this section. The student will learn the fundamental mechanisms of skin disease and the basis of the various treatment modalities. The course will cover the most common skin diseases and some of the more important communicable diseases.

In this section the relationship between structure and function becomes apparent to the student. The genesis of skin disorders and the principles of therapy are taught in the context of the underlying mechanisms involved.

### Section Three Basic - Clinical Skin Care (620 Hours)

The objective of this section is to provide the student with a fundamental understanding of the principles of skin care. Basic techniques in giving facials, cleansing, extraction, moisturizing, and facial massage are taught. The common conditions seen by skin care specialists are explained and demonstrated. Special attention is given to sterile technique and the do's and dont's of basic skin care. Basic electrotherapy, hair removal, and make-up are taught in this section. The student is introduced to client handling and client care. Mask therapy and the use of special plant extracts in certain skin conditions are introduced in this section as well. The professional relationship is developed in this section and the importance of this relationship is stressed throughout the remainder of the course. In this period the student must master the techniques and principles of therapy for the common skin disorders together with an understanding of emotional effects of any skin disorder on the client. The student is taught a holistic approach to skin care that encompasses both mind and matter as well as the influence of a positive attitude of the skin care specialist.

### Section Four - Advanced Clinical Skin Care (620 Hours)

The objective of this section is to provide the student with the knowledge and the skills that prepares her/him to work in the field of medicine. The training builds on basic skills and extends this knowledge while adding new information in the areas of pre and post-operative care, wound healing and surgical procedures. Extensive training in camouflage make-up and enhancement of appearance for radical surgical cases is taught. Actual patient contact and experience is needed to make this an effective course. Facial peels at various levels using a variety of chemicals and techniques is covered. Advanced electrical techniques and surgical procedures used with or under the direction of a physician are part of this section. Time and effort must also be expended in teaching the student the complexities of cosmetic surgery, patient selection and expectations, how to handle patients' problems, and problem-patients. The new methods of treating aging skin will be an important part of this section.

Finally, the training needed to operate a successful skin care business is extremely important for the student. A knowledge of fundamental accounting procedures and office management along with sales and marketing skills is essential to a good business orientation. Methods of building a practice and maintaining clients, keeping files and records, the legal aspects of skin care, and the need for professionalism in all aspects of the business is stressed.

These are skills best taught by professionals well trained in these arts. It is a tragedy that many skilled professionals are unsuccessful financially because they have not learned how to operate the business side of their profession. It has always been a mystery to me that this area is so neglected by the schools that train professionals. Earning a living, being happy in your chosen occupation, and being financially secure depends on how you manage your resources.

## THE NEW FRONTIER - THE TOTAL PERSON

At this stage in this textbook I would like to venture into an area that I feel holds promise for the skin care specialists, the area of mind-matter. I know that this is a controversial area and many readers may label this a cracked-pot idea, but nevertheless, I feel strongly about the subject. Anyone who practices medicine for a long time will encounter cases with outcomes that he or she does not understand: patients who have rapid healing of wounds, spontaneous cures of cancer and other fatal diseases, visions and even extra-corporeal experiences. You can ignore all these things or else you can look for some explanation beyond what you can physically know. Anyone who deals with individuals on a basis of trust exercises considerable power over that person. How you use this power depends to a large measure on your personal integrity which relates ultimately to your basic principles or beliefs. These principles or beliefs may be termed your philosophy or religion. Both are based on belief on nonmaterial entities such as truth, honor, etc, things you can not see but know exist.

If I said to you that at any given moment there were hundreds of voices in the air and hundreds of pictures in the air you would think that I am a bit balmy. Yet with a simple $5.00 radio I can pull many of these voices out of the air into the radio and thus into the physical world of sound. Without the radio I am totally unaware of these sounds, yet they exist as real entities just beyond my limits of physical perception. The same is true of television and its countless images. (In a way this is a blessing. Can you imagine being plagued with televison all day and night?) The images are there but mercifully just beyond are perception.

We are lost to know what mind or soul is, in fact ,we can not even define matter with any agreed upon parameters. Is it not amazing when we speak of mind and soul that suddenly the doubters have absolute knowledge that there is no mind or soul? If we only look a little bit at this area we soon become astounded not only with what we do not know but also with what we do know and can know.

A relatively new branch of science called **psychoneuroimmunology** now relates the action of the brain to the immune system. In fact, the brain, along with other elements of the nervous system, is thought to have an immune system of its own. How this system interacts with the regular immune system is still unknown, but the presence of a link between the immune system and the nervous system may account for some of the unexplained phenomenon observed in all walks of life, not just medical practice. Look at the effects of fragrance for example. With the very same odor, the limbic system may produce in different individuals quite a variable number of responses. One could experience anything from joy, sorrow, love, hate, or even diarrhea. The effects of will or mind over matter can also be profound. I shall give you a few examples from my own experiences while practicing medicine many years ago. These happenings made me aware that there are many areas of life that I do not understand which, nonetheless, have an effect on our daily living.

### The Telephone Phenomenom

In the early days of my rural practice we still had a central switchboard which had to be connected by a human operator. You simply turned a crank and asked the operator for your number. Not infrequently the operators would listen in on calls (most likely to check the line). At times in the first year of practice calls would come in from a frantic mother who would neither identify herself or tell me where she lived before she hung up. The only thing I had to do was to dial the operator, ask her who had called, and then ask for directions. It was a small town and most people knew each other. One afternoon just as I was leaving for the hopsital to make rounds, I received a call from a young mother who informed me that she "was going to throw her three children in the well." I did not recognize her voice and frankly did not know what to do, so I told her not to do anything until I saw her and that I would come to see her immediately. She said. "Alright, Doctor." In my excited state, I hung up, forgetting to ask her name and address. I rang the operator who gave me the patient's name and directed me to the farm. When I arrived I found her in the yard near the house standing over the uncovered well with the three children - a new baby, a two year old girl and a three year old boy. She had opened the well and was standing by waiting for my arrival. She was haggard, and looked exhausted, pale as a ghost, and with a flat expression. My impression was that she had a post-partum psychosis. She was concerned about not being able to get supper for her husband because the kids took so much of her time. It seemed logical to her to get rid of the kids so her husband would not be angry with her. She was staying with her parents, both of whom were working in the city. As I spoke with her I learned that her grandmother lived nearby and that she had called the woman that morning. I suggested that we all go to her grandmother's house until her husband came home, and she agreed. Once at her grandmother's home we arranged for her hospitalization and treatment.

The strange aspect of this case was this woman had never been seen by a physician. Her family did not believe in doctors, her three children were delivered at home by a midwife, there was no pre-natal or postnatal care. Mental problems in this rural area were considered as "a notion" and not accounted as an illness. Following this episode she and her family became regular patients. Over the next twenty years she had no recurrence of psychotic episodes, but her children developed several serious medical problems that would have been fatal without treatment. Why had she called a doctor on this particular day and at this time?

In that case I had the name and directions to the farm. Some years later with progress we had a modern telephone system installed with a dial and all. No longer did we have operators who knew everyone and where they lived. One night at about 2 AM I receive a call from a frantic wife that her husband "was turning blue and dying." "Hurry!" she said and hung up. I did not recognize her voice for she was a first time caller. I dressed rapidly, drove my car out of my lane and turned right. I had no idea where I was going or who had called me. The back roads of rural Pennsylvania are twisted and branch frequently; there were so many choices of roads yet I seemed to make turns as if I knew where I was going. I felt very foolish, yet compelled to continue this trip. In one of the valleys I saw a lighted farm and drove towards it, looking for an entrance. A lane appeared and there was a car and driver at the end of the lane who urged me excitedly to follow him. We sped down the dirt road into a farm yard, then into the house and up the stairs where a very large man was gasping for breath, apparently in pulmonary edema.

After treating the patient and arranging for his admission to the hospital I sat with the family and had a cup of coffee. Only then did the wife realize that she had not given me directions, or told me who she was. How did I find the farm? To this day even with good directions it would take some doing to find that farm at 2 AM.

**Space and Time**

Even more difficult to explain was the time a retired auto dealer came to see me accompanied by his wife. They had moved into our area from an adjacent state several years before and were regular patients. A handsome couple in their late sixties, they were obviously very much in love and devoted to each other. She was quite concerned about an experience her husband had two days ago.

He was somewhat reluctant to talk about this experience even though we had good rapport. As his wife started to explain why they had come to see me he interrupted gently and said that he would tell me about what had happened. In his retirement he had decided to try farming and to this end he purchased a large tractor and other basic farm equipment. One evening he finished plowing a field, drove the tractor into the shed, went into the house, washed and dressed for dinner. As dinner was not quite ready he decided to sit on his porch and look over his fields, until his wife called him. As he was looking at the field he had just plowed *he saw himself on the tractor coming out of the field toward the house.* Startled, he called his wife and tried to relate what he had just "seen." His wife was baffled and concerned; she suggested he come in and lie down but he insisted he felt all right, only he was shaken by this. His first thought was that he was going insane and hallucinating. In way of background, this man had severe arterial disease. Two years prior to this episode he had surgery for a blocked carotid artery, but had made a good recovery and had a good post-operative result. On physical examination there were no signs of a stroke, no blood pressure change, no weakness, no sensory loss (to use a colloquial phrase "no nothing"). To him this episode was very real, not an hallucination. He related how he followed the tractor with his eyes right into the yard and into the shed. What was going on? My first thought was that he had "a little stroke", that is, small vessel rupture or closure that impedes brain function for a short time, often only a few minutes. In his case, there was no apparent physical dysfunction, only this visual phenomenon. He was rational and alert showing no obvious signs of a psychosis. My first thought was to pass this off as something that was not explainable, one of many things that happen to us in a lifetime that we can not understand. He would have none of that. He wanted a medical explanation, but I had none. Let's look at this episode. The man saw himself and the tractor after the event had occured, just like a video tape replay. There was perhaps a 30 minute time gap between the real episode and what he relates he saw. Remember, he could in no way have "seen" himself while he was on the tractor, so there was no prior visual imprint. Next, he felt that he was actually on the porch and on the tractor at the same time. This phenomenon is called **bilocation**. At the time, he was conscious and fully aware of his surroundings and of the real time, that is, before dinner. Somehow he had been translocated in both time and space back into the field and on the tractor. A very tough act to explain, but this was my explanation.

Both space and time are not absolute "things", they are both relative to each other. We can not have space without time and vice versa. The world as we see it is a world as no one else sees it. What is beautiful or ugly is truly in the eye of the beholder, and what is real or not real may also be in the eye of the beholder. Who then can say that what he saw was not real? Can we say because it sounds weird that it did not happen? I like to believe that he had a liitle stroke which messed up his brain pathways so that all those thousands of messages became scambled and produced this phenomenon. This is the most likely cause, even though I can not explain why that particular event was played back to him. Later in my practice I had two other men and one woman with similar experiences, all of whom had various types of arterial disease. We actually never see anything. What we perceive as an object is the reflected light from an object, hitting our retina and then being conveyed to an area of our brain via electrical and chemical signals that we interpret as a specific "thing". This means that we must use some system to interpret the input, place it into a category of time and place, soft or hard, friend or foe, all in an instant! Are we so sure of what is going on about us all the time?

Each of us lives in a world of his or her making, colored by our perceptions and our beliefs. This is the real part of you that relates to your client. The "real you" comes through to your client in your touch, for your touch conveys more than just the pressure and warmth of your hands.

## Touch and You

One of the most positive aspects of skin care is the touching of the client. There is no human activity that has such a powerful effect as touch. As a skin care specialist you will feel this power and convey it to your client. The importance of holistic care and the mind-matter effect is centered on your ability to communicate in a non-verbal manner through touch. Now, this is the crucial point to be made - you must be a real person to have a positive effect on your client. You must be a whole person who has confidence and security. To be a whole person you need conviction and committment, then you can convey these qualities to your client as you render your services. It makes a real difference in how you approach the client, how you convey your professionalism, how your personality comes through.

The magic of the healing hand has been a topic of discussion from the earliest times. The touch of hands has a profound effect when done with an emotional overlay. We are often repelled by a simple handshake; some individuals try to impress you with vigor and strength during a handshake, but the phoniness of their character comes through nevertheless. We all remember the hand-holding experience of our first love affair, the security of holding our parent's hand the first day of school, or a visit to the dentist as a child. These are powerful effects which last forever. Now you are able to transfer this power to your client by the magic of your hands, your presence and your skills. Do not forget that you are a whole person, and that your client is a person who trusts you and is in your care to be helped and nurtured. Beyond all the science and secular knowledge you have a power inherent in your soul that can reach out to other souls and to help. Inner beauty can be manifested outwardly only when all negative obstacles are removed. No one can appear beautiful with fear, hate, envy, and anger chewing at their fiber. This is why you need the holistic approach to each client, to know them and to help them. The immune system has incredible powers to heal and protect the body and you have the power to help activate that immune system in your clients simply by relating to them in a positive manner. It is well known observation that depressed individuals are more susceptible to organic disease than happy individuals. Depressed immune function can be objectively demonstrated in depressed individuals. It requires a receptive mind to appreciate these things. No one will ever understand the mind of God, but the sanctity of mankind must be a given.

I wish to leave the reader with one last thought about a subject which that I feel will assume a greater importance in our lives in the near future. This is the world of quantum theory. I raise this subject because you will be reading more about it every year. In fact, a recent book entitled Quantum Healing by Dr. Depak Choppra made quite a stir in many health areas. The impact is here already, my aim is only to introduce the reader to this subject.

## Quantum Theory and Life

There is a great deal written about quantum theory these days and I would like to share a few thoughts with the reader on the quantum theory and how it may affect our lives. You need not be a mathematicianto appreciate or even understand the basics of quantum theory, you need only an open mind and the will to learn. A good basic book is Taking The Quantum Leap by Fred Allan Wolf published by Harper and Row in 1989. This book was followed by the very thought provoking The Body Quantum also by Dr Wolf. As you read about the quantum theory you will become aware of many aspects of the so called physical world that will grip you and hold you in wonder. Why do I think this is important for skin care specialist to look into quantum theory? Without question it will broaden your interest and raise your horizons. It will also help you to appreciate the mind-matter relationship.

I have listed some books in the Appendix that will be a helpful starting point for those readers interested in pursuing this subject. This study will also introduce you to the almost limitless ability of man to explore both inner and outer space. Most likely some questions will be answered for you but many more will be raised. Quantum theory will also help you to appreciate the vast difficulty in understanding each other. Finally it will show you a small aspect of the majesty of God and the wonderous Universe created by God from nothing.

With your new skills and renewed confidence, faith in yourself and in humanity you are in a good position to make a major contribution to society.

One of the great privileges of working in medicine and in skin care is that you have the opportunity to meet so many wonderful and challenging people. If you are able to help even one of these people you will have a rewarding life.

# Hirsutism, Body Hair, and Skin Types

Of all the body features, the two that receive the most attention are **the hair and the skin**. These two structures are interrelated genetically, physically, and biochemically. While we know and understand a great deal about hair and skin we still have a great deal to learn about the **interaction of these two structures**. In this addendum I shall present some data on excessive or unwanted hair outlining how this condition comes about and what may be done to correct it. We shall need to discuss the male hormones and the role they play in body hair and body type. These hormones are called **androgens** as you will recall from Chapter 4. The level of circulating androgen is responsible for terminal hair, or the absence of it, on most areas of the body. Subtle changes in the level of androgens and changes in the metabolism of androgens can lead to a number of different skin types and physical apppearances which are called **phenotypes**. First, we need to define certain conditions associated with unwanted body hair and androgens. Then, we shall enter into a brief discussion of androgen chemistry, as we need this knowledge to understand the effects of androgens on the body.

## BACKGROUND ON BODY HAIR AND HAIR GROWTH IN FEMALES

Hair is derived from the epidermis of the skin. The vellus hairs, those light colored, fine, delicate hairs that cover most of the body surface, are precursors of the larger, dark terminal hairs. About three months before birth **all of the hair follicles that will ever exist are present in the skin**. There will be no new follicles after that period. These fine vellus hairs are destined to become the terminal hairs of the future. If you look carefully on a newborn or a young child you will see these fine hairs all over the body. They are awaiting a signal from the brain to develop into terminal hairs at puberty. The body chemicals that make this change are the androgens.

We know that masculine and feminine patterns are set before birth but the expression of these patterns requires further action by the brain and associated glands. We have defined three major conditions associated with unwanted hair growth.

**HIRSUTISM** is a condition of excessive facial hair. *Hirsutus* is the Latin word for **shaggy**. There are several varieties of this condition, most of which are benign and need not indicate a lack of femininity. This is called **idiopathic hirsutism**, meaning the cause is unknown. If the condition is associated with hair loss on the head, deepening of the voice, increased muscle mass, and clitoral enlargement, the condition is then called **VIRILISM**. *Vir* is Latin for man. **HYPERTRICHOSIS** is a term applied to excess hair on the arms, thighs, legs, and back. This condition may or may not be associated with hirsutism or virilism. Keep these three conditions in mind as we go along and it will prevent any confusion in terms.

## ANDROGENS AND THE BASIC BIOCHEMISTRY OF SEX HORMONES

There is a certain uniformity in nature that allows established pathways to produce more than one substance. In the case of the male hormones, called **androgens,** the exact same pathway is followed for the production of female hormones and the cortisone family of hormones. All of these hormones belong to a group called **steroid hormones**. The major difference in these glands is the quantity of the specific hormone produced by the ovary, adrenal gland, or the testicle. Keep in mind that these **glands all produce the same types of hormones**.

The pathway starts with **cholesterol,** proceeds stepwise to **progesterone,** and then to **17-OH progesterone.** From there by a series of steps it produces **estrogen, testosterone, or cortisone**. I have outlined these steps so you can see the uniformity and association of the various hormones from each gland.

**ANDROGENS** are a series of hormones of the steroid family that induce, regulate, and maintain the growth and development of the male reproductive organs and sexual characteristics. These hormones have certain effects on the skin including hair, muscle, bone, and the production of body proteins. In the female, they regulate sexual and axillary hair and stimulate the female libido.

There are **two glands in women that produce male hormones, or androgens: they are the ovary and the adrenal gland**. Now, it seems strange that a female should produce male hormones, but it is true. Similarly, males produce female hormones called estrogens. Let us take a careful look at how these hormones arise and function, for it is the key to understanding the appearance of hair and body types.

### Names of the Androgen Hormones

We shall deal with only four of the androgens produced by women. They are the most important ones. **Testosterone (T), dihydrotestosterone (DHT), androstenediol (A) and** dehydroepiandrosterone (DHEA). One of the interesting aspects of hormones is that they are **derived from precursors**. That means they have a common ancestor and are often interconvertible. Now we shall see from where these hormones come and what they do. The ovary and adrenal gland are the original two precursor sources but we may have **other hormones produced by cells in the skin**. This is an important and exciting part of this subject for the skin care specialist. Paying close attention to what follows will help you to understand the whole process. Here we go!

### The Great Scheme of Androgen Hormone Production

An overview of this scheme is as follows. **The hormones are produced in the ovaries and the adrenal glands and then circulate in the blood stream, bound to a special protein called sex hormone binding protein (SHBP)**. Only a very small fraction of the hormones are free or unbound, but it is this free portion, about 1% to 2% of all the androgens, that accounts for the effects. When the hormone reaches the skin cells, or hair cells, it must enter the cell and be bound to a receptor protein. It is then **transported to the nucleus** where it interacts with the DNA molecule to produce the hormonal effect. This is the fundamental action of all sex hormones on all cells. What is produced by the DNA molecule under the influence of the androgen is not fully understood. (In most cases special proteins are produced that have specific effects on the cells.)

In the ADRENAL GLAND the sequence is the same for the production of testosterone and estradiol. Cortisone, which is the major hormone produced by the adrenal gland, branches off from the precursor 17-OH PROGESTERONE. Now that we have testosterone, let's see what happens to it in the great scheme.

After testosterone enters the blood stream and is bound to the SHBP it is circulated about the body to various tissues, in our case the skin and hair. At this point a curious thing happens in which the testosterone is converted to a more active form called **DIHYDROTESTOSTERONE (DHT)** by a special enzyme known as **5 alpha reductase**. This enzyme is present only in the target organs like the skin and hair cells. DHT is 2-3 times more potent as an androgen than is testosterone. All of the DHT is produced in the peripheral tissue, skin, and hair, with virtually none produced by the ovaries or the adrenals. Now, this is an extremely important concept for what is to follow, for **without the enzyme 5 alpha reductase there would be no visible expression of the androgens in females or males.** In fact, there is a condition in which males and females have plenty of androgens but no manifestation of maleness, such as pubic hair and so forth. So keep in mind that this specific enzyme is responsible for some of the effect of testosterone in the skin and hair.

ANDROSTENEDIONE is produced by the adrenal glands and the ovaries as a by-product of testosterone. It may be interconverted to testosterone and vice versa. The level of androstrenedione fluctuates with the menstrual cycle and can account for changes in body hair on a cyclic fashion. While androstenedione is itself a weak androgen, being only about one-tenth as potent as testosterone, it is nevertheless a factor in hair and sebum production since it is interconvertible. About 5 to 10% of the hormone is produced in the peripheral tissues and the rest is secreted by the adrenals and the ovaries. This androgen is frequently found to be elevated in women with hirsutism.

**DHEA, or dehydroepiandrosterone,** is a very weak androgen, only 1/20 of that of testosterone. It is mainly produced in the adrenals with only about 5-10% being produced by conversion from androstenedione. This is an extremely important hormone for it has a great deal to do with prevention of breast cancer and has an important relationship to the aging process.

We are now ready to see how the hormones affect hair growth in the female. It is necessary to keep in mind all of the factors that we have covered above: how the androgenic hormones arise from the ovaries and the adrenals, how the hormone is transported to the cells in the blood stream on the SHBP, how only free hormone is able to enter the cell, and how the cell can convert certain hormones and produce an effect on the DNA. The altered DNA, in turn, produces a protein that has a major effect on the cell. This is diagrammed in **Figure A-1**.

### THE UNWANTED HAIR PROBLEM IN WOMEN

Women are pictured as smooth skinned with a large crop of flowing thick hair, streaming about their face and reflecting radiantly in the sunlight. We do not think of women with hair on their faces, legs, and chests. Unfortunately,

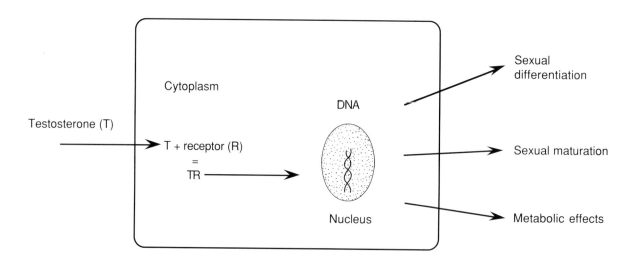

1. Testosterone enters cell
2. Testosterone combines with receptor
3. TR interacts with DNA
4. Effects produced by new proteins

**FIGURE A-1** Cellular mechanism showing action of hormone, receptor and DNA action.

| DESCRIPTION | CAUSE |
|---|---|
| 1. Idiopathic hirsutism or end-organ hypersensitivity | No endodrine abnormalities are found. The hair bulb is very sensitive to androgens. Often the hirsutism is localized. |
| 2. Hirsutism associated with ovarian disease | Polycystic ovarian disease also known as Stein-Leventhal syndrome, is associated with increased ovarian production of androgens, with testosterone being the main male hormone. Ovarian tumors and complications of pregnancy are also causes. |
| 3. Hirsutism associated with adrenal abnormalities. | The adrenal genital syndrome is an inherited trait and is the cause of hirsutism in 10 percent of cases. Cushing's syndrome and adrenal tumors are additional adrenal causes. |
| 4. Other causes | Hyperprolactinemia from stress or pituitary tumors, thyroid disease, drugs, and rarely, liver disease. Excessive growth hormone and other pituitary hormone can result in secondary androgen production. |

**TABLE A-1**

this occurs, but how, and is there help? The ultimate cause of this condition is circulating androgens. We know that there is great deal of difference in the amount of body and facial hair that characterizes various ethnic groups. In some countries hairy skin in the female is not considered a detriment to beauty. In our Western society it is in most cases a catastrophe. For ease in helping the skin care specialist decide whether or not to refer the client to a physician for help I have outlined a program to follow. I believe the best policy is a referral to an **endocrinologist** in all cases where there is evidence of virilism and/ or an abnormal menstrual history. Recently though, the use of sensitive laboratory tests have enabled many women to benefit from specific treatment for their condition.

We know that acne, male pattern baldness, and idiopathic hirsutism are androgen dependent disorders (1). When sections of skin were studied from areas of the body a considerable difference in 5 alpha reductase activity was found in sexual skin versus nonsexual skin. This study indicates a regional variation in the level and distribution of the enzyme 5 alpha reductase and the important role it plays in the expression of secondary sex characteristics (2).

Here are the most common causes of hirsutism:

1. Increased serum levels of testosterone or increased production rates.
2. Increased free levels of androgens due to decreased levels of SHBP
3. Increased levels of 5 alpha reductase activity.

It is not our purpose to go into the mechanism of each of these conditions but it is important for the skin care specialist to know the signs that indicate referral. Here they are: **rapid increase in hair growth, stopping of menstrual cycle or no menstrual cycle, and virilism**. In most cases the appearance of hirsutism is benign, and can be treated by a skin care specialist. In those cases associated with increased hormone production, there are specific treatments to reduce the hormone production and activity. In these cases you will need to work with a physician, specifically an endocrinologist. **Table A-1** shows an outline of the causes of hirsutism.

It has been found that hirsute women secrete about four times as much androstanediol, a metabolite of androstenedione, as do normal women. Skin taken from the pubic area of hirsute women produces four times as much DHA as normal women indicating an increase in 5 alpha reductase activity. A deficiency of this enzyme is associated with the absence of seborrhea and acne.

## TREATMENT OF HIRSUTISM

Management of hirsutism requires a combination of therapeutic measures, often in conjunction with the skin care specialist. The treatment plan revolves around 1. reducing the secretion of ovarian and adrenal androgens, 2. decreasing the androgen activity of the hair follicle by preventing the binding of DHT to the androgen receptor, and 3. mechanically removing the existing terminal hairs. Treatment by appropriate medications takes 6 to 24 months, so it is very slow.

**REMOVAL OF HAIR is best accomplished by shaving.** Why so many women are opposed to shaving is a mystery but it appears to stem from the masculine association of the morning beard. Women do not recognize that they have fewer facial hairs and that the rate of growth is slower than males. In addition, shaving will stimulate the skin and produce a better epidermis, activate fibroblasts, and strengthen the dermis. Other measures include **waxing and depilatories.** If you are trained in **electrolysis** this is a good technique for a limited number of facial hairs. The **result is permanent only if the total follicle is destroyed, including the germinal cells.**

## BODY TYPES ASSOCIATED WITH HAIR PATTERNS

**Sexual hair in the female includes the pubic hair, the axillary hair, and the eyebrow.** There is a very close association, if not a direct correlation, between the eyebrow pattern and the pubic hair pattern. Furthermore, the various patterns of eyebrows and pubic hair are associated with different skin types. It will come as a revelation to most readers that the eyebrow is partly sexual hair, but it is true. It has long been known that the eyebrow is very responsive to thyroid hormone and, in fact, the absence of the outer one-third of the eyebrow is a classic sign of hypothyroidism (low level of thyroid hormone.) First, let us review the sequence of sexual development in females and then we shall relate this development to the various skin types that I shall define later. Physical sexual development is called **puberty.**

**Puberty** in the female is a complex affair. It is initiated by an increased output of **gonado-**tropins by the pituitary gland. This action is the result of instructions sent by a part of the brain called the hypothalamus. Recall that the gonadotropins are the hormones that specifically target the ovaries and the breasts. The sexual organs respond to increased levels of estrogen and other hormones secreted by the ovaries. The first sign of onset of puberty in the female is the change in vaginal superficial cells as seen in the vaginal smear. In response to estrogen the vagina begins to lengthen and continues this action until the menstrual cycle begins and even later. **We recognize three major sexual characteristics in female at puberty: breast development, pubic hair development, and axillary hair development.** We shall look at each characteristic separately.

### Breast Development - The Five Stages

**Stage 1.** This is an infantile stage with only a tiny breast bud. It lasts from birth to puberty.

**Stage 2.** This is the stage of the enlarged breast bud in which the breast and papilla are elevated and the areola is increased in diameter. It represents the first visible sign of puberty changes in the breast.

**Stage 3.** The breast further increases in size and begins to round, like the adult breast.

**Stage 4.** The areola and the papilla increase in size to form a secondary mound projecting above the remainder of the breast. This may be the last stage in some females as the breast may not progress to Stage 5. A few girls will, however, skip Stage 4 and go directly to Stage 5.

**Stage 5.** The breast rounds, becomes smooth, and the elevation of Stage 4 disappears.

The ages of breast development are quite variable. Some girls start at age nine and some at 13 years. In some girls full maturity of the breast is obtained by age 12, while in others it may not be reached until age 19 or later. Classification is by J.M. Tanner in Endocrine and Genetic Diseases of Childhood. W.B Saunders 1969

### Pubic Hair Development - The Five Stages

**Stage 1.** No true pubic hair, but downy vellus hairs that may resemble those on the abdomen.

**Stage 2.** Sparse growth of long hair, slightly pigmented, either on the labia or on the mons pubis.

**Stage 3**. The hair becomes darker, coarser, and starts to curl. It spreads sparsely over the pubic symphysis.

**Stage 4.** The hair is adult in character but covers a smaller area. It does not spread to the thighs.

**Stage 5**. The hair is distributed in the inverse triangle, characteristic of the adult. It has spread to the thighs but not above the base of the triangle.

Pubic hair growth starts at any age from nine up to 12 years of age but the adult pattern may be attained from 12 to 17 years of age. It has been observed that pubic hair patterns and growth are also quite variable with no set relationship to breast development. Some girls may stay in Stage 2 or 3 for long periods of time before advancing to the next stage. Classification is from the same Tanner reference given above.

There was some controversy on the role of estrogen in the development of pubic hair. It is known now that only androgens are responsible for pubic hair growth in both males and females. We know that both the ovaries and the adrenal glands supply androgens to the pubic area.

**AXILLARY HAIR** appears usually two years after pubic hair, but again, there is a great variation in onset of growth of axillary hair.

**MENARCHE OR ONSET OF MENSES** is a variable event not necessarily related to the external signs of puberty. On an average, 95% of girls will experience their first period between the ages of 11 and 15 years of age. A few start as early as eight or nine and some as late as 19.

## VARIATION IN SEXUAL HAIR AND BODY TYPES

The androgen hormones control or express sexual hair and the action of these hormones depends to some measure on the level of associated enzymes in the skin. We expect that a strong interrelationship exists between the expression of the hormones and the location of the enzymes in the skin, the level of circulating hormone, both free and bound, and the level of SHBG. As a result of these variables we see differences in the phenotypic expression of sexual hair in the female.

Since the level of androgens also effects the fibroblasts in the dermis we shall notice differ-

ences in the texture of skin as well as changes in the hair patterns.

The following classification of skin types based on eyebrow pattern, pubic hair pattern, and skin characteristics was developed over thirty years of observation of over 500 adult females. The application of this classification covers ages 18 to 65 years. It includes only Caucasian females, but from a wide ethnic population.

### Eyebrow - Pubic Hair-Skin Types

Type I - The Most CommonType

**The eyebrow** is heaviest in the inner canthus and tails off to a sharp point at the outer canthus. It may or may not extend to the outer edge of the eye. There may be a clump of hair near the inner canthus which is not uniformly distributed over the rest of the eyebrow. The general shape is a gentle smooth arch with no breaks.

**The pubic hair** is a classic triangular pattern with most of the hair centering on the area of the clitoris. The mons is rarely heavily haired and the lateral extension may or may not reach the thighs. The extension down the labial will grow more sparse as it reaches the perineum. Little, if any, pubic hair extends posteriorly to the anus. There is often late onset of pubic hair development during puberty.

**The skin** is generally of fair complexion and smooth, with a tendency toward increased vellus hairs on the cheeks and outer lips. This type will show signs of aging rather quickly, usually in the thirties. Facial lines and telangiectasia is common. Acne will occur but it is usually not a problem with this type. The neck is vulnerable to early wrinkling. This group tends to have large breasts as young adults but the breasts sag after pregnancy. They have poor connective tissue.

Type I - A

**The eyebrow** is slightly heavier with a distinct increase in thickness in the inner one-third. The outer one-third is the same as in Type I.

**The pubic hair** pattern is essentially triangular with a middle clumped arrangement at the top of the labia. Hair on the lower labia is often more sparse than Type I.

**The skin** is usually fair and smooth but there

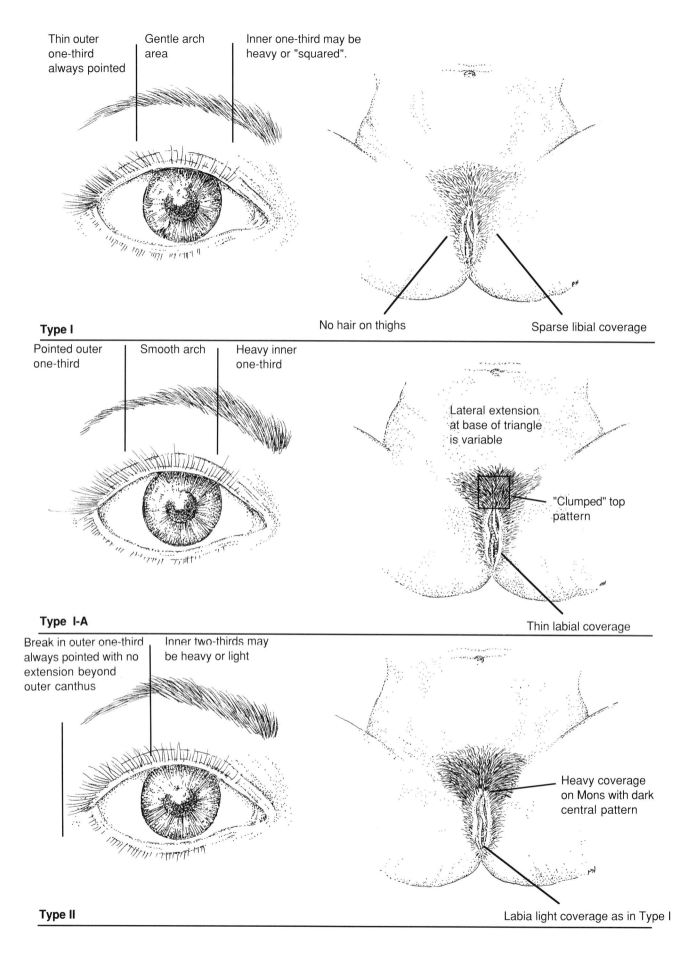

Thin outer one-third always pointed

Gentle arch area

Inner one-third may be heavy or "squared".

No hair on thighs

Sparse libial coverage

**Type I**

Pointed outer one-third

Smooth arch

Heavy inner one-third

Lateral extension at base of triangle is variable

"Clumped" top pattern

Thin labial coverage

**Type I-A**

Break in outer one-third always pointed with no extension beyond outer canthus

Inner two-thirds may be heavy or light

Heavy coverage on Mons with dark central pattern

Labia light coverage as in Type I

**Type II**

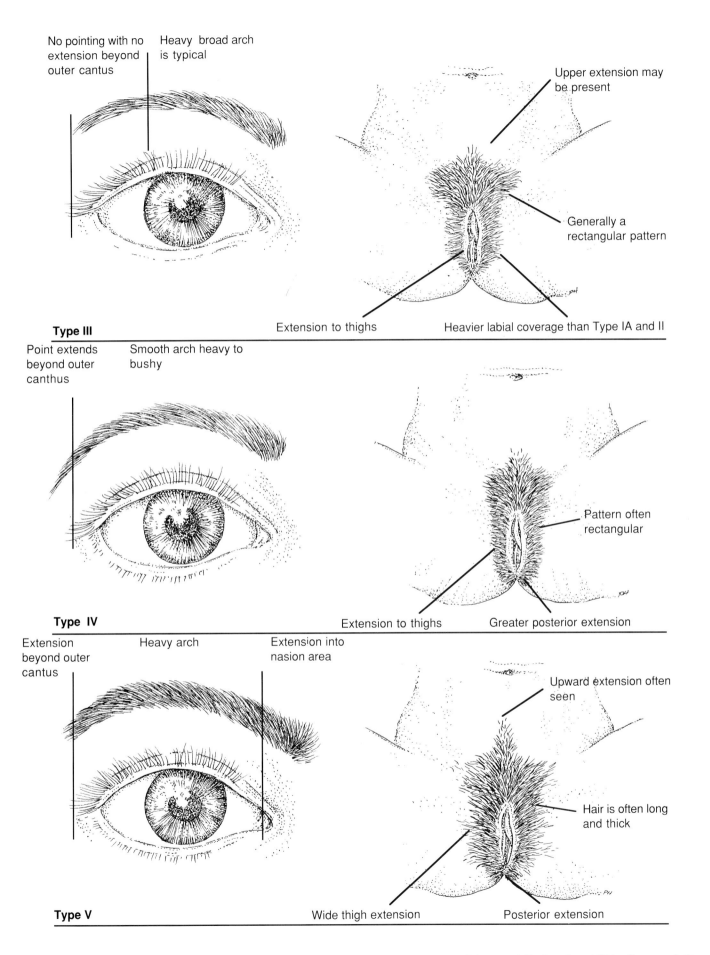

No pointing with no extension beyond outer cantus

Heavy broad arch is typical

Upper extension may be present

Generally a rectangular pattern

Extension to thighs

Heavier labial coverage than Type IA and II

**Type III**

Point extends beyond outer canthus

Smooth arch heavy to bushy

Pattern often rectangular

Extension to thighs

Greater posterior extension

**Type IV**

Extension beyond outer cantus

Heavy arch

Extension into nasion area

Upward extension often seen

Hair is often long and thick

Wide thigh extension

Posterior extension

**Type V**

Advanced Professional Skin Care   **A-9**

is often an underlying masculine feature to the face. Most of these women are quite attractive. Facial lines are frequent early in life (25-30). The breasts tend to be small to medium size with fairly good tone over the years. For some reason this type tends to be tense and nervous.

### Type II (Break in Arch)

**The eyebrow** exhibits a center peak rather than a true arch. Usually the medial portion is thicker than the lateral portion. The lateral or outer portion will tail off at times into a point but may be irregular. The extension is rarely beyond the outer canthus. Almost any hair color can have this type but it appears most often in non-Latin brunettes.

**The pubic hair** is characteristically heavy on the upper labia and the mons. It rarely extends laterally and has only a modest presence on the lower labia. The labia tend to be thin.

**The skin** is very much like TYPE I except it is usually of a finer texture. Aging progresses about as fast as in TYPE I but it is seen most often in the lower portion of the face, particularly about the mouth. The neck will wrinkle early if exposed to sun, but is less prone than Type I. Large to average breasts that withstand aging and pregnancy are seen.

### Type III

**The eyebrow** is a broad arch with an even expansion extending from the inner canthus to the outer canthus. There is no tailing and no breaks. There may be a smooth flow or occasionally a few larger hairs are seen to interrupt the curve but no frank break is seen.

**The pubic hair** assumes a rectangular pattern with only slight extension on to the thighs. In some cases thigh extension may be absent. The most marked characteristic of this pattern is its uniformity of density from the mons to the perineum. Early onset of puberty is frequent.

**The skin** of this type is quite variable. Depending on the ethnic origin it may be smooth or coarse with a slight tendency to acne. The skin is firm with a moderately strong mouth line. There is a tendency for early wrinkles in the forehead and outer cheeks. The neck is usually slow to wrinkle without sunbathing, but is not immune. Average breast size.

### Type IV

**The eyebrow** is broad as in Type III but extends over the edge of the upper orbit to the outer canthus of the eye. Usually it extends down the outer corner. There are no breaks in the arch but the appearance may be bushy or heavy. These women are usually brunette but all hair colors and ethnic groups share this type.

**The pubic hair** pattern is heavy and extends from the mons down to the anus and sometimes further posteriorly. Lateral extension is variable but occurs frequently in this type. The labia are usually thick and large, but variations occur. Early onset of pubic hair appearance at puberty with later onset of breast development.

**The skin** is usually oily with moderate pore size. These women are of moderate to large frame, and show more muscular development than the other types listed. They are more prone to acne but less prone to show signs of early aging. They are subject to idiopathic hirsutism, which is usually mild. As they get older they have more trouble with facial hair then they do with wrinkles. Breasts tend to be slightly below average size but not small.

### Type V

**The eyebrow** is very characteristic of this type. It is heavy as in Type IV but the inner canthus portion will show extension into the nasion area. In some rare cases the eyebrows actually meet. The hair is usally very dark brown, black or auburn, but some blondes also have this pattern. Lateral extension is the same as in Type IV. Often they will have a slight male-type supraorbital ridge over the eyes.

**The pubic hair** pattern is similar to Type IV only it is heavier and extends far to thighs and far posteriorly. The texture is often coarse and the length of the hair is frequently quite long.

**The skin** may be coarse and oily with a tendency to acne, but this is not always an attendant characteristic of this type. The women are as a rule "big boned" or large framed. The are subject to idiopathic hirsutism with excessive lip hair being a real problem for this type. They age slowly even though they tend to "bloom" early. Breasts are frequently smaller than average with dark areolae.

There are, of course, **subtypes** of these five

major types, for in nature very few features are clear cut and sharply demarcated. **No system of classification is perfect so expect only about 70 to 80% correlation** of the various signs presented here. Most of us are really shades of gray rather than black or white. By observing the eyebrow and the skin you can define a skin type that will assist you in the overall clinical appraisal of your client.

# Plants and Natural Plant Materials

This list represents only a small fraction of the natural materials which are available. When you purchase natural materials such as extracts of plants and essential oils you need to rely on the integrity of the source for guarantee of purity and potency. So much junk (garbage is the better word) is on the market that you must be knowledgeable about the quality of the material which you purchase.

Manufacturers of finished products who buy these materials rarely go into an extensive quality control process to be assured of the purity and potency of these starting materials. I urge you, therefore, to ask the manufacturer for his quality control checks on both the raw materials and the finished goods. Cosmetic companies are not obligated to do this but drug manufacturers are required. Since many companies are making claims that their products are active, that is, they do this or that to the skin, you have every right to ask, **"What is your proof for that statement?", "Show me your supportive data."** These two questions alone would eliminate just about everyone now selling so-called natural skin care products to the skin care specialist. Be wary and be demanding. It is both your right and your obligation to your client.

## COSMETIC AND SKIN CARE PRODUCTS

When you begin the study of plants and how to use them it is best to have a course first in botany and then in pharmacognosy, the study of the medicinal use of plants. There is no real short cut to learning this science, therefore, I can only hope to introduce you to some of these plant materials. An easy way to start is to look at individual plants and see what properties and uses they have. The selection is not comprehensive and in many ways reflects my personal interests or preferences.

**1. Aloe.** Aloe is complex material derived from the leaves of the plant *Folia Aloe Succinata.* It is a tropical plant which has quite a variable composition year to year based on weather conditions. The major ingredients are mucopolysaccarides, resins, and bitter principles (alkaloids). It finds use as an anti-inflammatory agent and is formulated, therefore, in soothing and healing preparations. The freezed dried form is most active and the most dependable form that I have used.

**2. Anise.** Anise is widely used as a flavor. The major active ingredient is anethole, a phenylpropanoid, in the essential oil fraction. Anise is a stimulant, or carminative: that is, it makes the skin red by dilating the capillaries. It is used in mouthwashes and dental care products. I like the fragrance but have found little use for it in skin care. The plant name is *Pimpinella anisum Linne.*

**3. Arnica.** Arnica is derived from the flowers of the *Arnica montana*, a member of the

Family Composita, a very large medicinal plant group. The active substances are arnidiol and faradiol, two dihydric alcohols. In addition, there are tannin, phytosterines, azulen and some alkaloids. This plant extract is used in treating bruises, sprains, and minor abrasions. Their actions appear to come from a counter-irritant effect. Other ingredients include several sequiterpene lactones that have anti-inflammatory and analgesic effects. There is also an anti-bacterial effect present due to other ingredients such as helenalin. Arnica should never be used internally as it is quite toxic. There is little clinical evidence to support the use of arnica but long historical use seems to warrant its continuence.

**4. Balm Mint.** *Melissa officinalis* or lemon balm is another name for this plant. It is one of my favorites. The leaves yield essential oils which have germicidal and fungicidal properties, chiefly terpines, but alkaloids and tannins are also present. Melissa is an excellent fragrance and an effective topical antiseptic. In acne, a tiny drop on a pimple is helpful. Do not use it all over large areas or in high concentrations.

**5. Butcher's Broom.** Butcher's broom has been used for treatment of dilated capillaries. The roots of this plant contains saponines, essential oils, and complex glycosides. It should be used as fresh as possible or as a freeze dried preparation.

**6. Camomile.** Camomile may be of two forms, *German camomile, Matricaria camomilia Linne and Roman camomile Anthemis nobilis*. This most popular plant needs little introduction. The essential oils are anti-inflammatory and anti-microbial. It may be used on inflammed skin. Again, do not use over extensive areas. Remember that since camomile is an extract derived from the flowers of the plant there may be pollen grains present that produce allergy in some individuals.

The major anti-inflammatory agent is bisabolol while the flavanoids account for other properties of the plant.

**7. Comfrey**. Comfrey is being studied more intensively these days. The plant is called by many names throughout the world but it is *Symphytum officiale* to botanists. Both the leaves and the roots contain allantoin and mucilage, while tannin is present mainly in the leaves. Comfrey tea is popular but it should not be taken internally as it contains toxic products called **pyrrolizidine alkaloids**. This group includes **symphytine, echimidine and lasiocarpine**. Liver disease, pancreatic damage, and cancer in animals has been reported from teas containing comfrey. There is not a great deal of scientific information on the use of comfrey as a topical agent. Most likely it is safe in small areas but until there is more evidence as to its safety and effectiveness **I would not recommend using comfrey.**

**8. Coneflower.** Coneflower is *Echinacea augustifolia,* one of the best plants in nature. Products obtained from the roots include echinaco-side, a microbicidal agent, echinacin B, an immune stimulant and an oil pentadecadiene that has antitumor properties. More research is needed on the properties of this plant to fully understand its uses. It makes a good mask for acne and for inflamed skin. It can be used in topical preparations as an immune stimulant.

**9. Glycyrrhiza.** The plant produces licorice from the rhizomes and roots. Licorice has many therapeutic properties as well as being an excellent confectionary. Glycyrrhizic acid is 50 times sweeter than sugar but when it is hydrolysed it becomes an aglycone called glycyrrhetic acid. Glycyrrhetic acid is an excellent anti-inflammatory agent. The plant name is *Glycyrrhiza glabra Linne.*

**10. Gotu Kola.** Gotu Kola is known as *Centella asiatica* to botanists. The leaves and stems of this plant contains two glycosides that inhibit bacteria and act as an anti-inflammatory agent. Do not confuse Gotu Kola with *Kola nut (Cola nitida)* which is also a very good anti-inflammatory. Kola nut extract contains caffeine while Gotu kola does not. Gotu Kola may be used in acne masks and acne treatment products and on inflamed skin.

**11. Witch hazel.** This material is extracted from the leaves of the *Hamamelis virginiana Linne*. The major property of witch hazel is its astringency attributed to the large amount of tannins present in the extract. It makes an excellent toner and skin smoothing agent. Also., it is useful to calm inflammation and swelling in mucous membranes

**13. Horsechestnut.** Horsechestnut is known as *Aesculus hippocastanum*. It must never be eaten as it is quite toxic. There is a substance contained in this nut called aesculin which has both anti-oxidant, and anti-inflammatory properties. In addition, it is effective in treating varicose veins and dilated capillaries. I do not know of an effective commercial source (finished product) since most spray dried preparations contain only small quantities of aesculin. Some companies will provide an analysis of their product for you. Ask for "thin layer chromatograph study" results.

**13. Hibiscus.** Hibiscus has red flowers that yield many exfoliative agents. If the flowers are ground or mashed, when the extract is applied to the skin it will produce a mild exfoliation of the skin. Many citric type acids are present in this plant. The scientific name is *Hibiscus sabdariffa Linne*.

**14. Parsley.** Parsley is a rich source of many vitamins including vitamins C and A, along with carotene, iron, and other essential minerals. It is pleasant to take orally and makes a good refreshing and stimulating mask for aging skin. Botanical name is *Petroselinum cris-pum*.

**15. Sarsaparilla.** The flavor of sarsaparilla is excellent but the plant also contains many sterol compounds. These compounds have certain hormone effects primarily as precursors of biologically active agents. It is an excellent topic anti-aging plant. The dried root is used as the active part. **Do not confuse this plant with sassafras which contains safrole, which is a known carcinogen** .The botanical name for sarsaparilla is *Smilax aristolochiaefolia Miller*.

**16. Flavanoids.** A classification of active agents in a variety of plants, they are classified as the aglycone derivatives of flavanol glycosides. The major flavanoids are rutin, quercitin, hersperidin, hesperetin, diosmin, and naringen. The last four are called bioflavanoids. Most are bright yellow in color and all seem to have some effect in healing or preventing bleeding due to capillary fragility.

Used with high doses of vitmain C (1 gram/day) it helps to reduce tiny veins on the face and legs.

**17. Yeast.** Yeast has been given a bad rap lately but most of it is nonsense. Take away yeast and the doughnut lovers of the world would rise up in universal rebellion! Yeast contains growth factors and metabolic stimulators, the cell wall also contains immune stimulants.

Brewers yeast can be taken orally every day and it can also be used topically in a mask formula. The most common form of yeast used in baking and brewing is *Saccharamyces cerevisiae Hansen*. Yeast contains protein and a high quantity of B vitamins. The recommended dose is 10 grams a day of dried yeast. Live yeast extract, also know as skin respiratory factor (SRF), is an effective wound healer and antiaging product. It can be used in masks and creams and is effective at 2000 units per ounce.

## WHERE TO GET SOME OF THESE NATURAL ITEMS

Active Organics
6849 Hayvenhurst Avenue
Van Nuys, Calif. 91406
Phone 818 786-3310

Bell Flavors and Fragrances
500 Academy Road
Northbrook, Ill. 60062
800-323-4387

Cosmetochem U.S.A. Inc
Industrial West
Clifton, N.J. 07012
201-471-8301

Nuherbs Co.
3820 Penniman Ave
Oakland, Calif. 94619
800-233-4307
415-534-Herb (In Calif)

Tri-K Industries, Inc
466 Old Hook Road
P.O Box 312
Emerson, N.J. 07630
201-261-2800

Red Star Division (For yeast extract)
Universal Foods
Milwaukee, Wis.
414-271-6755

# Satistical Data

## OFFICE VISITS TO U.S. PHYSICIANS IN 1979

| SPECIALTY | NO. OF VISITS | % ADMITTED TO HOSPITAL |
|---|---|---|
| All visits | 556,313,000 | 2.1 |
| Family practice/ general practice | 190,194,000 | 1.3 |
| Internal medicine | 66,908,000 | 2.1 |
| Podiatry | 58,126,000 | 0.5 |
| General surgery | 33,740,000 | 6.4 |
| Obstetrics/gynecology | 50,823,000 | 2.8 |
| Orthopedic surgery | 31,081,000 | 3.3 |
| Ophthalmology | 30,483,000 | 0.9 |
| **Dermatology** | **17,536,000** | **<0.1** |
| Psychiatry | 17,093,000 | 0.4 |
| Otolaryngology | 9,864,000 | 3.6 |
| Urology | 9,601,000 | 8.5 |
| Allergy | 7,626,000 | 0.1 |

Modified from NAMCS, United States, 1979.

## VISITS TO DERMATOLOGISTS FOR SELECTED DISEASES OF THE SKIN AND CONNECTIVE TISSUE

| DISEASE | NO. OF VISITS | % OF ALL SPECIALTIES |
|---|---|---|
| Acne | 4,639,000 | 78 |
| Infectious warts | 1,784,000 | 46 |
| Psoriasis | 936,000 | 67 |
| Eczema | 814,000 | 45 |
| Keratoderma | 902,000 | 60 |
| Disease of hair follicles | 540,000 | 63 |
| Seborrheic dermatitis | 532,000 | 63 |
| Lichenification | 415,000 | 58 |
| Pruritus | 524,000 | 36 |
| Rosacea | 248,000 | 73 |

Data from National Disease and Therapeutic Index, 1982.

## DERMATOLOGIC REASONS FOR VISITING PHYSICIANS

| REASONS | BY RANK | NO. OF VISITS | % | CUMULATIVE |
|---|---|---|---|---|
| Skin rash | 9 | 20,053,000 | 1.74 | - |
| Acne | 28 | 10,239,000 | 0.89 | 2.63 |
| Skin lesions | 39 | 7,455,000 | 0.65 | 3.28 |
| Warts | 59 | 4,492,000 | 0.39 | 3.67 |
| Skin irritations | 61 | 4,470,000 | 0.39 | 4.06 |
| Skin growths | 85 | 3,153,000 | 0.27 | 4.33 |
| Swelling of skin | 87 | 3,113,000 | 0.27 | 4.60 |
| Discoloration/pigmentation | 110 | 2,329,000 | 0.20 | 4.80 |
| Carbuncle, furnicle, boil | 114 | 2,252,000 | 0.20 | 5.0 |
| Symptom of skin mole | 118 | 2,070,000 | 0.18 | 5.18 |
| Infection of skin | 119 | 2,059,000 | 0.18 | 5.36 |
| Eczema/dermatitis | 164 | 1,323,000 | 0.11 | 5.47 |
| Symptoms referrable to hair and scalp | 166 | 1,310,000 | 0.11 | 5.58 |
| Skin cancer | 180 | 1,175,000 | 0.10 | 5.68 |
| Symptoms of nails | 198 | 1,082,000 | 0.09 | 5.78 |
| Psoriasis | 232 | 789,000 | 0.07 | 5.85 |
| Fungus infections | 245 | 710,000 | 0.06 | 5.91 |

Modified from NAMCS, 1977-1978.

Reprinted with permission from the Journal of the American Academy of Dermatology, article titled Prevalence, morbidity, and cost of dermatologic diseases, volume 11, Number 5, part November 1984, pp. 930-936, by Johnson et. al.

## ANNUAL VISIT RATE PER 1000 PERSONS BY AGE, SEX, AND RACE OF PATIENT IN THE U.S.,1979

| DIAGNOSIS | ALL | AGE | | | | | SEX | | RACE | |
|---|---|---|---|---|---|---|---|---|---|---|
| | | <15 | 15-24 | 25-44 | 45-64 | 65- | Female | Male | White | Black/other |
| Viral warts | 15 | 15 | 30 | 15 | 7 | 4 | 14 | 16 | 17 | 1 |
| Mycoses | 18 | 11 | 22 | 26 | 20 | 5 | 23 | 13 | 19 | 16 |
| Malignant neoplasm of the skin | 9 | - | 2 | 5 | 13 | 45 | 8 | 10 | 11 | - |
| Infection of skin and subcutaneous tissue | 23 | 28 | 21 | 23 | 21 | 22 | 21 | 26 | 24 | 16 |
| Contact dermatitis/eczema | 26 | 29 | 23 | 29 | 25 | 24 | 28 | 25 | 28 | 18 |
| Acne | 24 | 12 | 82 | 20 | 1 | 3 | 30 | 17 | 26 | 14 |

Modified from NAMCS, United States, 1979.

## CHARACTERISTICS OF PATIENT VISITS TO DERMATOLOGISTS

BY AGE

| | |
|---|---|
| Under 15 | 8.5% |
| 15-24 | 29.8% |
| 25-44 | 27.9% |
| 45-64 | 19.6% |
| Over 64 | 14.3% |

BY REFERRAL

| | |
|---|---|
| From another physician | 6.9% |

BY PROBLEM

| | |
|---|---|
| New patient | 26.1% |
| Old patient, new problem | 7.2% |
| Old patient, old problem | 66.7% |

OTHER

| | |
|---|---|
| Mean duration of visit | 11.9 min. |

Modified from NAMCS, United States, 1979.

## DISTRIBUTION OF PATIENTS' VISITS TO DERMATOLOGISTS BY AGE, SEPT. 19 TO AUG. 1983

| AGE (YR) | DERMATOL-OGISTS (%) | ALL OTHER PHYSICIANS (%) |
|---|---|---|
| 0-2 | 1 | 7 |
| 3-9 | 2 | 7 |
| 10-19 | 17 | 9 |
| 20-39 | 34 | 26 |
| 40-59 | 20 | 21 |
| 60-64 | 6 | 7 |
| 65-99 | 20 | 23 |

Unpublished data from National Disease and Therapeutic

## OVER-THE-COUNTER DRUG SALES (MILLION OF DOLLARS) IN 1981

| | |
|---|---|
| Moisturizing creams | 624.6 |
| Moisturizing lotions | 267.9 |
| Dandruff medicated shampoo | 214.5 |
| Sun oils and lotions | 207.4 |
| Astringents and cleansers | 192.8 |
| Acne preparations | 150.6 |
| Lip protectors | 93.9 |
| Salves, ointments and balm | 92.0 |
| Jock itch treatments | 82.0 |
| Hydrocortisone | 74.3 |
| Sun screens | 71.2 |
| Talcum and body powder | 65.3 |
| Poison ivy preparations | 31.4 |
| Pediculicide | 16.6 |
| Medicated soap | 10.9 |

Adapted from Drug Topics, Vol. 126, No. 13.

## MORTALITY FIGURES FOR SKIN-RELATED DISEASE, 1978

| DISEASE | NO. OF DEATHS |
|---|---|
| Malignant melanoma | 4,452 |
| Other malignant neoplasms | 1,596 |
| Infections of the skin | 602 |
| Other inflammatory conditions | 425 |
| Pemphigus | 89 |
| Herpes zoster | 133 |
| Other skin disease | 1,578 |
| Ulcers | 1,556 |
| Decubitus ulcers | 1,494 |

Modified from National Center for Health Statistics, Vital Statistics of the United States, 1978. Vol. II.,Mortality, Part A. DHHS Pub. No. (PHS) 83-1101, Public Health Service, Washington, DC, Government Printing Office, 1982.

## 1988 TREATMENT LOCATIONS AND FEE RANGES FOR ASPRS PATIENTS

| PROCEDURE | AVERAGE FEES | | | TREATMENT LOCATION | | |
|---|---|---|---|---|---|---|
| | Low | High | Office | Free-Standing | Hospital Outpatient | Hospital Inpatient |
| Breast augmentation | $1,900 | $2,500 | 50% | 19% | 27% | 4% |
| Breast lift (mastopexy) | 2,000 | 3,200 | 42% | 13% | 27% | 18% |
| Breast reduction | 3,000 | 5,200 | 9% | 47% | 34% | 10% |
| Cheek augmentation | 1,400 | 2,200 | 64% | 16% | 13% | 7% |
| Chemical peel | 1,200 | 2,500 | 77% | 9% | 9% | 5% |
| Chin Augmentation (mentoplasty) | 800 | 2,000 | 56% | 15% | 21% | 8% |
| Collagen injections | 200 | 400 | 99% | <1% | 0% | 0% |
| Dermabrasion | 600 | 1,500 | 56% | 11% | 26% | 7% |
| Ear pinning (otoplasty) | 1,500 | 2,400 | 37% | 15% | 41% | 7% |
| Eyelid (blepharoplasty) | 2,000 | 2,800 | 62% | 11% | 22% | 5% |
| Facelift (rhytidectomy) | 2,500 | 5,800 | 58% | 11% | 14% | 17% |
| Fat injections | 300 | 700 | 90% | 3% | 7% | 0% |
| Forehead lift | 1,200 | 2,400 | 61% | 16% | 16% | 7% |
| Hair replacement | 800 | 5,000 | 70% | 7% | 17% | 6% |
| Liposuction | 800 | 4,000 | 46% | 15% | 30% | 9% |
| Nose reshaping (rhinoplasty) | 1,700 | 2,900 | 35% | 14% | 33% | 18% |
| Retin-A* | 30 | 60 | 100% | 0% | 0% | 0% |
| "Tummy tuck" (abdominoplasty) | 2,500 | 4,500 | 33% | 8% | 24% | 35% |

NOTE: Fees listed represent **average** highs and lows for the entire country. Costs could vary significantly from these estimates depending on the geographic location, complexity of the particular operation, etc. Treatment locations represent those surgeries performed in the doctors' offices, free-standing surgi-centers and hospitals.
*Estimated fees for Retin-A are based on the **per visit** cost, excluding the expense for the medication itself.

## 1988 SEX AND AGE DEMOGRAPHICS FOR ASPRS AESTHETIC SURGERY PATIENTS

| PROCEDURE | SEX | | AGES | | | |
|---|---|---|---|---|---|---|
| | Male | Female | <18 | 19-34 | 35-50 | 50+ |
| Breast augmentation | 0% | 100% | 2% | 65% | 30% | 3% |
| Breast lift (mastopexy) | 0% | 100% | 1% | 62% | 31% | 6% |
| Breast reduction | 0% | 100% | 9% | 47% | 34% | 10% |
| Cheek augmentation | 24% | 76% | 3% | 45% | 42% | 10% |
| Chemical peel | 12% | 88% | <1% | 5% | 44% | 50% |
| Chin augmentation (mentoplasty) | 24% | 76% | 9% | 48% | 32% | 11% |
| Collagen injections | 9% | 91% | 1% | 19% | 53% | 27% |
| Dermabrasion | 22% | 78% | 7% | 48% | 27% | 18% |
| Ear pinning (otoplasty) | 53% | 47% | * (see note below) | | | |
| Eyelid (blepharoplasty) | 23% | 77% | <1% | 8% | 49% | 43% |
| Facelift (rhytidectomy) | 12% | 88% | 0% | 2% | 37% | 61% |
| Fat injections | 22% | 78% | 1% | 28% | 46% | 25% |
| Forehead lift | 10% | 90% | 0% | 4% | 47% | 49% |
| Hair replacement | 100% | 0% | 8% | 44% | 43% | 5% |
| Liposuction | 13% | 87% | 2% | 44% | 39% | 15% |
| Nose reshaping (rhinoplasty) | 28% | 72% | 16% | 54% | 25% | 4% |
| Retin-A | 13% | 87% | 1% | 16% | 43% | 40% |
| "Tummy tuck" (abdominoplasty) | 7% | 93% | 1% | 27% | 58% | 14% |

NOTE: Overall, 16% of aesthetic plastic surgery patients in 1988 were males (22% when only facial surgery is considered). Top 4 aesthetic surgeries for males in 1988--rhinoplasty (20,720), blepharoplasty (17,950), liposuction (13,530) and facelift (5,870). Top 4 aesthetic surgeries for females in 1988--liposuction (87,460), breast augmentation (71,720), blepharoplasty (60,540) and facelift (42,610).
*Otoplasty: Newborn to 2 -- 1%, 3 - 6 -- 21%, 7 - 12 -- 31%, 13 - 18 -- 16%, 19 - 34 -- 22%, >34 -- 9%.

Printed with permission from the American Society of Plastic and Reconstructive Surgeons, Inc.

## ESTIMATED NUMBER OF AESTHETIC SURGERY PROCEDURES PERFORMED BY ASPRS MEMBERS

| PROCEDURE | 1988 | 1981 | % INCREASE |
|---|---|---|---|
| Breast augmentation | 71,720 | 72,000 | - |
| Breast lift (mastopexy) | 12,440 | 12,800 | - |
| Breast reduction | 35,500 | 32,000 | 11% |
| Cheek augmentation (malar augmentation) | 3,140 | N/A | N/A |
| Chemical peel | 9,430 | 9,700 | - |
| Chin augmentation | 12,730 | N/A | N/A |
| Collagen injections* | 68,880 | N/A | N/A |
| Dermabrasion | 20,250 | 17,000 | 19% |
| Ear pinning (otoplsty | 9,930 | 11,500 | -14% |
| Eyelid surgery (blepharoplasty) | 78,490 | 56,500 | 39% |
| Facelift (rhytidectomy) | 48,480 | 39,000 | 24% |
| Fat injections* | 9,680 | N/A | N/A |
| Fibrel injections* | 1,540 | N/A | N/A |
| Forehead lift | 14,800 | N/A | N/A |
| Hair replacement | 2,220 | 4,200 | -47% |
| Liposuction | 101,000 ** | 55,900 (1984 figure**) | 81% |
| Nose reshaping (rhinoplasty) | 73,250 | 54,500 | 34% |
| Retin-A* | 59,360 | N/A | N/A |
| "Tummy-tuck" (abdominoplasty) | 22,260 | 15,300 | 45% |
| **ESTIMATED TOTALS** | 619,565 | 380,400 | 63% |

Liposuction breakdown:

| Face | 21% | Buttock | 13% |
|---|---|---|---|
| Hips/thighs | 34% | Legs | 9% |
| Abdomen | 23% | | |

NOTES: * The number quoted for injectables (including collagen, fat and Fibrel) represents the total patients treated, since more than one injection is often required to obtain the desired result. Likewise, the total quoted for Retin-A also reflects the number of patients, since more than one doctor's visit may be required for each individual.

** The totals for liposuction are estimated based on the number of different procedures performed, with each body site considered a seperate operation. For example, if one patient had both the abdomen and thighs suctioned during the survey year, this is counted as two procedures. Also, the number of liposuctions was quoted only for 1988 and 1984, since the procedure was not introduced to the United States until 1982 -- a year after the first ASPRS survey.

## DID YOU KNOW...

...that when asked about their attitude towards aesthetic plastic surgery, a random sample of consumers (mostly women older than 25) said:

| | 1988 | 1982 | % CHANGE |
|---|---|---|---|
| Approve of aesthetic sugery for themselves and others | 48% | 32% | +50% |
| Approve of aesthetic sugery for others but not themselves | 16% | 19% | -16% |
| Were undecided | 32% | 39% | -18% |
| Disapprove of aesthetic sugery | 3% | 9% | -66% |

...that research shows these patient demographics:

- - Slightly more than half (51%) are currently married.

- - 83% have completed at least some college education, and 58% of those have some graduate education (persons with at least some college education are 13% more likely to choose aesthetic plastic surgery)

- - 30% have household incomes of $25,000 or less, 35% earn $25,000 - $50,000, and 23% make $50,000 or over

...that when asked how long they had considered aesthetic surgery before taking action, a random sample of patients said:
Under one year - - 43%, 1 - 2 years - - 25%, 2 - 3 years - - 11%, 3 - 5 years - - 7%, and 5 - plus years - - 14%.

(For more information on how these studies were conducted, call the ASPRS Communications Department, 708-228-9900.)

# The Metric System

| UNIT | MEASURE | SYMBOL | ENGLISH EQUIVALENT |
|------|---------|--------|--------------------|
| **LINEAR MEASURE** | | | |
| 1 kilometer | = 1,000 meters | km | 0.62137 mile |
| 1 meter | | m | 39.37 inches |
| 1 decimeter | = 1/10 meter | dm | 3.937 inches |
| 1 centimeter | = 1/100 meter | cm | 0.3937 inch |
| 1 millimeter | = 1/1,000 meter | mm | |
| 1 micrometer (or micron) | = 1/1,000,000,000 meter | μm (or μ) | English equivalents |
| 1 nanometer | = 1/1,000,000,000 | nm | infrequently used |
| **MEASURES OF CAPACITY (For fluids and gases)** | | | |
| 1 liter | = 1/1,000 liter | L | 1.0567 U.S. liquid |
| 1 millimeter | = volume of 1 g of water at standard temperature and pressure (stp) | ml | quarts |
| 1 millimeter | | | |
| **MEASURES OF VOLUME** | | | |
| 1 cubic meter | | $m^3$ | |
| 1 cubic decimeter | = 1/1,000 cubic meter<br>= 1 liter (L) | $dm^3$ | |
| 1 cubic centiimeter | = 1/1,000,000 cubic meter<br>= 1 milliliter (mL) | $cm^3$ = ml | |
| 1 cubic millimeter | = 1/100,000,000 cubic meter | $mm^3$ | |
| **MEASURES OF MASS** | | | |
| 1 kilogram | = 1,000 grams | kg | 2.2046 ponds |
| 1 gram | | g | 15.432 grains |
| 1 milligram | = 1/1,000 gram | mg | .01 grain (about) |
| 1 microgram | = 1/1,000,000 gram | μg (or mcg) | |

# Glossary

**A band (anisotropic)** Dark area of thick myofilaments within a sarcomere

**Acetylcholine (Ach)** A neurotransmitter

**Actin** Muscle protein comprising most of the myofilament

**Actinic** Relating to electromagnetic (sun damaging) rays

**Action potential** Change in the membrane's state of tension in muscle tissue when excitation occurs

**Acute** Said of a disorder that comes on suddenly, lasting less than a week

**Adipose tissue** Fatty tissue

**Adventitia** The outer covering of an artery or organ, not actually part of the artery or organ

**Ala** The wing of the nostril

**Albino** An individual with a deficiency or absence of melanin in skin, eyes, and hair

**All-or-nothing principle** Says that a muscle will contract only if the threshold stimulation is reached

**Alopecia** Loss of hair

**Alternating current** Flow of electricity periodically changing direction and intensity

**Ameboid** Having an irregular shape with projections

**Amorphous** Without shape

**Ampere** A unit measure of current flow

**Anabolism** The process of combining simple compounds into more complex ones

**Anaerobic** Without oxygen; said of metabolic pathways

**Anagen** The growth phase of the hair cycle

**Anaphylaxis** A severe allergic reaction

**Anastasmosis** A connection of two nerves, blood or lymph vessels, either directly or indirectly

**Anion** A negatively charged particle (ion)

**Anode** A positively charged pole which attracts anions

**Antecubital fossa** The depressed area in front of the elbow

**Antibody** A substance formed or evoked in response to a foreign body or antigen

**Anticholinergic** Refers to the inhibition of acetylcholine in nerve transmissions

**Anticoagulant** A substance which prevents blood from clotting

**Antigen** A foreign body, such as bacteria, which can stimulate the immune system

**Antioxidant** A substance which prevents oxidation from occurring

**Apocrine gland** A coiled gland which contributes part of its cells in its secretion

**Appendage** Any part attached to a main structure, such as an arm

**Arachidonic acid** A fatty acid which is a precursor of prostaglandins

**Arteriole** A tiny artery

**Artery** A blood vessel which carries blood to the heart

**Atrophy** The wasting of cells or tissues and organs

**Auricular cartilage** Cartilage of the outer ear

**Axilla** The underarm area

**Axon** The tail-like projection of a nerve cell which carries impulses from one cell to another

**Basal lamina** The basement membrane

**Basal layer** The innermost layer of epidermis; contains livingand dividing cells

**Basophil** A white blood cell which forms heparin

**Benign** A mild form of illness, as opposed to fatal or malignant

**Benzyl benzoate** A topical compound used in the treatment of scabies

**Beta 1,3 glucan** A substance extracted from the yeast cell wall, capable of stimulating the immune system

**Bradykinin** A potent vasodilator

**Buccal mucosa** The inner lining of the cheek

**Calor** Heat

**Calorie** A unit measure of heat

**Canthus** The corner of the eye, inner and outer

**Capacitance** The quantity of electrical charge that may be stored per unit electric potential

**Capacitor** A device for holding a charge of electricity; condensor

**Capsid** The protein covering around the nucleoid of an elementary virus particle (See nucleocapsid)

**Carbonization** Charring

**Cartilage** Connective tissue characterized by lack of blood vessels and firm consistency

**Catabolism** The breakdown of complex compounds into simpler ones

**Catagen** The resting phase of the hair cycle

**Cecum** Part of the large intestine

**Cell cycle** The cell goes through a cycle of four stages: Interphase (GI period), DNA synthesis (S period), postsynthesis (G2 period), mitotic (M period)

**Cell membrane** The bilayer of lipids and protein surrounding the cell

**Centistoke** A measure of viscosity (thickness)

**Central nervous system** The brain and spinal column

**Cerumen** Ear wax

**Chalone** An inhibitory substance which acts on a specific tissue

**Chemotaxis** The migration of cells

**Cholesterol** A lipid, and the most abundant steroid in animal tissues

**Chondrocyte** A cartilage cell

**Chromosome** A body within the cell nucleus containing the biological units of heredity (genes)

**Chronic** Any symptoms or disorder lasting more than a month

**Cilia** Little hairs

**Circumscribe** To completely encircle with a line, or confine

**Cleave** Splitting or dividing, as of a molecule

**Coagulate** To clot

**Collagen** The major protein comprising connective tissue, bone, and cartilage

**Colloidal** Like a colloid; gluelike

**Columna** The fleshy end of the nose

**Complement system** A complex of components (C1-C9) combining with antibody-antigen complex in a specific sequence

**Conductor** Material connecting the two poles which offers resistance to the flow of current

**Configuration** A particular arrangement of (atoms, molecules, cells)

**Connective tissue** Fibrous tissue which functions as the supporting framework of the body; holds muscle to skin, muscle to bone, bone to bone, etc.

**Constitutive skin color** Skin color generated without exposure to radiation or hormones

**Contraindication** Any special circumstance or symptom that renders the use of a remedy inadvisable

**Cornified** Hardened, such as cornified cells of the stratum corneum

**Cortex** Outermost part of an organ

**Cortisone** An anti-inflammatory drug which blocks the action of prostaglandins

**Covalent** Said of two atoms bound together and sharing 2,4 or 6 electrons

**Cutaneous** Relating to the skin

**Cuticle** The outer thin covering of a hair

**Cyanosis** A condition caused by the blood not containing enough oxygen and too much carbon dioxide, resulting in a blue color to the skin

**Cytoplasm** The fluid part of a cell containing organelles

**Cytochemical** The chemistry of a cell

**Cytotoxicity** The condition of damaging or poisoning the cell

**Deep fascia** Lies between the superficial fascia and muscles; contains muscles and body organs

**Degenerated nucleus** A cell nucleus which has deteriorated

**Dendrite** A projection of a cell which receives and directs impulses to the cell body

**Dermatome** An area of skin supplied by a particular nerve branch

**Dermis** The lower layer of skin, beneath the epidermis

**Desmosome** A site of adhesion between two cells

**Desquammation** The sloughing off of cells from the surface of the skin

**Dessicate** To dry out

**Diapedesis** The migration of cells through blood vessel walls

**Diascope** A flat glass plate for examining superficial lesions

**Differentiation** The process of a cell acquiring a specialized function

**Diploid** Said of chromosomes which occur in pairs

**Direct current** Constant flow of electricity in one direction

**Discoidal** Disc-shaped

**Diurnal** Occuring and most active during the day

**DNA** A storehouse of genetic activity, master template of protein synthesis

**Dolor** Pain

**Dynamic** Constantly changing

**Dyne** A unit measure of force

**Eccrine gland** Any coiled tubular sweat gland that is not an apocrine gland

**Echinacea** The coneflower; believed to stimulate immune system

**Edema** An accumulation of excess fluid

**Elastin** The major connective tissue protein of elastic structures, such as large blood vessels

**Elastosis** A degenerative change in elastic tissue, mostly due to excessive sun exposure

**Electrocautery** Burning with electric current

**Electrodessication** The process of destroying tissue, usually hair, by removing all its moisture by means of electric current

**Electrolysis** Decomposition of a salt or certain tissue of the body by means of electricity

**Elective** Optional; said of a procedure chosen for esthetic rather than health reasons

**Electron transport cycle** (ETS) Cytochrome system, transfers electrons to oxygen

**Empirical** Experimental

**End cell** A cell which has reached its final form

**Endomysium** Fibrous connective tissue covering individual myofibers

**Endoneurium** Delicate connective tissue enveloping single nerve fibers in a peripheral nerve

**Endoplasmic reticulum** An organelle with the function of protein synthesis

**Endothelium** A lining made up of a layer of flat cells

**Endotoxin** A toxin from outside the organism

**Enzyme** A protein which acts as a catalyst to cause or speed up a chemical reaction during which the enzyme itself is not changed

**Eosinophil** A white blood cell which stains red with eosin

**Epidermal cell kinetics** The process of renewing cells

**Epidermal melanocyte unit** One melanocyte serving 36 keratinocytes

**Epidermis** The outer portion of the skin

**Epilation** Process of removing hair

**Epimysium** A fibrous membrane surrounding a muscle

**Epithelial** Pertaining to epithelium

**Erythema** Inflammation, redness of the skin

**Esterify** The elimination of water ($H_2O$) between the -OH group of an acid group and the -OH of an alcohol to form an ester

**Etiology** The cause, or the study of the cause, of disease

**Eukaryocyte** A cell with a nuclear membrane and complex organization of organelles

**Eumelanin** A brown-black pigment; true melanin

**Eunuch** A castrated male

**Exotoxin** A poison or toxin which is created outside the cell (see endotoxin)

**Extracellular fluid** Fluid (e.g. blood, water) found outside the cell

**Exudate** Fluid leaking out of a cell

**Gamma benzene hexachloride** A topical compound effective in the treatment of scabies

**Hallux** Big toe

**Hidrosis** Sweat

**Hydroquinone** A bleaching agent for skin

**Interdigital** Between the fingers

**Interphalangeal** Between the phalanges

**Facultative pigmentation** Pigmentation occuring by means of ultraviolet light, hormones or radiation; eg, tanning

**Fascicle** A bundle of myofibers (muscle fibers)

**Fatty acid** The basic unit of lipids; palmitic and stearic are the most common fatty acids in the body

    **free fatty acid** - not bound up in a lipid; the result of the break down of lipids

**Fibrillar** Threadlike

**Fibroblast** A cell capable of synthesizing collagen and elastin

**Fibrotic** Pertaining to the formation of fibrous tissue (usually a reparative process)

**Fluctuant** Soft feeling, wave-like motion indicating presence of fluid

**Fulgurate** To destroy tissue with sparks from a high frequency device

**Fungi** Plant-like organisms feeding on organic matter

**Galvanic current** Direct current

**Gamma benzene hexachloride** A parasitocide (bug killer)

**Genome** A complete set of chromosomes derived from one parent

**Germinative** Pertaining to reproduction

**Gestation** Pregnancy

**Galvanic current** Direct current

**Glabrous** Hairless

**Glands of Moll** A type of apocrine, sudoriferous gland in the eyelid with ducts which open into the eyelashes

**Glial cells** Supporting cells of the nervous system which protect and aid neurons

**Glycolipids** A molecule of sugar and fat

**Glycosoaminoglycan** The ground substance of the dermis in which components of the dermis are embedded

**Golgi complex** Concerned with intercellular formation of secretions

**Granular** Composed of, or resembling, granules

**Ground** A large conducting body used as a common return for current relative zero electrical potential

**Ground substance** Glycosoaminoglycans

**H zone** A region within the center of the A band which contains only thick myofilaments

**Haploid** A single chromosome; does not occur in pairs

**Hederiform** Ivy-shaped

**Hematuria** Blood in the urine

**Hemostasis** The arrest of bleeding

**Hexosamine** Any six carbon sugar with an amine group

**Hirsute** Having excessive hair

**Holocrine gland** A gland which secrete s its own cells; the sebaceous gland

**Humoral** Pertaining to extracellular fluid

**Hydrocarbon** A chain of carbon and hydrogen molecules linked together

**Hydrolysis** Breakdown of a compound into simpler components, by the uptake of water

**Hyaluronic acid** A gelantinous material which acts as an intercellular "cement" throughout the body

**Hyperkeratotic** Excessively producing keratin, resulting in rough, hard skin

**Hyperproliferate** To excessively reproduce (as in psoriasis)

**Hyperpigmentation** An excessive production of melanin

**Hyperplasia** Excessive growth of cells

**Hypha** A branched structure of fungi or plants

**Hypopigmentation** Deficiency or absence of melanin in skin

**Hypostome** The anchoring device of a tick

**Hypotonic** Having a lesser degree of tension (said of muscle)

**I band (isotropic)** Light area of thin myofilaments within a sarcomere

**Immunoglobulin** (IG) A class of proteins acting as antibodies; all antibodies are IG's

**Immunology** The study of the defenses of the body against disease, allergy, or other damage

**Innervated** Supplied with nerves

**Intercellular space** The space between the cells

**Intercellum canniculum** A little tunnel between cells

**Interfibrillar** Between fibrils, or tiny fibers

**Interferon** Large molecules produced in response to infection with active or inactivated viruses

**Interstial fluid** Fluid in spaces between cells or structures

**Intraepidermal** Within the epidermis

**Involution** The return of an enlarged organ to normal size; e.g., the uterus after pregnancy

**Iontophoresis** A delivery system which transfers medicaments intothe skin by direct current

**Ischemia** Lack of blood and oxygen

**Isoinertial** Constant load presented to muscle

**Isokinetic** Muscle moved at constant velocity

**Isometric** A static muscle contraction with no joint involvement

**Isotonic** Constant tension through a range of

motion

**Keloid** Hyperplastic scar tissue

**Keratin** A protein found in skin, hair, and nails

**Keratinocyte** A cell which produces keratin

**Ketone body** A substance produced when the body metabolizes fat, rather than glucose for energy

**Krause's end bulb** A sensory nerve ending, encapsulated within layers of connective tissue, which mediate sensations of touch and pressure (also called mucocutaneous corpuscles)

**Labyrinth** A maze

**Lamellar bodies** Complex lipids that for part of the corneocyte barrier

**Latency period** The time after a twitch and before tension in fibers begins to rise

**Leukocyte** A infection fighting white blood cell; basophils, neutrophils, monocytes, eosinophils are all leukocytes

**Leukotriene** A chemical derived from arachidonic acid, leukotrienes are secreted by leukocytes in response to an allergen, and produce the symptoms associated with an allergic reactions

**Lichenification** A thickening of the skin due to scratching or chronic inflammation

**Lipid** A group of substances not soluble in water

**Lipolytic** Capable of breaking down lipids

**Load** Resistance offered to a muscle

**Lumen** A cavity in a cell or organ

**Lymph** A clear fluid collected from the tissues of the body, whcih flows through the lymphatic vessels, and is added to the venous circulation; contains a clear fluid portion, some white and a few red blood cells

**Lymphocyte** A white blood cell which comprises approximately 25% of the leukocytes

**M line** A region within the center of the H zone

**Macrophage** A phagocyte involved in many immune functions

**Macromolecule** A large molecule

**Mast cell** A cell which releases histamine, causing the redness and swelling of a wound

**Malignant** A severe form of an illness, usually resistant to treatment (such as cancer)

**Mechanoreceptor** A sensory receptor stimulated by mechanical means, such as pressure

**Medicament** A medicine or remedy

**Meissner corpuscle** A sensory receptor, encapsulated by layers of connective tissue, which mediates feeling of touch and pressure

**Melanin** Brown pigment

**Melanocyte** A cell which produces the pigment, melanin

**Melanogenesis** The creation of melanin

**Melanosome** Melanin granules in the melanocyte

**Merkel disc** A sensory receptor in the skin, encapsulated by layers of connective tissue, which mediates feelings of touch and pressure

**Mesenchymal cell** Embryonic tissue which gives rise to connective tissue, smooth muscle, vascular endothelium, or blood cells.

**Metabolism** The chemical processes within the body which break down substances (fat, glucose) into smaller components to release energy, and use that energy and components to build other substances (such as protein)

**Metatasize** The spread or shifting of a disease from one part of the body to another

**Miconazole** An antifungal agent

**Milliamp** One thousandth of an amp

**Millicalorie** One-thousandth of a calorie

**Mitochondria** An organelle in nucleus of cell responsible for energy production

**Mitogen** Substance which causes mitosis and cell proliferation

**Mitosis** The process of dividing cells

**Moiety** Formally a half, now one of two or more parts into which something is divided

**Molecular weight** Indicative of the size of the chemical compound

**Monocyte** A macrophage in the blood stream

**Motor** Related to movement

**Motor end plate** An area where the axon terminal comes close to the sarcolemma

**Motor neuron** A cell within the nervous system which stimulates muscle

**Mucocutaneous corpuscle** Found in the transitional zones between the skin and a mucous membrane (e.g. lips, eyelids), these nerve endings are believed to be pressure receptors

**Mucoid** Having the characteristics of mucous

**Mucopolysaccharide** A complex of protein and polysaccharides; blood substances are mucopolysaccharides

**Muscle twitch** The lowest recordable activity of muscle response

**Myelin** The covering on certain nerve fibers,

made up of lipids

**Myerhoff pathway** Anerobic pathway of sugar metabolism

**Myoepithelium** Spindle-shaped contractile cells arranged around sweat glands and certain secretory glands

**Myofiber** A muscle fiber

**Myofibril** Comprise muscle fibers; hundreds to thousands per fiber

**Myofibroblast** A fibroblast cell with microfilaments that allow the cell to migrate by contracting

**Myofilament (thick and thin)** Comprise myofibrils

**Myoneural junction** The area of the motor end plate and axon terminal

**Nasolabial fold** The fold running from the corner of the nose to the corner of the mouth; deepens with age

**Neoplasia** A new growth of cells

**Nervous system** Subdivided into the central **(CNS)** and the peripheral **(PNS)** nervous systems; the CNS includes the brain and spinal column; the PNS includes the nerves which supply the outer or peripheral regions of the body (arms, legs, etc.)

**Neuron** A nerve cell

**Neutrophil** The most phagocytic of all leukocytes

**Nucleolus** The dark area within the nucleus believed to contain fibers that synthesize RNA

**Nuclear membrane** The thin tissue surrounding the nucleus of a cell

**Nucleocapsid** An elementary virus particle consisting of a nucleoid surrounded by a capsid

**Nucleus** The oval or rounded part of a cell (distinct from the cytoplasm) which contains the organelles and divides to reproduce the cell

**Ohm** A measure of electrical resistance

**Oncogenic** Inducing or suitable for development of a neoplasm

**Organelle** A body within the nucleus of a cell, with a specialized function

**Oxidation** The chemical reaction in which a molecule gains an atom of oxygen
beta oxidation - fatty acid oxidation

**Pacinian corpuscle** A sensory receptor in the skin which is encapsulated and mediates feelings of touch and pressure

**Palliative** Treatment that addresses the symptoms, but does not cure the disease

**Palpebrae** Eyelid

**Papilla** A hairlike projection

**Papillary dermis** Hairlike projections of the dermis that fit into the valleys of the epidermis, the top part of the dermis

**Papillomatous** Relating to papilloma, a circumscribed benign epitumor

**Pathogenicity** The condition of being able to cause disease

**Perineurium** Layer of cells surrounding a bundle of nerves

**Periungual** Surrounding the nail

**Perimysium** Fibrous tissue covering a fascicle

**Permeable** Allowing substances to flow into or out of

**Phaeomelanin** A yellow pigment similar to melanin but containing cysteine

**Phagocytosis** The process of cells consuming other cells, or foreign bodies, bacteria, etc.

**Phenothiazine** Also called thiodiphenylamine, dibenzothiazine; a compound used to treat intestinal worms

**Phospholipid** A lipid containing phosphorus

**Phosphorylate** Addition of a phosphate group to an organic compound

**Photobiology** Science of dealing with electromagnetic energy and life

**Photogenic** Produced by light, or producing light

**Photoimmunolgy** The science of light's effect on the immune system

**Pilomotor** Refers to moving the hair, as in pilomotor muscles

**Pilosebaceous apparatus** Consists of the hair, follicle, and sebaceous gland

**Pinocytosis** The process of a cell engulfing a liquid

**Pituitary gland** The "master gland", located at the base of thebrain; controls much of the hormonal activity of the body

**Plexus** A network of nerves and blood vessels or lymphatic vessels

**Polarity** the property of having two opposite poles; the possession of opposite characteristics

**Polydimethylsiloxane** A silicone compound

**Polymer** A substance made up of a chain of identical units, such as a chain of glucose molecules

**Polymorphonuclear cell** White blood cell which engulfs foreign matter

**Popliteal space** The space behind the knee

**Prepuce** The foreskin of the penis

**Pressure** Force per unit area

**Primary heating effect** The relationship of current strength, resistance, time of current flow

**Prokaryocyte** A simple cell with no nuclear membrane

**Proliferation** Growth and reproduction

**Properdin** A component of the complement system

**Prostaglandin** A class of physiologically active substances present in many tissues

**Proteoglycan** A component of ground substance

**Psychogenic** Caused by emotional or psychological factors

**Ptosis** The condition of falling, as in sagging eyelids or breasts

**Purulent** Containing or forming pus

**Pus** Fluid product of inflammation, containing dead white blood cells and other debris

**Pyoderma** A secondary infection

**Ovoid** Oval shaped

**Quantum** The smallest unit of energy

**Reduction** The process of a molecule giving up or losing an atom; e.g. hemoglobin losing an atom of oxygen

**Reflect** To throw back (a ray of light)

**Refract** To bend (a ray of light)

**Reflex arc** The route followed by a nerve impulse

**Relaxation time** Period in which a muscle will release tension and return to zero tension

**Resistance** The opposition that a material body offers to the passage of the flow of current (or blood)

**Rete** A network of small vessels or nerve fibers

**Reticular dermis** A layer of the dermis composed of a fine network of cells, and connective tissue fibers between cells

**Reticulum** A fine network of cells, or formed of certain structures within cells or of connective tissue fibers between cells

**Ribosome** Structure found on the rough endoplasmic reticulum which assist in the synthesis of protein

**RNA** Ribonucleic acid; involved in the replication of cells

**Rubor** Redness

**Ruffini corpuscle** Encapsulated nerve endings found just below the sebaceous duct; believed to be receptors of pressure

**Sarcolemma** The membrane surrounding a muscle fiber

**Sarcomere** A section of a myofibril, composed of myofilaments

**Sarcoplasmic reticulum** A network of tubes enclosed in membrane

**Sebaceous gland** A holocrine gland that usually opens into a hair follicle and secretes sebum

**Sebum** An oily, semifluid substance

**Septal cell** A round, pale cell found in the lungs

**Sequela** An after effect

**Sign** Objective evidence of a disorder, able to be observed by someone other than the patient

**Sinus** A hollow in bone or other tissue

**Smooth muscle** Muscle without the striations of skeletal muscle; found in internal organs and blood vessels

**SPF** Sun protection factor;the SPF number is the amount of time one can remain in the sun without burning; for example, if you burn in 15 minutes without protection, with a sunscreen with SPF 4 you can remain in the sun for 60 minutes before erythema occurs

**Specific heat** The amount of heat, measured in calories, needed to raise the temperature of one gram of material one degree Celsius

**Sphingolipid** Any lipid containing a long chain base

**Spindles** Receptors in muscles which monitor tone and relay messages to the brain

**Spiny layer** A layer of the dermis that gets its name from the many papillae or tiny hairs, which connect the cells

**Sterile technique** Practice of producing and maintaining a germ-free condition in a specific area

**Steroid** A large family of chemical substances comprising many hormones, vitamins, body constituents and drugs

**Sterol** A steroid

**Stratum corneum** The outermost layer of the skin consisting of cornified cells

**Subcutaneous** Under the skin

**Subacute** Said of condition lasting for a week or more

**Subchronic** Said of a condition lasting for a month

**Substrate** The substance an enzyme acts upon

**Sudoriferous gland** Sweat gland

**Summation** The accumulation of several action potentials

**Superficial fascia** A fine structure above surface muscle; contains blood vessels, nerves, fatty tissue. Stores fat and water to act as a buffer

**Sympathetic nervous system** The division of the nervous system that activates the body during a stressful situation

**Symptom** Evidence of a disorder as perceived by the patient

**Synaptic end bulb** Bulb-like structure at distal ends of axon terminal

**Syndrome** A collection of signs and symptoms indicating a particular disorder

**T tubule** Transverse tubule in the muscle

**Tactily** Using the fingers

**Telogen** The active phase of hair cycle

**Tension** Force exerted to overcome load

**Terminal cistern** Dilated sac

**Tetany** A continuous muscle contraction

**Thermal conductivity** The transfer of energy by interaction of single molecules

**Tolnafate** An antifungal agent

**Tone** A state of partial contraction in which some fibers are contracted and some are relaxed

**Toxic** Poisonous

**Triad** A T tubule and two cisterns

**Trigeminal nerve** The main sensory nerve of the face

**Tropomysin** Muscle protein in the thin myofilament which help regulate muscle contraction

**Troponin** Muscle protein in the thin myofilament which helps regulate muscle contraction

**Tugor; turgid** Swelling; stiff

**Urethritis** Inflammation of the urethra

**Vacuole** A cavity in the cytoplasm of a cell which may act as a stomach

**Vascular** Pertaining to, or containing, blood vessels

**Vasoconstriction** The constriction, or shrinking in diameter, of blood vessels

**Venule** A tiny vein

**Vellus hair** Very fine, soft, light hair, usually found on the body

**Violaceous** Purplish discoloration of the skin

**Virulent** Extremely poisonous

**Viscosity** The thickness or consistency of a fluid

**Volt** A measure of electrical pressure

**Wood's Light** A ultraviolet lamp used for diagnosis (320 nm to 400 nm)

**Zymosan** Anticomplementary factor; a carbohydrate found in the cell wall of yeast

# Bibliography

**Chapter 1**

Cohen MN: *Health and the Rise of Civilization*. Yale University Press, New Haven, 1989.
Patzer GL: *The Attractiveness Phenomena*. Plenum Press, New York, 1985.


**Chapter 2**

Anson BJ: *The Atlas of Human Anatomy*. W. B. Saunders, Philadelphia, 1950.
Atlas RM: *Microbiology, Fundamentals and Applicatons*. Macmillian, New York, 1984.
Benjamini E and Leskowitz S: *Immunology, A Short Course*. Alan R. Liss, Inc., New York, 1988.
Clark JOE : *The Human Body*. Arch Cape Press, New York, 1989.
Gray H: *Gray's Anatomy*. Bounty Books, New York, 1977.
Hyde BM, Montes LF, Wilborn WH: *Scanning Electron Microscopy of Normal and Abnormal Human Skin*. VCH Publishers, Deerfield Beach, 1985.
Landau BR: *Essential Human Anatomy and Physiology*. Scott Foresman and Company, Glenview, 1980.
Marieb EN: *Human Anatomy and Physiology*. Benjamin Cummings Co., Redwood City, 1989.
Marieb EN: *Human Anatomy and Physiology, Studyguide*. Benjamin Cummings Co., Redwood City, 1989.
Mason EB and Spense AP: *Human Anatomy and Physiology,*. Benjamin Cummings Co., Menlo Park, 1979.
Netter FH: *Atlas of Human Anatomy*. CIBA-Geigy Corp., West Caldwell, 1989.

**Chapter 3**

Champion RH, Gillman T, Rook, AJ, Sims RT (eds): *An Introduction to the Biology of Skin*. Blackwell Scientific Publications, Oxford, 1970.
Darnell J, Lodish H, Baltimore D (eds.): *Molecular Cell Biology* (a*Scientific American* Book). W. H. Freeman and Company, New York, 1990.
Fitzpatrick TB, Eisen AZ, Wolff K, Freedberg IM, Austen KF (eds.): *Dermatology In General Medicine*. McGraw-Hill, Inc., New York, 1987.

Jarrett A (ed.): *The Physiology and Pathophysiology of the Skin.* Academic Press, London, 1973.

Junqueira LC, Carneiro J, Kelley RO: *Basic Histology.* Appleton &Lange, East Norwalk, 1989.

Krstic RV: *Illustrated Encyclopedia of Human Histology.* Springer-Verlag, Berlin, 1984.

Maibach HI, and Boisits EK (eds): *Neonatal Skin.* Marcel Dekker, Inc., New York, 1982.

Mier PD, and Cotton DWK: *The Molecular Biology of Skin.* Blackwell Scientific Publications, Oxford, 1976.

Thody AJ, and Friedmann PS: *Scientific Basis of Dermatology.* Churchill Livingstone, Edinburgh, 1986.

Tregear, RT: P*hysical Functions of Skin.* Academic Press, London, 1966.

## Chapter 4

Bickers DR, Hazen PG, Lynch WS: *Clinical Pharmacology of SkinDisease.* Churchill Livingstone, New York, 1984.

Bier OG, Silva WD, Gotze D, Mota I: *Fundamentals of Immunology.* Springer-Verlag, Berlin, 1986.

Galli CL, Hensby CN, Marinovich M (eds): *Skin Pharmacology and Toxicology.* Plenum Press, New York, 1990.

Goldsmith LA (ed): *Biochemistry and Physiology of the Skin.,* Vol I, Oxford University Press, Inc., New York, 1983.

Marks R and Payne PA (eds): *Bioengineering and the Skin.* MTP Press Limited (International Medical Publishers), Lancaster, 1981.

Montagna W, Bentley JP, Dobson RL (eds): *The Dermis.* Appleton-Century-Crofts/Meredith Corporation, New York, 1970.

Stryer L: *Biochemistry,* W. H. Freeman and Company, New York, 1988.

## Chapter 5

Ackerman AB: *Histologic Diagnosis of Inflammatory Skin Diseases.* Lea & Febiger, Philadelphia, 1978.

Balin AK and Kligman AM (eds): *Aging and the Skin.* Raven Press, New York,1989.

Drill VA and Lazar P: *Cutaneous Toxicity.* Academic Press, New York, 1977.

Gallin JI, Goldstein IM, Snyderman, R: *Inflammation. Basic Principles and Clinical Correlates.* Raven Press, New York, 1988.

Goodman LS and Gilman A: *The Pharmacological Basis ofTherapeutics.* The Macmillan Company, London, 1970.

Jackson EM and Goldner R (eds): *Irritant Contact Dermatitis.* Marcel Dekker, Inc. New York, 1990.

Messmer K, Hammersen F: *Microcirculation and Inflammation: Vessel Wall-Inflammatory Cells-Mediator Interaction.* Karger, Basel, 1987.

Mitchell J and Rook A: *Botanical Dermatology.* Greengrass, Vancouver, 1979.

Pinkus H and Mehregan AH: *A Guide to Dermatohistopathology.* Appleton-Century-Crofts/Prentice-Hall, Inc., New York, 1976.

## Chapter 6

Adams RM and Nethercott JR (eds): *Dermatologic Clinics, Contact Dermatitis,* Vol. 8/No.1. W. B. Saunders Company, Philadelphia, 1990.

Callen JP and Jorizzo JL (eds): *Dermatologic Clinics, Skin Signs of Internal Disease,* Vol. 7/No. 3. W. B. Saunders Company, Philadelphia, 1989.

Fry L (ed): *Skin Problems in the Elderly.* Churchill Livingstone, Edinburgh, 1985.

Landau T: *About Faces* (an *Anchor* book). Doubleday, New York, 1989.

Lewis GM: *Practical Dermatology.* W. B. Saunders Company, Philadelphia, 1952.

Marks R: *Skin Disease in Old Age.* J. B. Lippincott Company, Philadelphia, 1987.

Moschella SL, Pillsbury DM, Hurley HJ: *Dermatology*, Vol. II. W. B. Saunders Company, Philadelphia, 1975.

Pillsbury DM and Heaton CL: *A Manual of Dermatology*. W. B. Saunders Company, Philadelphia, 1980.

Reeves JRT and Maibach H: *Clinical Dermatology Illustrated*. Williams & Wilkins and Associates Pty Limited, Sydney,1986.

### Chapter 7

Goldschmidt H (ed): *Physical Modalities in Dermatologic Therapy.* Springer-Verlag, New York, 1978.

Polk C and Postown E: *Handbook of Biological Effects of Electromagnetic Fields*. CRC, Chicago, 1986.

Regan JD and Parrish JA (eds): *The Science of Photomedicine*. Plenum Press, New York, 1982.

Sebben JE: *Cutaneous Electrosurgery*. Year Book Medical Publishers, Inc., Chicago, 1989.

Stacy RW, Williams DT, Worden RE, McMorris RO: *Essentials of Biological and Medical Physics*. McGraw-Hill Book Company, Inc., New York, 1955.

### Chapter 8

Berger TG, Elias PM, Wintroub BU: *Manual of Therapy for Skin Diseases,* Churchill Livingstone, New York, 1990.

Cunliffe WJ: *Acne*. Year Book Medical Publishers, Inc. Chicago, 1989.

Ely H and Thiers BH: *Dermatologic Clinics*. W. B. Saunders Company, Philadelphia, 1989.

Fitzpatrick TB, Eisen AZ, Wolff K, Freedberg IM, Austen KF: *Dermatology in General Medicine*. McGraw-Hill Book Company, New York, 1987.

Pierantoni H: *Basic Knowledge of Esthetics*, Vol. I. Les Nouvelles Esthetiques, Paris.

Pierantoni H: *Basic Knowledge of Esthetics*, Vol II. Les Nouvelles Esthetiques, Paris.

Thiers BH and Ely H: *Dermatologic Clinics* , Vol 6/Number 4. W. B. Saunders Company, Philadelphia, 1988.

### Chapter 9

Berger TG, Elias PM, Wintroub BU: *Manual of Therapy for Skin Diseases,* Churchill Livingstone, New York, 1990.

Michlovitz SL (ed): *Thermal Agents in Rehabilitation*. F. A. Davis Company, Philadelphia, 1986.

Neale D and Adams IM (eds): *Common Foot Disorders*. Churchill Livingstone, New York, 1989.

Norman L: *Feet First.* Simon & Schuster, Englewood Cliffs, 1988.

Otterness I, Capetola R, Wong S: *Therapeutic Control of Inflammatory Diseases.* Raven Press, New York, 1984.

Payton OD, DiFabio RP, Paris SV, Protas EJ, VanSant AF: *Manual of Physical Therapy*. Churchill Livingstone, Inc., New York, 1989.

Scher R and Daniel CR: *Nails: Therapy, Diagnosis, Surgery.* W.B. Saunders, Philadelphia, 1989.

Weil A: *Natural Health, Natural Medicine*. Houghton Mifflin Company, Boston, 1990.

Weiss RF: *Herbal Medicine*. Medicini Bio., Portland, 1988.

### Chapter 10

Hershman JM: *Endocrine Pathophysiology.* Lea & Febiger, Philadelphia, 1988.

Linder MC: *Nutritional Biochemistry and Metabolism*. Elsevier, New York, 1985.

Paige DM: *Clinical Nutrition*. The C.V. Mosby Company, St. Louis, 1988.

Tepperman J: *Metabolic and Endocrine Physiology.* Year Book Medical Publishers, Inc. Chicago, 1980.

Townsend CE: *Nutrition and Diet Therapy.* Delmar, Charlotte, 1985.

### Chapter 11

Dicker RL and Syracuse VR: *Consultation with a Plastic Surgeon.* Nelson-Hall, Chicago, 1975.

Moynahan PA: *Cosmetic Surgery for Women.* Crown Publishers, Inc. New York,1988.

### Chapter 12

Aly R and Maibach HI: *Clinical Skin Microbiology.* Charles C. Thomas Publisher, Springfield, 1978.

Atkinson LJ and Kohn ML: *Operating Room Technique, Introduction.*

Berman WE: *Rhinoplastic Surgery.* The C.V. Mosby Company, St. Louis, 1989.

Cocke WM, White RR, Lynch DJ, Verheyden CN: *Wound Care.* Churchill Livingstone, New York, 1986.

Fuerst E, Wolff L, Weitzel M: *Fundamentals of Nursing.*

Gonzalez-Ulloa M, Meyer R, Smith JW, Zaoli G (eds): *Aesthetic Plastic Surgery.* The C. V. Mosby Company, St. Louis,1988.

Kaye BL: *Facial Rejuvenative Surgery.* Lippincott Medical, Philadelphia, 1987.

McGregor IA: *Fundamental Techniques of Plastic Surgery and Their Surgical Applications.* Churchill Livingstone, New York, 1989.

Morris AM, Stevenson JH, Watson ACH: *Complications of Plastic Surgery.* W. B. Saunders, New York, 1989.

Nelson GD and Krause JL: *Clinical Photography in Plastic Surgery.* Little Brown, Boston, 1987.

Stegman S, Tromovitch R, Glogau R: *Cosmetic Dermatologic Surgery .* Year Book Medical Publishers, Chicago, 1989.

Thomas JR, Holt RG: *Facial Scars, Incision,, Revision, & Camouflage.* The C. V. Mosby Company, St. Louis, 1988.

Westaby S (ed): *Wound Care.* The C. V. Mosby Company, St. Louis, 1986.

### Chapter 13

Ackerman D. *Natural History of the Senses.* Random House, New York, 1990.

Finger TE and Silver WL (eds): *Neurobiology of Taste and Smell.* John Wiley & Sons, New York, 1987.

Goodman M and Morehouse F: *Organic Molecules in Action.* Gordon and Breach Science Publishers, New York, 1973.

Knobloch IW (ed): *Selected Botanical Papers.* Prentice-Hall, Inc., Englewood Cliffs, 1963.

Shepard GM: *Neurobiology.* Oxford University Press, New York, 1988.

Valnet, J: *The Practice of Aromatherapy.* Healing Arts Press, Rochester, 1989.

### Chapter 14

Balsam MS, Sagarin E, Gershon SD, Rieger MM, Strianse SJ: *Cosmetics, Science and Technology.* Wiley-Interscience/John Wiley & Sons, Inc., New York, 1972.

Buchman DD: *Herbal Medicine.* Crown, New York, 1980.

Clayman CB (ed): *AMA's Guide to Prescription and Over-the-Counter Drugs.*

Der Marderosian A: *Natural Product Medicine,* George F. Stickley Co., Philadelphia, 1988.

Erichsen-Brown C: *Medicinal and Other Uses of North American Plants.* Dover, New York, 1989.

Goldemberg, R: *Advances in Cosmetic Technology.* Harcourt Brace Jovanovich, Inc., New York,

1978.

Grieve M: *Modern Herbal,* Vol. I. Dover, New York, 1971.

Grieve M: *Modern Herbal,* Vol. II. Dover, New York, 1971.

Homburger F, Hayes JA, Pelikan EW (eds): *A Guide to General Toxicology.* Karger, Basel, 1983.

Katzung BG: *Basic and Clinical Pharmacology.* Appleton & Lange, East Norwalk, 1989.

deNavarre MG: *The Chemistry and Manufacture of Cosmetics.* Continental Press, Orlando, 1975.

Matoren GM (ed): *The Clinical Research Process in the Pharmaceutical Industry.* Marcel Dekker, Inc., 1984.

Meyer JE: *The Herbalist.* Meyerbooks, Glenwood, 1986.

Middleton AW: *Cosmetic Science.* Butterworths Scientific Publications, London, 1959.

Millspaugh C: *American Medicinal Plants.* Dover, New York, 1974.

Peterson N: *Herbs and Health.* Viking Penquin, New York, 1990.

Reid DP: *Chinese Herbal Medicine.* Shambhalo, Boston.

Tyler VE, Brady LR, Robbers JE: *Pharmacognosy.* Lea & Febiger, Philadelphia, 1981.

Wilkinson JB and Moore RJ: *Harry's Cosmetology.* Chemical Publishing, New York, 1982.

**Chapter 15**

Achterberg J: *Imagery in Healing.* New Science Library, Boston, 1985.

Bloch M: *The Royal Touch.* Dorset Pr., New York, 1990.

Chardin PT: *Hymn of the Universe.* Harper & Row, New York, 1965.

Chopra D: *Quantum Healing.* Bantam Books, New York, 1989.

Dossey L: *Space, Time & Medicine.* New Science Library, Boston, 1985.

Dyson F: *Disturbing the Universe.* Basic Books, Inc., New York, 1979.

Hawking SW: *A Brief History of Time.* Bantam Books, Toronto, 1988.

Kippenhahn R: *Light from the Depths of Time.* Springer-Verlag, Berlin,1987.

Marsh P: *Eye to Eye.* Salem House Publishers, Topsfield, 1988.

Montagu A: *Touching.* Harper & Row, New York, 1978.

Morris R: *Time's Arrows* (a*Touchstone* book). Simon & Schuster, Inc., New York, 1985.

Sambursky S: *Physical Thought* . PICA Press, New York, 1975.

Thommen GS: *Biorhythms.* Crown, New York, 1986.

Thompson CJS: *Magic and Healing.* Crown, New York, 1989.

Wolf FA: *The Body Quantum.* MacMillan Publishing Company, New York, 1986.

Wolf FA: *Parallel Universes* (a*Touchstone* book). Simon & Schuster, Inc., New York, 1988.

Wolf FA: *Taking the Quantum Leap.* Harper & Row, New York, 1981.

**Appendix**

Abraham GE: Ovarian and adrenal contribution to the peripheral androgens during the menstrual cycle. *J. Clin Endocrinol Metab* 39:340, 1974.

Agnew LRC, Aviado DM, Brody JI, Burrows W, Butler RF, Combs CM, Gambill CM, Glasser O, Hine M, Shelley W, Daly LW (eds): *Dorland's Medical Dictionary.* W. B. Saunders Company, New York,1965.

Bardin CW and Lipsett MB: Testosterone and androstenedione blood production with idiopathic hirsutism or polycystic ovaries. *J Clin Invest* 46:235, 1967.

Bierich JR: *Clinics in Endocrinology and Metabolism,* Vol 4/Number 1, W.B. Saunders Company Ltd, London, 1975.

Bonner C, et al: Androgen receptors in human skin. *Br J Dermatol* 97:501, 1977.

Givens JR: Hirsutism and hyperandrogenism. *Adv Intern Med* 21:221, 1976.

Hershmann JM (ed): *Endocrine Pathophysiology.* Lea and Febiger, Philadelphia, 1988.

Klein HA: *The World of Measurements.* Simon and Schuster, NewYork, 1974.

Kuttenn F, et al: Androgen production and skin metabolism in hirsutism. *N Eng J Med* 294:637,

1977.

Mahesh VB and Greenblatt RB: *Hirsutism and Virilism. Pathogenesis, Diagnosis and Management.* John Wright/PSG, Inc., Boston, 1983.

Price VH: Testosterone metabolism in the skin. *Arch Dermatol* 111:1496, 1975.

Stedman LT: *Stedman's Medical Dictionary.* The Williams & Wilkins Company, Baltimore, 1976.

Schweikert HU: Regulation of human hair growth by steroid hormones. Testosterone metabolism in isolated hairs. *Clin Endocrinol Metab* 38:811, 1974.

Wilson JD and Walker JD: The conversion of testosterone to 5 alpha androstane-17 beta ol-3-one by skin slices in man. *J Clin Invest* 48:371, 1969.

# Index